Volume 43   CLINICAL EPIDEMIOLOGY OF CHRONIC OBSTRUCTIVE
PULMONARY DISEASE
Edited by Michael J. Hensley and Nicholas A. Saunders

CLINICAL EPIDEMIOLOGY OF CHRONIC OBSTRUCTIVE PULMONARY DISEASE

Edited by

Michael J. Hensley

Nicholas A. Saunders

Faculty of Medicine
University of Newcastle
Newcastle, New South Wales, Australia

MARCEL DEKKER, INC.   New York • Basel

Library of Congress Cataloging-in-Publication Data

Clinical epidemiology of chronic obstructive pulmonary disease /
  [edited by] Michael J. Hensley, Nicholas A. Saunders.
      p.   cm. -- (Lung biology in health and disease ; v. 43)
    Includes bibliographies and indexes.
    ISBN 0-8247-8087-6
    1. Lungs--Diseases, Obstructive--Epidemiology.   I. Hensley,
Michael J.   II. Saunders, Nicholas A.   III. Series.
    [DNLM: 1. Lung Diseases, Obstructive--epidemiology. W1LU62 v.
43 / WF 600 C641]
RA645.L84C58   1989
616.2,4-dc20
DNLM/DLC
    for Library of Congress   89-11839
                                                                    CIP

MARCEL DEKKER, INC.
270 Madison Avenue, New York, New York 10016

Current printing (last digit):
10 9 8 7 6 5 4 3 2 1

PRINTED IN THE UNITED STATES OF AMERICA

INTRODUCTION

Epidemiology is the study of the distribution and determinants
of disease frequency in man

MacMahon and Pugh, 1970

If this quotation defines epidemiology, this volume is indeed a treatise on the epidemiology of chronic obstructive pulmonary disease (COPD). Although epidemiology is a scientific approach that may have begun in the late 17th century, probably in France, the term "epidemiology" seems to have been used first by the Spaniard, Don Joaquin de Villalba, in 1802 (Epidemiologia Española). Subsequently, epidemiology as a science and as a tool of medicine has become a preponderant discipline intimately tied to public health; as stated by A. and D. Lilienfeld, "For without public health, there is no epidemiology." However, the same two authors remarked in 1981 that "During the last two decades, the discipline of epidemiology has become increasingly divorced from those activities in the real world that result in the improvement of public health. . . ."

Well, where does this leave our current volume? *Clinical Epidemiology of Chronic Obstructive Pulmonary Disease* is the 43rd volume of the series of monographs Lung Biology in Health and Disease. Is this volume divorced from the real world of researchers and clinicians? I believe the answer to this question is to be found in the blend and breadth of subjects that are examined by the authors and editors. The book utilizes epidemiology to describe and assess the burden of COPD, its causation, its preventive and therapeutic interventions, and its health care implications.

Twenty-five years ago, COPD was a disease that we could only describe and helplessly comment about. Since then we have seen considerable progress relative to its etiology, its pathophysiology, and its pathogenesis. Because research approaches have advanced from descriptive physiology to cellular and molecular biology, there is new hope that creative intervention may soon become available. Meanwhile COPD continues to pose a major, worldwide public health problem.

Greenwood (1935) said that epidemiology "differs from the study of disease by a clinician primarily in respect of the unit of investigation . . . The physician's unit of study is a single human being, the epidemiologist's unit is not a single human being but an aggregate of human beings." What this volume does is to bridge the two units of study. It is both a text of individual medicine and also a text of population medicine.

Chronic obstructive pulmonary disease is not a new topic to the Lung Biology in Health and Disease series. Three prior volumes are exclusively devoted to this subject, which is also included in several other volumes. Michael Hensley and Nick Saunders have assembled here an international authorship that brings new ideas, issues, and points of view to the study of COPD. This volume will enrich the students of this disease, and also challenge those who investigate it, be they concerned with single individuals or with populations.

As the editor of the series, I wish to express my deepest appreciation to the editors and the authors of this new addition.

Claude Lenfant, M.D.
Bethesda, Maryland

PREFACE

The application of information derived from the study of groups of sick and healthy people to the management and prevention of disease in individuals forms the basis of clinical epidemiology (Sackett et al., 1985). Such information may concern the diagnosis, occurrence, prognosis, and cause of disease or the efficacy, effectiveness, and efficiency of preventive and therapeutic interventions. Although the phrase clinical epidemiology was coined more than 50 years ago (Paul, 1938), and the tools of the discipline have been used by many critically thinking and rational physicians, it is only in the last two decades that clinical epidemiology has been recognized as a science with something to contribute to the practice of medicine. This recognition is reflected in the recent publication of four excellent books on the principles and practice of clinical epidemiology (Fletcher et al., 1988; Sackett et al., 1985; Feinstein, 1985; Weiss, 1986).

A framework for the application of clinical epidemiology has been set out by members of the Department of Clinical Epidemiology and Biostatistics of McMaster University in Canada (Tugwell et al., 1985). They propose a number of logical steps for "the critical appraisal of need, benefits and costs of health interventions." The steps include measurement of the incidence, prevalence, mortality, and morbidity from a disease (so-called burden of illness); identification, if possible, of the cause; evaluation of whether an intervention works in an ideal setting (efficacy) or in the real world where provider and patient compliance are important (effectiveness); economic analysis of the intervention (efficiency); description of the synthesis and planning of its implementation; and finally, evaluation of the impact of an intervention on the burden of illness.

We have used the McMaster model to plan the structure of this book. The first five chapters address issues related to the diagnosis and occurrence of chronic obstructive pulmonary disease (COPD): definitions and research methods; incidence, prevalence, and mortality; measurement of morbidity and quality of life; small airways disease; and the analysis of longitudinal lung function data.

Chapter 6 summarizes a current view of the natural history of COPD and the next five chapters deal with accepted and proposed causal factors for this disorder: cigarette smoking, genetic and prenatal factors including those related to atopy and asthma, bronchial reactivity, acid air pollution, and occupation. This list of possible causal factors is not exhaustive. The notable omissions are the role of acute and chronic bronchial infection, the possible contribution of early childhood respiratory illness, and the molecular and cellular biology of lung damage. Excellent reviews are available on some of these topics (Tager and Speizer, 1975; Samet et al., 1983; Snider et al., 1986).

The final chapters concern interventions to reduce the occurrence of COPD by reducing cigarette smoking and to improve the outlook for those with COPD by pharmacological and physical agents. An economic analysis of smoking reduction is also presented. Again there are omissions such as the economics of home oxygen prescribing, which has been reviewed elsewhere (Lowson et al., 1981), and the cost of screening for COPD.

We would like to acknowledge our gratitude to: all the authors who contributed to this volume; Kyla Stevenson, Mandy Holley, and Peter Powers, who provided secretarial and indexing assistance; Paul Dolgert and Della McEneaney from Marcel Dekker Inc., who ensured that an idea for a volume in the series was realized; and Claude Lenfant, who provided advice and support during the development of this book.

References

Feinstein, A. R. (1985). *Clinical Epidemiology. The Architecture of Clinical Research.* W. B. Saunders, Philadelphia.

Fletcher, R. H., Fletcher, S. W., and Wagner, E. H. (1988). *Clinical Epidemiology. The Essentials.* Second Ed. Baltimore, Williams and Wilkins.

Lowson, K. V., Drummond, M. F., and Bishop, J. M. (1981). Costing new services: long-term domicilary oxygen therapy. *Lancet* 1:1146–1149.

Paul, J. R. (1938). Clinical epidemiology. *J. Clin. Invest.* 17:539.

Sackett, D. L., Haynes, R. B., and Tugwell, P. (1985). *Clinical Epidemiology: A Basic Science for Clinical Medicine.* Boston, Little, Brown, and Company.

Samet, J. M., Tager, I. B., and Speizer, F. E. (1983). The relationship between respiratory illness in childhood and chronic air-flow obstruction in childhood. *Am. Rev. Resp. Dis.* 127:508–523.

Snider, G. L., Lucey, E. C., and Stone, P. J. (1986). Animal models of emphysema. *Am. Rev. Resp. Dis.* 133:149–169.

Tager, I. B., and Speizer, F. B. (1975). Role of infection in chronic bronchitis. *N. Engl. J. Med.* **292**:563–571.

Tugwell, P., Bennett, K. J., Sackett, D. L., and Haynes, R. B. (1985). The measurement iterative loop: a framework for the critical appraisal of need, benefits, and costs of health interventions. *J. Chron. Dis.* **38**:339–351.

Weiss, N. S. (1986). *Clinical Epidemiology: The Study of the Outcome of Illness*. New York, Oxford University Press.

Michael J. Hensley

Nicholas A. Saunders

CONTRIBUTORS

Margaret R. Becklake National Centre for Occupational Health and Department of Community Health, University of the Witwatersrand, Johannesburg, South Africa; Department of Epidemiology and Biostatistics, McGill University, Montreal, Quebec, Canada

Benjamin Burrows, M.D. Chalfant-Moore Professor of Medicine, Director, Division of Respiratory Sciences, University of Arizona College of Medicine, Tucson, Arizona

Graham A. Colditz, M.B., B.S., D.P.H. Instructor in Medicine, Department of Medicine, Harvard Medical School, Brigham and Women's Hospital, Boston, Massachusetts

David B. Coultas, M.D. Assistant Professor, Pulmonary Division, Department of Medicine, University of New Mexico School of Medicine, Albuquerque, New Mexico

Douglas W. Dockery, M.D. Assistant Professor of Environmental Science and Physiology, Harvard School of Public Health; Associate Epidemiologist, Harvard Medical School, Brigham and Women's Hospital, Boston, Massachusetts

Eric Garshick, M.D., M.O.H. Brockton/West Roxbury VA Medical Center; Instructor in Medicine, Brigham and Women's Hospital, Harvard Medical School, Boston, Massachusetts

Hennie T. Groeneveld Institute for Biostatistics of the South African Medical Research Council, Johannesburg, South Africa

Michael J. Hensley, M.B., B.S., Ph.D., FRACP Associate Professor in Clinical Epidemiology, Centre for Clinical Epidemiology and Biostatistics,

Faculty of Medicine, University of Newcastle, Newcastle, New South Wales, Australia

Millicent W. Higgins, M.D., D.P.H. Associate Director for Epidemiology and Biometry Program, Division of Epidemiology and Clinical Applications, National Heart, Lung and Blood Institute, National Institutes of Health, Bethesda, Maryland

Les M. Irwig, M.B., B. Ch., Ph.D., F.F.C.M. Associate Professor in Epidemiology, Department of Public Health, University of Sydney, Sydney, New South Wales, Australia

John W. Kusek, Ph.D. Prevention, Education, and Research Training Branch, Division of Lung Diseases, National Heart, Lung and Blood Institute, National Institutes of Health, Bethesda, Maryland

David C. Levin, M.D., F.C.C.P. Professor of Medicine, University of Oklahoma Health Sciences Center; Pulmonary Disease and Critical Care Section, and Director, Outpatient Chest Medicine, Veterans Administration Medical Center, Oklahoma City, Oklahoma

Louis Levin, M.D., M.A. (Int. Med.) Adjunct Professor of Internal Medicine, University of New Mexico School of Medicine; Medical Director, Pickard Presbyterian Convalescent Center, Albuquerque, New Mexico

James L. McKeon, M.B., B.S., FRACP Professorial Registrar, Department of Thoracic Medicine, Royal Newcastle Hospital, Newcastle, New South Wales, Australia

Sydney R. Parker, Ph.D. Chief, Prevention, Education, and Research Training Branch, Division of Lung Diseases, National Heart, Lung and Blood Institute, National Institutes of Health, Bethesda, Maryland

Susan Redline, M.D., M.P.H. Assistant Professor of Medicine, Division of Pulmonary Medicine, Roger Williams General Hospital, Brown University Medical School, Providence, Rhode Island

Jonathan M. Samet, M.D., M.S. Professor, Pulmonary Division, Department of Medicine, University of New Mexico School of Medicine, Albuquerque, New Mexico

Nicholas A. Saunders, M.D., B.S., FRACP Professor of Medicine, Faculty of Medicine, University of Newcastle, Newcastle, New South Wales, Australia

Marc B. Schenker, M.D., M.P.H. Associate Professor and Division Chief, Division of Occupational and Environmental Medicine, University of California School of Medicine, Davis, California

Frank E. Speizer, M.D. Professor of Environmental Science, Harvard School of Public Health; Professor of Medicine, Harvard Medical School, Brigham and Women's Hospital, Boston, Massachusetts

Ira B. Tager, M.D., M.P.H. Associate Professor of Medicine and Epidemiology, University of California, San Francisco; Division of Infectious Diseases, VA Medical Center, San Francisco, California

Thomas Thom, B.A. Division of Epidemiology and Clinical Applications, National Heart, Lung and Blood Institute, National Institutes of Health, Bethesda, Maryland

Scott T. Weiss, M.D. Associate Professor in Medicine, Harvard Medical School, Brigham and Women's Hospital; Pulmonary Division, Beth Israel Hospital, Boston, Massachusetts

Joanne L. Wright, M.D. Department of Pathology, University of British Columbia, Health Sciences Center Hospital, Vancouver, British Columbia, Canada

CONTENTS

CLINICAL EPIDEMIOLOGY OF CHRONIC OBSTRUCTIVE PULMONARY DISEASE

1

Definitions and Methodology in COPD Research

JONATHAN M. SAMET

University of New Mexico School of Medicine
Albuquerque, New Mexico

In the 1950s, as the burden of morbidity and mortality posed by chronic respiratory diseases was recognized, epidemiological investigations were undertaken to determine the frequency and causes of these disorders. The need for uniformly applied definitions and for standardized methods of data collection was quickly recognized. The 1958 Ciba Guest Symposium represented the first attempt to achieve a consensus on definitions and methods for the study of chronic bronchitis, emphysema, and disorders associated with chronic airflow obstruction (Ciba, 1959). At this symposium a group of British investigators were brought together to develop definitions and terminology, and to consider research needs. Their report provided definitions (Table 1) that have been widely applied and that are still generally accepted in their original form (Fletcher, 1978; Fletcher and Pride, 1984). The Medical Research Council questionnaire on respiratory symptoms, first published in 1960 (Medical Research Council, 1960), filled the need for a standardized method for collecting subjective symptom data (Samet, 1978). The emphasis on standardized definitions and methods for data collection has been maintained in subsequent research on chronic obstructive lung disease.

When the first studies of chronic obstructive lung disease were implemented, little was known about the frequency, causes, or natural history of

1

Table 1 Definitions of Respiratory Disorders from the 1958 Ciba Guest Symposium (1959)

Emphysema: A condition of the lung characterized by increase beyond the normal in the size of air spaces distal to the terminal bronchiole either from dilatation or from destruction of their walls

Chronic bronchitis: The condition of subjects with chronic or recurrent excessive mucus secretion in the bronchial tree

Irreversible or persistent obstructive lung disease: The condition of subjects with widespread narrowing of the bronchial airways, which has been present for more than 1 year and which is unaffected by bronchodilator drugs (including corticosteroids)

Asthma: The condition of subjects with narrowing of the bronchial airways which changes its severity over short periods of time either spontaneously or under treatment

this disease (Stuart-Harris, 1954). However, clinical observations and the results of prevalence surveys soon suggested an etiological sequence that has been referred to as the "British hypothesis" (Fletcher et al., 1976). The definitions and standardized questionnaire developed by the early British investigators largely reflected the pathogenetic mechanisms of the "British hypothesis" (Ciba, 1959; Medical Research Council, 1965; Samet 1978; Fletcher and Pride, 1984). In this hypothesis, mucus hypersecretion, secondary to cigarette smoking and other environmental factors, was considered to represent the initial stage of chronic obstructive lung disease. The development of mucus hypersecretion was postulated to increase the occurrence of respiratory infections and lead to changes in the lung including airways obstruction and emphysema. An alternative hypothesis advanced by Dutch investigators (Orie et al., 1961) emphasized the role of endogenous susceptibility in determining the development of chronic obstructive lung disease. The longitudinal study of male patients in west London (Fletcher et al., 1976) and other prospective studies (U.S. DHHS, 1984) have now disproved the "British hypothesis." Nevertheless, current methodology for investigating chronic obstructive lung disease remains heavily influenced by the definitions of the Ciba symposium and the original Medical Research Council questionnaire.

Chronic obstructive lung disease has been intensively investigated since the 1950s and many of the original questions concerning its frequency, natural history, and causes have now been answered (Speizer and Tager, 1979; Burrows et al., 1981; U.S. DHHS, 1984). Cigarette smoking has been identified as the cause of most cases, but the factors that place individual smokers at risk remain largely unknown. Current epidemiological research emphasizes the determinants of risk in cigarette smokers; the degree of airways reactivity and childhood respiratory illness experience are of particular interest at present. For the purpose of prevention, methods for detecting the earliest stages of chronic obstructive lung disease have also been emphasized.

This chapter reviews the definitions and methods used for research on chronic obstructive lung disease. It emphasizes the limitations of conventional methodology for addressing contemporary research questions and offers suggestions for changes.

I. Definitions

A. Introduction

The difficulties in defining chronic obstructive lung disease and related disorders were acknowledged at the Ciba Symposium in 1958 and were, in fact, an impetus for holding the symposium (Ciba, 1959). The symposium report proposed that a group with a disease might be identified on a clinical, morbid anatomical, functional, or etiological basis. Scadding (1959, 1963) elaborated on the difficulty of establishing definitions for bronchopulmonary diseases and the untoward consequences of not doing so. Definitions have been written for each of the most common chronic respiratory diseases including chronic bronchitis, emphysema, chronic obstructive lung disease, and asthma; among these definitions, the diagnostic criteria are variably based on clinical, pathological, and physiological information.

B. Chronic Bronchitis

The Ciba Symposium (1959) proposed that "chronic bronchitis refers to the condition of subjects with chronic or recurrent excessive mucous secretion in the bronchial tree." Appropriate responses to a symptom questionnaire have been used to meet this clinically based definition, which makes no specifications for the simultaneous presence of airflow obstruction (Medical Research Council, 1965). The histopathological counterpart of chronic bronchitis has been considered to be mucus gland enlargement, although the morphological data derive largely from populations of smokers (Thurlbeck, 1976). The term *chronic bronchitis* has been criticized because it implies inflammation rather than mucus hypersecretion (Fletcher and Pride, 1984). However, a recent study showed that inflammation of the cartilaginous airways was more severe in patients with chronic bronchitis than in patients without chronic bronchitis and that measures of mucus gland size in the central airways were comparable in the two groups (Mullen et al., 1985).

In 1962 the American Thoracic Society (1962) adopted a definition similar to that of the Ciba symposium. However, subsequently, both the World Health Organization (1975) and a joint committee of the American College of Chest Physicians and the American Thoracic Society (1975) proposed definitions that included functional, morphological, and etiological components without clinical criteria. These newer definitions cannot be readily applied in the context of an epidemiological study nor in clinical practice and should not replace the original Ciba symposium recommendations.

The term *chronic obstructive bronchitis* has been proposed to describe chronic bronchitis accompanied by persistent abnormalities of airflow (Medical Research Council, 1965; World Health Organization, 1975). In the Medical Research Council's (1965) definition, narrowing of the intrapulmonary airways was assumed to be responsible for increased resistance to airflow; the World Health Organization's (1975) definition attributed the reduced expiratory flows to mechanisms other than loss of lung recoil. These definitions assume the pathogenetic sequence of the "British hypothesis" and cannot be readily used for epidemiological purposes. Fletcher and Pride (1984) have correctly suggested that the term *chronic obstructive bronchitis* be abandoned.

Clinicians may apply the term chronic bronchitis to symptom complexes not identical to chronic sputum production as ascertained by questionnaire. In Tucson, for example, Burrows and Lebowitz (1975) examined the symptoms reported by adults with physician-confirmed chronic bronchitis and found that 28% denied chronic cough, 35% denied chronic sputum production, and 22% denied either symptom. A physicians' diagnosis of chronic bronchitis was associated with the symptoms of dyspnea and wheezing, with the diagnoses of asthma and emphysema, with cigarette smoking, and with ventilatory impairment. In children, another study in Tucson (Taussig et al., 1981) showed that physician diagnoses of chronic bronchitis and asthma overlap considerably. Taussig et al. (1981) questioned physicians in Tucson about criteria for the diagnosis of chronic bronchitis in children. Wheezing and allergies were important considerations for most of the physicians and bronchodilator therapy was frequently given to children diagnosed with chronic bronchitis. These results demonstrate that physicians' diagnoses of chronic bronchitis in children and in adults are not equivalent to those based on the questionnaires generally used by epidemiologists.

C. Emphysema

Although the term *emphysema* has been used by some clinicians to refer to chronic obstructive lung disease, formal definitions have always been based on morphological findings (Thurlbeck, 1976). The definitions of emphysema by the Ciba symposium participants (1959) included airspace enlargement due to either dilatation or destruction. Subsequent definitions have limited emphysema to airspace enlargement associated with destructive changes (American Thoracic Society, 1962; World Health Organization, 1975; American College of Chest Physicians–American Thoracic Society, 1975). The definition of emphysema has been further clarified by a recent workshop that defined it as including airspace enlargement and destruction of respiratory airspaces (National Heart, Lung and Blood Institute, 1985).

D. Chronic Obstructive Lung Disease

A widely varying set of terms and definitions have been proposed for persistent airflow obstruction (Table 2). The Ciba symposium (1959) applied the definition *irreversible or persistent obstructive lung disease* to the persistent form of *generalized obstructive lung disease*. The definition emphasized a structural change, airways narrowing, rather than physiological abnormality. Definitions proposed by the World Health Organization (1975) and the committee of the American College of Chest Physicians and the American Thoracic Society (1975) included reduced expiratory airflow but did not specify the extent of reduction required to meet the definition. The latter group also proposed the terms *chronic obstructive bronchitis* and *chronic obstructive emphysema*. Thurlbeck (1976) also emphasized physiological change whereas Snider (1983) inferred a disease process. Unfortunately, none of these definitions can be readily applied for either clinical or epidemiological purposes.

Development of a satisfactory definition of chronic obstructive lung disease has been hindered by the variable histopathological findings in the lungs of patients with this condition (Thurlbeck, 1976). The extent of expiratory flow limitation does not depend in a simple fashion on the severity of emphysema or of airways changes. For example, Nagai and colleagues (1985a,b) recently described structure–function correlations in 48 patients with a clinical diagnosis of chronic obstructive lung disease and evidence of airflow obstruction on spirometry. Although the patients were relatively homogeneous clinically, the extent of abnormalities in bronchi, bronchioles, and parenchyma was highly variable. While smokers with chronic airflow obstruction generally have more severe morphological abnormalities than unaffected smokers, qualitatively similar lesions are present

Table 2 Definitions of Chronic Obstructive Lung Disease

Source	Term	Definition
Ciba Symposium (1958)	Irreversible or persistent obstructive lung disease	The condition of subjects with narrowing of the bronchial airways, which has been present for more than 1 year and which is unaffected by bronchodilator drugs (including corticosteroids)
World Health Organization (1975)	Chronic generalized airways obstruction	The term "airways obstruction" refers to slowing of forced expiration . . . "chronic" is used when airways obstruction persists . . . or when it has been demonstrated in at least two examinations over a period of at least 3 months . . .
American College of Chest Physicians– American Thoracic Society (1975)	Chronic obstructive pulmonary disease	Diseases of uncertain etiology characterized by persistent slowing of airflow during forced expiration
Thurlbeck (1976)	Chronic obstructive lung disease	Those conditions that may be accompanied by chronic or recurrent obstruction to airflow with the lung
Snider (1983)	Chronic obstructive pulmonary disease	A process characterized by nonspecific changes in the lung parenchyma and bronchi that may lead to emphysema and airflow obstruction

in the lungs of obstructed and nonobstructed smokers (Hale et al., 1984). Thus, criteria for the diagnosis of chronic obstructive lung disease cannot be readily validated against morphological findings.

Clinicians have applied many different labels to patients with chronic obstructive lung disease. In the past, the term *chronic bronchitis* was frequently used in the United Kingdom and the term *emphysema* used in the United States. More recently, chronic obstructive pulmonary disease (COPD), chronic obstructive lung disease (COLD), chronic airflow obstruction (CAO), and similar labels have been used by clinicians. The preference for these terms is confirmed by trends of reporting diagnoses on death certificates; since the introduction of a code for chronic obstructive lung disease into the International Classification of Diseases, there has been a progressive shift of cause of deaths into this category from those for chronic bronchitis and emphysema (National Heart, Lung and Blood Institute, 1980). Nevertheless, clinicians continue to use the terms *chronic bronchitis* and *emphysema*, but the use of these terms depends on the gender, the age, and the smoking habits of the patient (Dodge et al., 1986).

Epidemiologists have also used diverse labels and definitions for chronic obstructive lung disease (Table 3) (U.S. DHHS, 1984). The criteria have been most often based on physiology but consistency has not been maintained among investigations. Some investigators have used reports of a physician's diagnosis of chronic bronchitis or emphysema as a measure of chronic obstructive lung disease (Lebowitz et al., 1975; Samet et al., 1982).

Although numerous definitions and terms for the presence of chronic airflow obstruction have been published, confusion persists among clinicians and epidemiologists with regard to terminology and criteria for diagnosis. Definitions have variably emphasized structure and function (Table 2) and epidemiologists have created their own terminology and criteria (Table 3).

E. Asthma

As for chronic obstructive lung disease, numerous definitions of asthma have been published, but none lead to specific criteria for differentiating asthmatic from nonasthmatic persons (Samet, 1987). In fact, participants in the 1971 Ciba Study Group on the Identification of Asthma (1971) concluded that the information available at that time was inadequate for defining asthma. The 1958 Ciba symposium (1959) defined asthma as ". . . the condition of subjects with widespread narrowing of the bronchial airways, which changes its severity over short periods of time either spontaneously or under treatment. . . ." Subsequent definitions by other groups have emphasized airways hyperresponsiveness (American Thoracic Society,

Table 3 Criteria for Chronic Obstructive Lung Disease in Selected Epidemiological Studies

Study/Source	Terms	Criteria
Belen, NH, 1961 Ferris (1962)	Irreversible obstructive lung disease	Wheezing most days or nights, sufficient dyspnea, or $FEV_1/FVC < 60\%$
Tecumseh, MI, 1962-1979; Higgins (1983)	Obstructive airways disease	$FEV_1 < 65\%$ predicted and $FEV_1/FVC < 80\%$
Glenwood Springs, CO, 1967; Mueller (1971)	Chronic airway obstruction	$FEV_1/FVC < 60\%$
East Boston, MA, 1973-1974; Tager (1978)	Obstructive airways disease	$FEV_1 < 65\%$ predicted

1962; American College of Chest Physicians–American Thoracic Society, 1975; World Health Organization, 1975). Some patients with chronic obstructive lung disease may display a varying degree of airflow obstruction over time and thus partially fulfill the criteria for asthma. The appropriate terminology for such patients is problematic (Medical Research Council, 1965; Fletcher, 1978; Fletcher and Pride, 1984).

F. Conclusions

Research on chronic obstructive lung disease has been facilitated by the early efforts to develop consensus definitions. The definitions proposed by the Ciba symposium (1959), however, intrinsically reflect a concept of disease pathogenesis that has been disproven. Neither the Ciba symposium's nor subsequent definitions of chronic obstructive lung disease have proved satisfactory for epidemiologists. In view of the extensive data now available on the epidemiology of chronic obstructive lung disease, reevaluation of the standard definitions appears appropriate and timely. Changing emphasis in research on chronic obstructive lung disease provides a further rationale for this reevaluation.

Individuals with chronic obstructive lung disease can be identified by the finding of persistent ventilatory impairment, by the measurement of excessive functional loss over time, or by a physician's diagnosis (U.S. DHHS, 1984). A physician's diagnosis, however, is inherently unstandardized and is also influenced by patterns of medical care access and usage. For epidemiological purposes, the adoption of a definition of chronic obstructive lung disease based on the demonstration of ventilatory impairment seems appropriate. Both epidemiologists and clinicians rely on spirometry for the diagnosis of this disease and any new definition should be expressed in terms of levels of the FEV_1 and of the FEV_1/forced vital capacity (FVC) ratio. A definition in these terms would merely formalize an accepted epidemiological practice. The choice of any particular degree of abnormality to establish the presence of chronic obstructive lung disease would be arbitrary; categories of severity should be established with physiologically meaningful boundaries. Excessive decline of ventilatory function should not be considered equivalent to chronic obstructive lung disease, but as indicating the presence of the disease process that leads to chronic obstructive lung disease.

The term *chronic bronchitis* has less relevance for present research than for earlier studies conducted to test the "British hypothesis." Use of this term has emphasized a particular pattern of chronic cough and sputum production, but this focus appears to have been unwarranted. The use of the term in different ways by epidemiologists and clinicians has unnecessarily complicated research on chronic obstructive lung disease. I suggest that *chronic bronchitis* be replaced by use of appropriate descriptive terms such as chronic cough and sputum, which do not carry etiological, pathological, or clinical implications.

II. Methods

A. Introduction

As epidemiological research on chronic obstructive lung disease began in the 1950s, the problem of observer variation in obtaining a history of respiratory symptoms was quickly recognized (Cochrane et al., 1951). Subsequently, a standardized questionnaire on respiratory symptoms was developed and published by the British Medical Research Council. The 1958 Ciba symposium (1959) advocated use of a version of this questionnaire and made recommendations on lung function testing. Subsequently, revisions of the Medical Research Council questionnaire have been made (Samet, 1978).

In the United States, an American Thoracic Society committee adopted the Medical Research Council questionnaire in 1969 and also made recommendations on study design for epidemiological surveys and lung function testing (American Thoracic Society, 1969). Questionnaires and survey methods were the subject of a 1971 workshop held by the Division of Lung Diseases of the National Heart and Lung Institute. Subsequent Division of Lung Diseases workshops led to additional recommendations but problems with the standards were evident (Ferris, 1978). As a result, the American Thoracic Society contracted with the Division of Lung Diseases to develop standardized methods for assessing respiratory symptoms, for lung function testing, and for chest radiography. The report of the American Thoracic Society's Epidemiology Standardization Project was published in 1978 (Ferris, 1978); revisions have not yet been undertaken.

Other groups have also made recommendations on methods for epidemiological research on chronic obstructive lung disease. The 1975 report of a World Health Organization Committee (World Health Organization, 1975) addressed methods of data collection. Florey and Leeder (1982) have written a monograph for the World Health Organization on methods for longitudinal studies of chronic obstructive lung disease that reviews methodology. The European Economic Community has prepared its own version of the Medical Research Council questionnaire (van der Lende and Orie, 1972) and made recommendations on standardizing physiological testing (Quanjer, 1983). The International Union Against Tuberculosis has devised a standardized questionnaire for research on asthma (Burney and Chinn, 1987).

Epidemiological research on chronic obstructive lung disease has been accomplished primarily using symptom questionnaires and spirometry. Other physiological tests, such as the diffusing capacity and measures of small airways function, have been used in epidemiological research but have generally proved to be uninformative. Examination by a clinician and use of chest radiography have been used infrequently and both approaches are sensitive only to more advanced chronic obstructive lung disease (Fletcher, 1952). Accordingly, this review emphasizes questionnaires and spirometry, although some other methods for data collection will also be addressed.

B. Questionnaires

The Medical Research Council questionnaire and modifications developed by other groups have now been used extensively in epidemiological research and substantial information has become available on the characteristics of respiratory symptom questionnaires (Samet, 1978; Florey and Leeder, 1982). The questionnaires for adults contain a core set of items (Table 4), which may be supplemented. Both the Medical Research Council

Table 4 Core Items in a Standard Respiratory Symptom Questionnaire for Adults

---

Cough

Phlegm

Periods of cough and phlegm

Wheezing

Dyspnea

Chest illnesses

Past illnesses

Tobacco smoking history

---

and American Thoracic Society questionnaires are published with instructions for their administration and for the training of interviewers.

A questionnaire's utility is determined by its validity—the extent to which it measures what it was designed to measure—and by its reliability—the extent to which responses are repeatable. Bias—the intrusion of an unplanned or unwanted influence—may reduce both its validity and reliability.

With regard to validity, assessment has been limited to the phlegm, dyspnea, and chest illness questions because appropriate standards for comparison are not available for other items (Samet, 1978). In a series of reports based on a survey of London post office workers, Fletcher and colleagues (Fairbairn et al., 1959; Fletcher et al., 1959; Elmes et al., 1959) addressed the validity of a prototype of the Medical Research Council questionnaire. Questions about the extent of daily expectoration correlated well with morning sputum volume. For questions about chest illnesses, only 82% of men and 54% of women gave responses that were confirmed by their work sickness records. The indirect maximal breathing capacity correlated poorly with the breathlessness questions. Other studies have confirmed the validity of the questions about phlegm for assessing sputum production (Fletcher and Tinker, 1961; Holland et al., 1966).

The reliability of standard respiratory symptom questionnaires has also been assessed (Samet, 1978). As reviewed by Samet (1978), the repeatability of the phlegm questions varied from 80 to 90% in studies in the United Kingdom, but was only 62% in a study of shipyard workers in the United States (Samet et al., 1978). For other symptoms, the repeatability ranges from 70 to 90% (van der Lende et al., 1972; Lebowitz and Burrows, 1976; Samet et al., 1978).

Bias from the observer, the season of administration, questionnaire modification, and the method of administration have been examined. In early British respiratory disease surveys, the observer was a major source of bias (Cochrane et al., 1951; Schilling et al., 1955). However, correct use of a standardized questionnaire has been shown to prevent observer bias (Samet, 1978). An influence of the season in which the questionnaire is completed on both the reporting of symptoms and the severity of symptoms is plausible. Consistent effects of season on response patterns have not been found, however (Samet, 1978). With regard to questionnaire modification, major changes in wording affect responses (Holland et al., 1966; Lebowitz and Burrows, 1976; Helsing et al., 1979; Comstock et al., 1979) and should not be made by individual investigators. Method of administration (by interviewer in person, by telephone, or by self-completion) has little effect on responses (Lebowitz and Burrows, 1976; Samet, 1978; Samet et al., 1978; Helsing et al., 1979). Other potential sources of bias include "training effects" with repetitive administration and subjects' attitudes toward the questionnaire (Samet, 1978). The validity of responses from surrogate sources, such as next of kin, has not been examined.

The Medical Research Council questionnaire has satisfied the need for a standardized survey instrument that led to its development. The questions about phlegm have demonstrated validity and have proved adequate for testing the "British hypothesis." However, the current versions of the Medical Research Council and American Thoracic Society questionnaires are less suitable for current research on chronic obstructive lung disease, which emphasizes potential determinants of susceptibility to cigarette smoke such as childhood history of respiratory illness and airways hyperreactivity (U.S. DHHS, 1984). Neither questionnaire adequately covers wheezing and other manifestations of airways hyperreactivity (Samet, 1987). The Medical Research Council questionnaire does not include a question on childhood respiratory illness and the single question included in the American Thoracic Society questionnaire is not sufficiently specific. Family history is not included in the Medical Research Council questionnaire and is obtained only for parents in the American Thoracic Society questionnaire. Furthermore, neither questionnaire obtains a sufficiently detailed history of cigarette smoking to profile lifetime consumption of cigarettes of different types. The questions on inhalation of cigarette smoke have never been validated physiologically.

The dyspnea questions have changed little from the form originally proposed by Fletcher and colleagues (1959). Newer approaches for assessing dyspnea have been advocated (Mahler et al., 1984; Stoller et al., 1986) and questionnaries are now available for assessing physical activity (Washburn and Montoye, 1986). The present dyspnea questions capture the minimum level of activity that produces breathlessness; the questions neither rate the effort involved in performing that task nor describe the extent of functional impairment. The standard dyspnea questions should be revised to address these deficiencies.

The need for other revisions is also obvious. The Medical Research Council questionnaire does not adequately cover past respiratory illnesses and neither the Medical Research Council nor the American Thoracic Society questionnaire inquires about chronic obstructive lung disease or related diagnostic terms. In the design of the standardized respiratory symptom questionnaires, emphasis has been placed on maintaining brevity. However, brevity must be sacrificed if adequate information is to be obtained to address current research questions.

C. Spirometry

Spirometric testing has been recommended by all groups that have considered methodology for epidemiological studies of chronic obstructive lung disease. Spirometry is simple, inexpensive, and noninvasive, but sensitive to the physiological abnormalities that develop in chronic obstructive lung disease (Mead, 1979). In comparison with many other tests of lung function, spirometric measures have less variability, particularly the FEV_1 and the FVC. A spirometer integrated with a microprocessor can measure flow rates at various lung volumes and store data for transmission to a computer.

Standardization of spirometric testing has long been advocated (Table 5). However, in spite of the attempts of several expert groups to establish procedures for testing, controversy remains concerning the number of tracings that should be obtained and the selection of values from particular tracings for data analysis.

With regard to the number of blows into the spirometer, Hutchinson in 1846 advocated that three observations should be made. He considered that the first is for practice and that fatigue follows the third. More recent recommendations have called for three to five FVC maneuvers (Table 5). The Epidemiology Standardization Project of the American Thoracic Society recommended that three acceptable tests should be routinely obtained. As rationale for this choice, this report cited Hutchinson's arguments as well as the results of several analyses of contemporary data sets. A similar recommendation was made by the Working Party of the European Coal and Steel Community (Quanjer, 1983).

Most of the relevant analyses indicate that the choice of three acceptable tests is arbitrary but appropriate and not likely to introduce bias in comparison with alternative test procedures. When five tests are obtained,

Table 5 Recommendations for Performance of Spirometry

Source	Number of Blows	Selection of Values
Hutchinson (1846)	Three	Not discussed
Medical Research Council (1965)	For FEV_1, two practice, then three more. For FVC, three additional	Not discussed
American Thoracic Society (1969)	Three to five	Mean of last three
National Heart and Lung Institute (1971)[a]	Five	Mean of best two
American Thoracic Society, 1978 (Ferris, 1978)	Three	Best FVC and FEV_1
European Community, 1983 (Quanjer, 1983)	At least three	Best FVC and FEV_1

[a]Unpublished memorandum based on a workshop held by the National Heart and Lung Institute in 1971.

the best test for the FEV_1 and for the FVC is not more often the fourth or fifth than one of the first three (Knudson et al., 1976). Furthermore, the mean and maximum values change little as the number of tests is increased from three to five (Freedman and Prowse, 1966; Stebbings, 1971; Nathan et al., 1979). Nathan et al. (1979) comprehensively assessed the effect of tracing number in data from the Tucson epidemiological study and from subjects studied by Edward A. Gaensler, M.D. In the Tucson population, cross-sectional comparison showed only small mean differences for the FEV_1 and for the FVC when the first three were compared with five tracings. Variation during the first 3 years of follow-up was comparable for three and five tracings. The cross-sectional findings were confirmed with Gaensler's data. Obtaining more than five blows may introduce bias (Ferris et al., 1978).

Algorithms for the selection of data from a set of spirometric tracings have been even more controversial and recommendations have been variable (Table 5). The most recent recommendations by the American Thoracic Society and the European Community are for selection of the maximum FEV_1 and FVC, regardless of whether they occur on the same blow. This algorithm is supported by some but not by all relevant analyses.

The extent of reproducibility has been considered the most appropriate criterion for evaluating alternative algorithms (Stebbings, 1971; Fletcher et al., 1976). Ferris and colleagues (1965) found a slightly larger standard deviation for the maximum of five FEV_1 values in comparison with the mean of the last three trials. In contrast, Stebbings (1971) found lesser intraindividual variation with the maximum FEV_1 than with the mean. In a study of steel workers, Lowe et al. (1968) found slightly smaller standard deviations for the maximum of two FEV_1 values in comparison with the mean of the two values. The results of analysis of the longitudinal data from working men in London were similar (Fletcher et al., 1976). Other investigators have found trivial differences between the maximum and the mean and also concluded that the maximum is preferable, in part for the sake of simplicity (Nathan et al., 1979; Sorenson et al., 1980). Analyses by Tager et al. (1976) and by Ferris et al. (1978) imply that mean values may be most reproducible, but neither analysis fully evaluated the maximum.

Two recent reports also led to recommendations for selection of mean values. Ullah and colleagues (1983) obtained 20 spirometric curves, the blows being separated by 1 min intervals, from 30 normal, 49 asthmatic, and 26 chronic bronchitic subjects. The distributions of the replicates were consistent with a normal frequency distribution and the authors therefore concluded that the mean provides the best estimate of the true value. It is interesting that there was no evidence of fatigue with repeated testing in either the normal subjects or the patients. For epidemiologists, this report has little utility, however, because the test situation is not at all comparable to the usual circumstances of field data collection.

Oldham and Cole (1983) also concluded that a mean value from a set of tracings is preferable to the maximum, but their analyses indicate that the choice of index is of little consequence. In one study, these investigators compared variance components for nine different FEV_1 indices calculated from data collected by repeat testing of 40 normal subjects on six separate days. While the mean of the largest three of five tracings was optimal, the differences among the nine indices were small and of no practical consequence. In the second study, the investigators compared the nine indexes as the dependent variable in a regression of FEV_1 on age and extent of pneumoconiosis in data from 335 dust-exposed men. As in the first study, the differences among the indices were small.

This continued debate over selection of values from a series of spirometric tracings seems unnecessary; its perpetuation emphasizes the need for standardization. The preponderance of evidence suggests that the choice of a mean or of a maximum value has little consequence either for estimating lung function level or for minimizing variability. Adherence to the current recommendations of the American Thoracic Society and the European Community is warranted.

Recent analyses of data from occupational populations indicate that application of repeatability criteria, such as those of the Epidemiology Standardization Project, may introduce bias by differentially excluding subjects with a greater likelihood of developing disease (Eisen, 1987). Eisen and colleagues (1983 and 1984) examined rate of decline of FEV_1 in a cohort of Vermont granite workers evaluated for a 5-year period. At each survey, about 11% of subjects could not meet the repeatability criterion of two FEV_1 values within 200 ml. Subjects who persistently did not meet this criterion had a more rapid decline of FEV_1 than those who did. Kellie et al. (1987) reported similar findings concerning the consequences of standardization based on analysis of data from 7,790 U.S. coal miners. This same source of bias may affect epidemiological studies of chronic obstructive lung disease. In cross-sectional surveys, the anticipated bias would differentially exclude subjects with lower levels of function and in longitudinal studies slopes would be biased toward lesser rates of decline.

D. Other Physiological Tests

Other tests of lung function can be used in the context of an epidemiological investigation of chronic obstructive lung disease. Assessment of airways responsiveness, which is relevant for current hypotheses related to susceptibility, is addressed elsewhere in this volume. Noninvasive measurement of oxygenation represents an approach for assessing the spectrum of severity of chronic obstructive lung disease in the community. The arterial oxygen pressure can be estimated by transcutaneous measurement or by oximetry. For example, Williams and Nichol (1985) made transcutaneous measurements to estimate the prevalence of persons with chronic obstructive lung disease and hypoxemia requiring oxygen therapy. Walking tests might be used in the context of an epidemiological study to assess functional status (Guyatt et al., 1985).

E. Chest Radiography

Epidemiologists have rarely used chest radiography in field studies of chronic obstructive lung disease; feasibility, subject acceptance, cost, and technical considerations weigh against its use (Ferris, 1978). Furthermore, the relationships among radiographic findings, lung function, and morphological abnormalites are extremely complex (Thurlbeck, 1976) and interpretations may be affected by observer bias (Ferris, 1978). For these reasons, the American Thoracic Society did not recommend chest radiography for epidemiological studies of chronic obstructive lung disease (Ferris, 1978). Recent studies suggest that computed tomographic (CT) scanning can detect emphysema (Hayhurst et al., 1984; Bergin et al., 1986). This technique might be applied to selected subjects from epidemiological studies.

III. Conclusions

The standardized methods and definitions that were developed during the 1950s have pervaded epidemiological studies on chronic obstructive lung disease. Studies based on these definitions and methods have identified the cause of most cases of chronic obstructive lung disease as cigarette smoking, and indicated directions for new research. The newer hypotheses on the origins of chronic obstructive lung disease might be more effectively tested if the traditional methods and definitions were comprehensively reevaluated and modified. Regardless of whether such revisions are undertaken, the emphasis on a standardized approach must be maintained.

References

American College of Chest Physicians–American Thoracic Society (1975). Pulmonary terms and symbols. *Chest* **67**:583–593.

American Thoracic Society (1962). Chronic bronchitis, asthma and pulmonary emphysema. A statement by the committee on diagnostic standards for nontuberculous respiratory disease. *Am. Rev. Respir. Dis.* **85**:762–768.

American Thoracic Society. Committee on Standards for Epidemiologic Surveys in Chronic Respiratory Disease (1969). *Standards for Epidemiologic Surveys in Chronic Respiratory Disease*. New York, National Tuberculosis and Respiratory Disease Association.

Bergin, C., Muller, N., Nichols, D. M., Lillinton, G., Hoggs, J. C., Mullen, B., Grymaloski, M. R., and Pare, P. D. (1986). The diagnosis of emphysema. A computed tomographic–pathologic correlation. *Am. Rev. Respir. Dis.* **133**:541–546.

Burney P., and Chinn, S. (1987). Developing a new questionnaire for measuring the prevalence and distribution of asthma. *Chest* 91 (Supplement):79S–83S.

Burrows, B., and Lebowitz, M. D. (1975). Characteristics of chronic bronchitis in a warm, dry region. *Am. Rev. Respir. Dis.* **112**:365–370.

Burrows, B., Halonen, M., Barbee, R. A., and Lebowitz, M. D. (1981). The relationship of serum immunoglobulin E to cigarette smoking. *Am. Rev. Respir. Dis.* **124**:523–525.

Chochrane, A. L., Chapman, P. J., and Oldham, P. D. (1951). Observers' errors in taking medical histories. *Lancet* 1:1007–1009.

CIBA Foundation Guest Symposium (1959). Terminology, definitions and classification of chronic pulmonary emphysema and related conditions. *Thorax* 14(4):286–299.

CIBA Foundation Study Group No. 38 (1971). *Identification of Asthma.* Edinburgh and London, Churchill Livingstone.

Comstock, G. W., Tockman, M. S., Helsing, K. J., and Hennesy, K. M. (1979). Standardized respiratory questionnaires: comparison of the old with the new. *Am. Rev. Respir. Dis.* 119:45–53.

Dodge, R., Cline, M. G., and Burrows, B. (1986). Comparisons of asthma, emphysema, and chronic bronchitis diagnoses in a general population sample. *Am. Rev. Respir. Dis.* 133:981–986.

Eisen, E. A. (1987). Standardizing spirometry: problems and prospects. In *Occupational Medicine. State of the Art Reviews. Occupational Pulmonary Disease.* Edited by L. R. Rosenstock. Philadelphia, Hanley and Belfus, pp. 213–225.

Eisen, E. A., Wegman, D. H., and Louis, T. A. (1983). Effects of selection in a prospective study of forced expiratory volume in Vermont granite workers. *Am. Rev. Respir. Dis.* 128:587–591.

Eisen, E. A., Robins, J. M., Greaves, I. A., and Wegman, D. H. (1984). Selection effects of repeatability criteria applied to lung spirometry. *Am. J. Respir. Dis.* 120:734–742.

Elmes, P. C., Dutton, A. A. C., and Fletcher, C. M. (1959). Sputum examination and the investigation of "chronic bronchitis." *Lancet* 1:1241–1244.

Fairbairn, A. S., Wood, C. H., and Fletcher, C. M. (1959). Variability in answers to a questionnaire on respiratory symptoms. *Br. J. Prev. Soc. Med.* 13:175–193.

Ferris, B. G. (1978). Epidemiology standardization project. *Am. Rev. Respir. Dis.* 118(6, part 2):1–120.

Ferris, B. G., Jr., and Anderson, D. O. (1962). The prevalance of chronic respiratory disease in a New Hampshire town. *Am. Rev. Respir. Dis.* 86:165–177.

Ferris, B. G., Anderson, D. O., and Zickmantel, R. (1965). Prediction values for screening tests of pulmonary function. *Am. Rev. Respir. Dis.* 91:252–261.

Ferris, B. G., Speizer, F. E., Bishop, Y., Prang, G., and Weiner, J. (1978). Spirometry for an epidemiologic study: deriving optimum summary statistics for each subject. *Bull. Eur. Physiopathol. Respir.* 14:145–155.

Fletcher, C. M. (1952). The clinical diagnosis of pulmonary emphysema-an experimental study. *Proc. R. Soc. Med.* 45:577–584.

Fletcher, C. M. (1978). Terminology in chronic obstructive lung diseases. *J. Epidemiol. Commun. Health* 32:282–288.

Fletcher, C. M., and Pride, N. B. (1984). Definitions of emphysema, chronic bronchitis, asthma, and airflow obstruction: 25 years on from the CIBA symposium. Editorial. *Thorax* 39:81–85.

Fletcher, C. M., and Tinker, C. M. (1961). Chronic bronchitis: a further study of simple diagnostic methods in a working population. *Br. Med. J.* 1:1491–1498.

Fletcher, C. M., Elmes, P. C., Fairbairn, A. S., and Wood, C. H. (1959). The significance of respiratory symptoms and the diagnosis of chronic bronchitis in a working population. *Br. Med. J.* 2:257–266.

Fletcher, C., Peto, R., Tinker, C., and Speizer, F. E. (1976). *The Natural History of Chronic Bronchitis and Emphysema. An Eight-Year Study of Early Chronic Obstructive Lung Disease in Working Men in London.* Oxford, Oxford University Press.

Florey, C. du V., and Leeder, S. R. (1982). Methods for cohort studies of chronic airflow limitation. WHO Regional Publications, European Series No. 12.

Freedman, S., and Prowse, K. (1966). How many blows make an F.E.V.? *Lancet* 2:618–619.

Guyatt, G. H., Thompson, P. J., Berman, L. B., Sullivan, M. J., Townsend, M., Jones, N. L., and Pugsley, S. O. (1985). How should we measure function in patients with chronic heart and lung disease? *J. Chron. Dis.* 38:517–524.

Hale, K. A., Ewing, S. L., Gosnell, B. A., and Niewoehner, D. E. (1984). Lung disease in long-term cigarette smokers with and without chronic air-flow obstruction. *Am. Rev. Respir. Dis.* 130:716–721.

Hayhurst, M. D., Flenley, D. C., McLean, A., Wightman, A. J. A., MacNee, W., Wright, D., Lamb, D., and Best, J. (1984). Diagnosis of pulmonary emphysema by computerized tomography. *Lancet* 2:320–322.

Helsing, K. J., Comstock, G. W., Speizer, F. E., Ferris, B. G., Lebowitz, M. D., Tockman, M. S., and Burrows, B. (1979). Comparison of three standardized questionnaires on respiratory symptoms. *Am. Rev. Respir. Dis.* 120:1221–1231.

Higgins, M. W., Keller, J. B., Becker, M., Howatt, W., Landis, J. R., Rotman, H., Weg, J. G., and Higgins, I. (1982). An index of risk for obstructive airways disease. *Am. Rev. Respir. Dis.* 125:144–151.

Holland, W. W., Ashford, J. R., and Colley, J. R. (1966). A comparison of two respiratory symptoms questionnaires. *Br. J. Prev. Soc. Med.* 20:76–96.

Hutchinson, J. (1846). On the capacity of the lungs; and on the respiratory functions, with a view of establishing a precise and easy method of detecting disease by the spirometer. *Trans. Med. Chir. Soc. Lond.* 29:137–252.

Kellie, S. E., Attfield, M. D., Hankinson, J. L., and Castellan, R. M. (1987). Spirometry variability criteria—association with respiratory morbidity and mortality in a cohort of coal miners. *Am. J. Epidemiol.* **125**:437–444.

Knudson, R. J., Slatin, R. C., Lebowitz, M. D., and Burrows, B. (1976). The maximal respiratory flow-volume curve. Normal standards, variability, and effects of age. *Am. Rev. Respir. Dis.* **113**:587–600.

Lebowitz, M. D., and Burrows, B. (1976). Comparison of questionnaires: the BMRC and NHLI respiratory questionnaires and a new self-completion questionnaire. *Am. Rev. Respir. Dis.* **113**:627–635.

Lebowitz, M. D., Knudson, R. J., and Burrows, B. (1975). Tucson epidemiologic study of obstructive lung diseases. I: Methodology and prevalence of disease. *Am. J. Epidemiol.* **102**:137–152.

Lowe, C. R., Pelmear, P. L., Campbell, H., Hitchens, R. A. N., Khosla, T., and King, T. C. (1968). Bronchitis in two integrated steel works. 1. Ventilatory capacity, age, and physique of non-bronchitic men. *Br. J. Prev. Soc. Med.* **22**:1–11.

Mahler, D. A., Weinberg, D. H., Wells, C. K., and Feinstein, A. R. (1984). The measurement of dyspnea. Contents, interobserver agreement, and physiologic correlates of two new clinical indexes. *Chest* **85**:751–758.

Mead, J. (1979). Problems in interpreting common tests of pulmonary mechanical function. In *The Lung in the Transition Between Health and Disease*. Edited by P. T. Macklem and S. Permutt. New York, Marcel Dekker, pp. 43–51.

Medical Research Council (1960). Standardized questionnaires on respiratory symptoms. *Br. Med. J.* **2**:1665.

Medical Research Council Committee on the Aetiology of Chronic Bronchitis (1965). Definition and classification of chronic bronchitis for clinical and epidemiological purposes. *Lancet* **1**:775–779.

Mueller, R. E., Keble, D. L., Plummer, J., and Walker, S. H. (1971). The prevalance of chronic bronchitis, chronic airway obstruction, and respiratory symptoms in a Colorado city. *Am. Rev. Respir. Dis.* **103**:209–228.

Mullen, J. B. M., Wright, J. L., Wiggs, B. R., Pare, P. D., and Hogg, J. C. (1985). Reassessment of inflammation of airways in chronic bronchitis. *Br. Med. J.* **291**:1235–1239.

Nagai, A., West, W. W., Paul, J. L., and Thurlbeck, W. M. (1985a). The National Institutes of Health intermittent positive-pressure breathing trial: pathology studies. I. Interrelationship between morphologic lesions. *Am. Rev. Respir. Dis.* **132**:937–945.

Nagai, A., West, W. W., and Thurlbeck, W. M. (1985b). The National Institutes of Health intermittent positive-pressure breathing trial: pathology studies. II. Correlation between morphologic findings, clinical findings, and evidence of expiratory air-flow obstruction. *Am. Rev. Respir. Dis.* **132**:946–953.

Nathan, S. P., Lebowitz, M. D., and Knudson, R. J. (1979). Spirometric testing. *Chest* **76**:384–388.

National Heart, Lung and Blood Institute (1980). Epidemiology of Respiratory Diseases. Task Force Report. U.S. Department of Health and Human Services, NIH Publication No. 81-2019, October.

National Heart, Lung and Blood Institute, Division of Lung Diseases Workshop (1985). The definition of emphysema. *Am. Rev. Respir. Dis.* **132**:182–185.

Oldham, P. D., and Cole, T. J. (1983). Estimation of the FEV. *Thorax* **38**:662–667.

Orie, N. G., Sluiter, H. J., DeVries, K., Tammeling, G. J., and Witkop, J. (1961). Bronchitis, an International Symposium, April 27–29, 1960. Royal Vangorcum Association, Assen, The Netherlands, pp. 43–59.

Quanjer, P. H. (editor) (1983). Standardized lung function testing. *Bull. Eur. Physiopathol. Respir.* **19**(Supplement):1–9S.

Samet, J. M. (1978). A historical and epidemiologic perspective on respiratory symptoms questionnaires. *Am. J. Epidemiol.* **108**:435–446.

Samet, J. M. (1987). Epidemiological approaches for the identification of asthma. *Chest* **91**(Supplement):74S–78S.

Samet, J. M., Speizer, F. E., and Gaensler, E. A. (1978). Questionnaire reliability and validity in asbestos exposed workers. *Bull. Eur. Physiopathol. Respir.* **14**:177–188.

Samet, J. M., Schrag, S. D., Howard, C. A., Key, C. R., and Pathak, D. R. (1982). Respiratory disease in a New Mexico sample of Hispanic and non-Hispanic whites. *Am. Rev. Respir. Dis.* **125**:152 157.

Scadding, J. G. (1959). Principles of definition in medicine with special reference to chronic bronchitis and emphysema. *Lancet* **1**:323–325.

Scadding, J. G. (1963). Meaning of diagnostic terms in broncho-pulmonary disease. *Br. Med. J.* **2**:1425–1430.

Schilling, R. S. F., Hughes, J. P. W., and Dingwall-Fordyce, I. (1955). Disagreement between observers in an epidemiological study of respiratory disease. *Br. Med. J.* **1**:65–68.

Snider, G. L. (1983). A perspective on emphysema. In *Clinics in Chest Medicine*. Vol. 4, No. 3. Edited by G. L. Snider. Philadelphia, W. B. Saunders, pp. 329–336.

Sorensen, J. B., Morris, A. H., Crapo, R. O., and Gardner, R. M. (1980). Selection of the best spirometric for interpretation. *Am. Rev. Respir. Dis.* **122**:802–805.

Speizer, F. E., and Tager, I. B. (1979). Epidemiology of chronic mucus hypersecretion and obstructive airways disease. *Epidemiol. Rev.* **1**:124–142.

Stebbings, J. H. Jr. (1971). Chronic respiratory disease among nonsmokers in Hagerstown, Maryland. *Environ. Res.* **4**:163–192.

Stoller, J. K., Ferranti, R., and Feinstein, A. R. (1986). Further specification and evaluation of a new clinical index for dyspnea. *Am. Rev. Respir. Dis.* **134**:1129–1134.

Stuart-Harris, C. H. (1954). The epidemiology and evolution of chronic bronchitis. *Br. J. Tuberc. Dis. Chest* **48**:170–178.

Tager, I., Speizer, F. E., Rosner, B., and Prang, G. (1976). A comparison between the three largest and three last of five forced expiratory maneuvers in a population study. *Am. Rev. Respir. Dis.* **114**:1201–1203.

Tager, I., Tishler, P. V., Rosner, B., Speizer, F. E., and Litt, M. (1978). Studies of the familial aggregation of chronic bronchitis and obstructive airways disease. *Int. J. Epidemiol.* **7**:55–62.

Taussig, L. M., Smith, S. M., and Blumenthal, R. (1981). Chronic bronchitis in childhood: what is it? *Pediatrics* **67**:1–5.

Thurlbeck, W. M. (1976). *Chronic Airflow Obstruction in Lung Disease.* Philadelphia, W. B. Saunders.

Ullah, M. I., Cuddihy, U., Saunders, K. B., and Addis, G. J. (1983). How many blows really make an FEV$_1$, FVC, or PEFR? *Thorax* **38**:113–118.

United States Department of Health and Human Services (1984). *The Health Consequences of Smoking. Chronic Obstructive Lung Disease.* Washington, D.C., U.S. Government Printing Office.

van der Lende, R., and Orie, N. G. M. (1972). The MRC-ECCS questionnaire on respiratory symptoms (use in epidemiology). *Scand. J. Respir. Dis.* **53**:218–226.

van der Lende, R., van der Muelen, G. G., and Wever-Hess, J. (1972). Investigation into observer and seasonal variation of the prevalence of respiratory symptoms at Schiermonnikoog. *Int. J. Epidemiol.* **1**:47–50.

Washburn, R. A., and Montoye, H. J. (1986). The assessment of physical activity by questionnaire. *Am. J. Epidemiol.* **123**:563–576.

Williams, B. T., and Nichol, J. P. (1985). Prevalence of hypoxaemic chronic obstructive lung disease with reference to long-term oxygen therapy. *Lancet* **2**:369–372.

World Health Organization (1975). Epidemiology of chronic non-specific respiratory diseases. Memorandum. *Bull. WHO* **52**:251–260.

2

Incidence, Prevalence, and Mortality: Intra- and Intercountry Differences

MILLICENT W. HIGGINS and THOMAS THOM

National Heart, Lung and Blood Institute
National Institutes of Health
Bethesda, Maryland

Estimates of morbidity and mortality from any disease depend on accurate diagnosis and complete ascertainment of affected individuals as well as on complete counting and correct classification of unaffected individuals in defined populations. Deaths must be registered and attributed correctly to specific causes; entries on death certificates must be classified and coded correctly. Accurate information on incidence of disease requires that new onsets be recognized and differentiated from patients developing the disease in the past and surviving into the present. When all these conditions are met, it is also possible to calculate case fatality rates (the proportion of cases dying in a specified period of time) and to devise other indices of the severity and duration of disease. Valid intra- and intercountry comparisons of morbidity and mortality rates can then be made and hypotheses related to cause or course of disease can be developed or tested. Even when these conditions are only partially met, estimates of the frequency and severity of disease can be used for setting priorities, allocating medical resources, identifying trends and determinants of the frequency and distribution of disease, estimating risks for individuals and groups, evaluating preventive and therapeutic interventions, and predicting and planning for the occurrence of disease in the future.

Aside from the problems that apply to all measurements of the frequency of disease and death in the population, some problems are specific to chronic obstructive pulmonary disease (COPD). There is no generally agreed upon definition of COPD. The term is used in a variable way to describe conditions that are sometimes labeled chronic bronchitis, emphysema, or other diseases associated with airway obstruction. Asthma is included sometimes but not always. The absence of a standard definition reflects and contributes to the difficulty of differentiating among conditions that give rise to some of the same symptoms and signs. The onset of COPD is insidious and its course slowly progressive with no dramatic clinical manifestations or highly sensitive and specific diagnostic tests to help in its recognition or to chart its early stages. Pulmonary function declines with age even in those without COPD and distinctions between normal and abnormal levels and rates of decline are based on arbitrarily selected cut-off points and values. Deaths from COPD are much less frequent than those from cardiovascular diseases and cancer but some of the causes and manifestations of coronary heart disease, lung cancer, and COPD are similar. Misclassification has a greater impact on COPD statistics than on more common conditions. COPD may be omitted from medical records and it is usually not included in vital statistics when it is judged to be a contributory but not the main cause of death.

It is, therefore, important to use what information is available but to interpret data on morbidity and mortality from COPD judiciously, giving appropriate weight to their strengths and weaknesses. In this overview, use will be made of information available from national sources, including vital statistics, health interview surveys, and hospital discharge records as well as from epidemiological studies of smaller geographically defined populations. Most of the statistics to be presented are for the population of the United States but international comparisons will be included based on information supplied by the World Health Organization (WHO) or reported in the medical literature.

In this report the abbreviation COPD is used to refer to chronic bronchitis, emphysema, and chronic airways obstruction (ICD/9 codes 490-492, 496). COPD plus asthma includes code 493 as well and COPD and allied conditions includes codes 490-496.

I. Magnitude of the Problem in the United States

A. Prevalence

COPD is more important as a cause of morbidity than as a cause of mortality but estimates of its frequency and distribution are inadequate and incomplete, as discussed above. Estimates of prevalence have been developed from responses to standard questions asked of representative samples of the civilian noninstitutionalized population of the United States in National Health Interview Surveys (NHIS) (National Center for Health Statistics 1974, 1986a, 1987). In 1986 there were estimated to be almost 11.4 million men and women with chronic bronchitis, almost 2 million with emphysema, and over 9½ million with asthma. Rates (unadjusted for age) of reporting emphysema were higher for men than women; 10.5 per 1,000 for men, and 6.5 per 1,000 for women, whereas rates of reporting chronic bronchitis were higher for women than men; 54.7 per 1,000 for women compared with 41.2 per 1000 for men (Table 1). Rates for asthma were approximately the same for men and women, namely 41 per 1000. Table 1 also shows larger numbers of affected persons and higher rates of reporting of these conditions in 1986 than in 1970, but the increases in chronic bronchitis were greater among women than among men and increases in emphysema were confined to women. The prevalence of COPD in total cannot be deduced from these figures since the number of people reporting more than one of these illnesses is not published. Age-adjusted prevalence rates are available for COPD and allied conditions for 55–84-year-old men and women; they were 110 and 119 per 1,000, respectively, in 1985 (Feinleib, 1987). The figures for individual conditions and total COPD depend on the frequency with which men and women report them. No attempt is made to check the accuracy of the diagnoses or the extent of under- or overreporting. Thus, age, race, socioeconomic, or other determinants of ascertainment and willingness to report disease influence these figures and may be different for men and women and may change over time.

Information on cumulative and current prevalence of bronchitis and/or emphysema, of chronic cough, and other conditions was collected in the National Health and Nutrition Examination Surveys in 1971-1974 and 1976-1980 (Table 2). These data also indicate higher rates of reporting bronchitis/emphysema among women than men but increases over time in these estimates are slight; rates of reporting chronic cough decreased among men but increased among women.

Estimates of prevalence of COPD vary depending on the diagnostic criteria used, the age and sex composition of the population, their exposure to cigarette smoke and possibly to other harmful environmental influences. A history of emphysema diagnosed by a physician or a measured level of impaired pulmonary function (usually FEV_1 less than 60 or 65% of predicted) has been found in 4–6% of adult white men and 1–3% of adult white women in a majority of population-based studies in the United States including Tecumseh, Michigan; East Boston; Albuquerque; and six cities.

Table 1 Estimated Prevalence of Chronic Obstructive Pulmonary Disease and Related Conditions; United States, 1970 and 1986

Condition	ICD/9 Code	Total				Men (No. per 1000)		Women (No. per 1000)	
		No. in thousands		No. per 1000					
		1970	1986	1970	1986	1970	1986	1970	1986
Chronic bronchitis	490, 491	6,526	11,379	32.7	48.1	31.2	41.2	34.0	54.7
Emphysema	492	1,313	1,998	6.6	8.5	10.3	10.5	3.1	6.5
Asthma	493	6,031	9,690	30.2	41.0	31.7	40.8	28.8	41.1
Bronchiectasis	494	116	139[a]	0.6	0.6[a]	—	0.7[a]	—	0.6[a]
Pneumoconiosis	495, 500–505	126	291[a]	0.6	1.3[a]	1.3	2.6[a]	—	0.1[a]
Other chronic interstitial pneumonia	515, 516.3	403	243[a]	2.0	1.1[a]	—	1.2[a]	—	1.1[a]

[a] 1979–1981.
Source: National Center for Health Statistics 1974, 1986a, 1987.

Table 2 Percentages of Subjects who Reported Selected Conditions: National Health and Nutrition Examination Survey, Adults 18–74 Years: 1971–1974 and 1976–1980

Condition	Total		Males		Females	
	Ever present	Still present	Ever present	Still present	Ever present	Still present
1971–1974						
Bronchitis/emphysema	6.3	4.1	5.5	3.9	7.0	4.3
Asthma	5.5	3.5	5.6	3.5	5.4	3.6
Hay fever	10.0	8.7	10.3	8.8	9.8	8.7
Chronic cough	3.1	2.5	3.6	3.0	2.6	2.0
1976–1980						
Bronchitis/emphysema	6.8	NA	6.0	NA	7.5	NA
Asthma	6.0	2.8	6.0	2.4	6.0	3.2
Hay fever	10.0	7.1	9.1	6.0	11.0	8.1
Chronic cough	3.1	2.4	2.9	2.2	3.3	2.7

NA: not available.
Source: Unpublished data from the National Health and Nutrition Examination Survey, National Center for Health Statistics.

Rates as high as 9–13% have been detected in men in Berlin, New Hampshire; Glenwood Springs, Colorado; and Tucson, Arizona; and as high as 8% in women in Berlin, New Hampshire (DHHS, 1984).

B. Visits to Physician

In 1985 over 17 million visits were made to doctors offices for COPD and allied conditions that were listed as the principal diagnosis. There were in addition several million office visits in which these conditions were listed as the second or third diagnosis. Among the first listed, or principal, diagnoses of chronic respiratory disease, bronchitis was the most frequent, asthma was second, and chronic airways obstruction was third. These numbers are based on the National Ambulatory Medical Care Survey and apply to office visits not individual patients (Table 3). Age-adjusted rates of office visits in 55–84-year-old men and women were estimated to be 164 and 125 per 1,000 population (Feinleib, 1987).

Table 3 Number of Office Visits for Chronic Obstructive Pulmonary Disease and Allied Conditions, United States, 1985

Diagnosis	ICD9 Code	Number of visits in thousands	
		Principal diagnosis	Second or third diagnosis
Total	490–496	17,774	—
Bronchitis, not specified as acute or chronic	490	7,563	2,750
Chronic bronchitis	491	659	262
Emphysema	492	430[a]	39[a]
Asthma	493	6,503	1,821
Bronchiectasis	494	64	17[a]
Extrinsic allergic alveolitis	495	[a]	12[a]
Chronic airways obstruction	496	2,555	2,323

[a]Estimate does not meet standards of reliability or precision.
Source: Unpublished estimates from the National Ambulatory Medical Care Survey, National Center for Health Statistics.

C. Hospital Discharges

The numbers of hospital discharges for COPD and allied conditions in 1986 are shown in Table 4. Hospital discharge data relate to numbers and rates of discharges for selected conditions, according to whether they are listed as the first or as a subordinate cause of hospitalization. Unfortunately, discharges for individual patients admitted more than once in the course of the year cannot be linked. For the entire group of conditions there were 923,000 discharges with COPD or allied conditions given as the first listed diagnosis. Five million seven hundred thousand days of hospitalization were attributed to these conditions, for which the average length of stay was 6.2 days. Asthma was the most frequently listed single condition; chronic airways obstruction was second and bronchitis third. Average length of stay was less than 5 days for asthma and ranged from 6 to over 8 days for bronchitis, emphysema, and chronic airways obstruction (National Center for Health Statistics, 1988a). Age-adjusted rates of hospitalization for all types of COPD considered together as the first listed diagnosis were 12.8 per 1000 for men and 9.4 per 1000 for women in 1985 (Feinleib, 1987).

Table 4 Estimated Numbers of Hospital Discharges for Chronic Obstructive Pulmonary Disease and Allied Conditions; United States, 1986

First-listed diagnosis	ICD9 code	Number of discharges (in thousands)	Length of stay (in days)	Number of days (in thousands)
Total	490–496[a]	923	6.2	5,680
Bronchitis, chronic and unqualified	490, 491	142	6.6	944
Emphysema	492	47	7.1	336
Asthma	493	477	4.8	2,279
Bronchiectasis	494	10	10.2	102
Extrinsic allergic alveolitis	495	0	0	0
Chronic airways obstruction	496	247	8.2	2,019

[a]Excludes cor pulmonale (code 415.0) for which there were an estimated 3,000 discharges, 26,000 days, and average stay of 8.7 days.
Source: National Center for Health Statistics, 1988a.

Table 5 Number of Deaths from Chronic Obstructive Pulmonary Disease and Allied Conditions; United States, 1985

Cause of death	ICD9 code	Number of deaths
Total	490-496	74,762[a]
Bronchitis, chronic and unqualified	490, 491	3,615
Emphysema	492	14,150
Asthma	493	3,980
Bronchiectasis	494	841
Extrinsic allergic alveolitis	495	19
Chronic airways obstruction	496	52,157

[a]Does not include 19 deaths from cor pulmonale (code 415.0).
Source: National Center for Health Statistics, 1988b.

D. Mortality

The numbers of deaths attributed to chronic obstructive pulmonary diseases in 1985 are shown in Table 5. These deaths amounted to 3% of all deaths and ranked fifth among causes of death in the United States (National Center for Health Statistics, 1988b). Death rates (age adjusted to the U.S. population in 1940) were 546 per 100,000 for all causes combined, 181 per 100,000 for heart diseases, 37 per 100,000 for lung cancer and 18 per 100,000 for COPD. Age-adjusted death rates for COPD and allied conditions in men and women aged 55–84 years were 196 and 81 per 100,000, respectively (age-adjusted to the total population in 1985) (Feinleib, 1987). The specific conditions entered on death certificates for COPD deaths in 1985 are shown in Table 5. In approximately 70% of the deaths, chronic airways obstruction was entered as the underlying cause and in nearly 19% emphysema was entered. These numbers and rates do not include deaths in which COPD was a contributory cause, but in studies of multiple causes of death these conditions were reported as contributory causes more often than as underlying causes. In 1985 74,800 deaths were attributed to COPD and allied conditions as the underlying cause and COPD was cited as a contributing cause in 83,000 deaths (National Center for Health Statistics) unpublished. In 1983 COPD and allied conditions were estimated to cause 130 million days of restricted activity, 72 million days of bed rest, and 7 million days of lost work (National Center for Health Statistics, 1986b). The economic cost of COPD (including asthma) was estimated to be 14.1 billion dollars in 1985, of which 7 billion was direct costs, 4 billion indirect costs associated with morbidity, and 3.1 billion indirect costs associated with premature mortality (unpublished estimates from the National Heart, Lung and Blood Institute).

II. Time Trends in Morbidity and Mortality from COPD in the United States

The increased recognition of COPD as an important cause of morbidity and mortality stems partly from its high rank among the leading causes of illness and death, but more recently from the contrast between its rising mortality rate and the decline in death rates for all causes combined, especially for most of the specific leading causes of death. Between 1966 and 1986 the age-adjusted death rates for coronary heart disease and stroke declined by 45% and 58%, respectively, whereas the death rate for COPD increased by 71% (Fig. 1). Between 1968 and 1986, the death rate for COPD increased by 52%. Recent trends in prevalence, hospitalization, and death rates for COPD among 65–74-year-old men and women are shown in Fig. 2. Between 1979 and 1985 prevalence rates fluctuated from year to year in men and increased in women. Hospitalizations have declined slightly since about 1982, but so have hospital discharge rates in total. Rates of hospitalization are influenced by trends in the practice of medicine, which have included increasing use of outpatient care and the use of new payment schedules. The impact of the use of diagnosis-related groups for reimbursement is not clear but one study has shown that errors in assigning codes for COPD are frequent (Kusserow, 1986). Death rates in 65–74-year-old men have not changed much since 1979, whereas death rates in women have increased progressively each year from 56 per 100,000 in 1979 to 95 per 100,000 in 1985. (Note that the scales for death rates are per 100,000, whereas those for prevalence and hospitalization are per 1000.)

There is some uncertainty about longer-term rates and trends for COPD mortality as revisions in the ICD codes, changing terminology, and diagnostic practices have influenced the numbers of deaths attributed to this cause. Chronic obstructive lung disease (COLD or COPD) or chronic airways obstruction have increasingly been entered on death certificates rather than the more specific terms, chronic bronchitis or emphysema. In 1970, 13% of all COPD deaths were certified as due to COLD (ICD8-code 519.3) whereas 70% were certified as chronic airways obstruction (ICD 9-code 496) in 1985. The marked declines in deaths attributed to chronic bronchitis and emphysema have been more than compensated for by the increased use of the broader COPD category (Fig. 3). If we compare the actual numbers of deaths at different times, aging of the population is a factor. For example, some of the difference between the 7,479 deaths attributed to chronic bronchitis, emphysema, and asthma in 1950 and the 74,762 attributed to COPD and allied conditions in 1985 is because there were more elderly people in 1985; further increases in the number of deaths

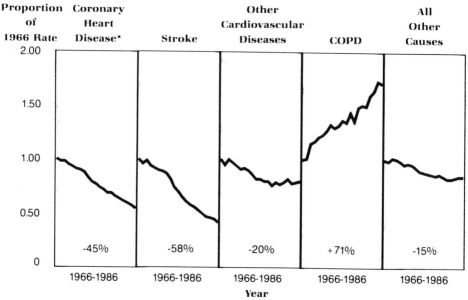

*Comparability ratios applied to rates for 1968-1978
Note: Data for 1986 are provisional.
Source: Vital Statistics of the U.S., NCHS.

Figure 1   Twenty year trends in age-adjusted death rates, United States 1966–1986 (expressed as a proportion of the rate in 1966).

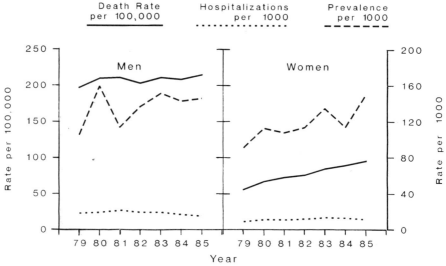

*ICD/9 codes 490–496
Sources: Vital statistics, the National Hospital Discharge Survey,
and the National Health Interview Survey. NCHS

Figure 2   Prevalence, hospitalizations and mortality for COPD for ages 65–74 by sex; United States 1979–1985.

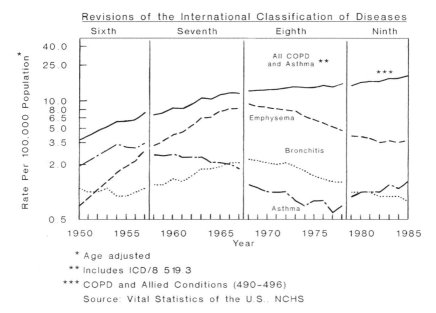

Figure 3 Death rates for bronchitis, emphysema, asthma, and other chronic obstructive lung disease; United States 1950–1985.

from COPD can be anticipated as the number and proportion of elderly people increase in the future. Although it is impossible to quantify precisely the extent to which the death rate for COPD has risen, it is clear that the rise is real and not solely an artifact resulting from increased frequency of diagnosis, changes in certification and coding of causes of death, aging of the population, and declining death rates from other causes. Relationships between COPD morbidity and mortality and cigarette smoking will be discussed below.

Levels and trends of death rates for COPD are shown for men and women separately in Figure 4. Trends in mortality over time are different for men and women and vary with age. Among men, death rates rose between 1960 and 1968 for all age groups over 45 years but they leveled off or declined in more recent years for men under 75. Death rates show a continuing rise among men aged 75–84 years. Among women, the rise in death rates has been much steeper throughout the period from 1960 to 1985 and a rising trend is continuing. In recent years it has been less steep among middle-aged than among elderly women. This figure shows that death rates in women are approximately equal to those in men 15–20 years younger at older ages, but the discrepancy is less at younger ages.

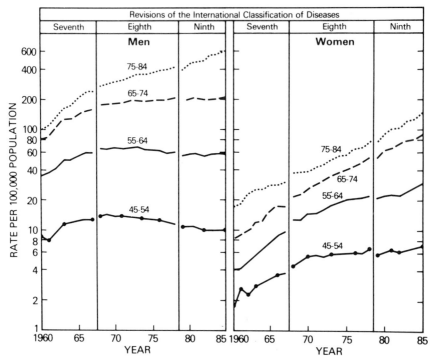

Figure 4 Death rates for chronic obstructive pulmonary diseases by sex for selected age groups; United States 1960–1985.

Trends in death rates for the entire population shown in Figure 3 combine trends in men and women but are influenced more by the higher rates in older men; these rose steeply in the early 1950s. In more recent years rising rates in women have contributed relatively more to the rising trends for the population as a whole. While recent trends suggest that COPD is no longer increasing in men except among those over 75 years of age, morbidity and mortality data indicate that COPD is increasing among women, but the rate of increase may be slowing among younger women.

III. Regional and Demographic Variation in COPD

A. Regional

Regional variation in mortality from COPD is apparent within the United States as shown in Figure 5. Each state compiles its own vital statistics, and

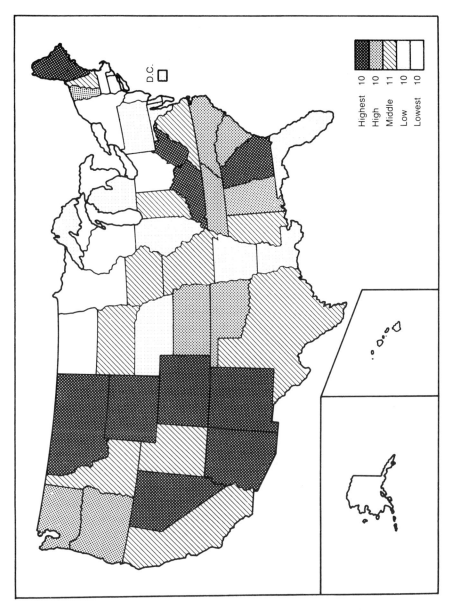

Figure 5 COPD death rates; white males, 55–75 years, 1979–1981. From vital statistics of the U.S. N.C.H.S.

differences in medical certification and coding practices probably account for some of the variability in regional death rates. Among white males aged 55–74 years the states with the highest rates were Arizona, Wyoming, Colorado, Nevada, New Mexico, and West Virginia. Rates were about twice as high as in states with the lowest rates, namely Alaska, Connecticut, Minnesota, and Massachusetts. Death rates in 1979–1981 ranged from 186 to 205 per 100,000 in the high-rate states and from 60 to 97 per 100,000 in the low-rate states; in Alaska the rate was only 60 per 100,000. Possible explanations for this regional variation include migration of patients with COPD into states with climates thought to be more beneficial, but differences may also be related to variations in exposure to cigarette smoke and other hazards, differences in altitude and climate, differences related to the practice of medicine or the completion or processing of death certificates, or other factors.

B. Demographic: COPD by Age, Sex, Race, and Socioeconomic Status

Relationships between COPD morbidity and mortality rates and sex are shown in Tables 1 and 2 and Figures 2 and 4; relationships between mortality rates and age are shown in Figure 4. Age- and sex-specific prevalence, hospitalization, and death rates in 1985 are shown in Figure 6. In both sexes, morbidity and mortality are higher at older ages but the rise with age is steeper in men than women. At ages over 60 years all three rates are higher in men than women but prevalence and hospitalizations were higher in women at younger ages. Clinical and epidemiological experience supports the associations of increased morbidity and mortality with male sex and older ages; although COPD has risen more in women than men in recent years, and the gap between male and female experience of COPD has narrowed, the apparently higher prevalence and hospitalization rates in younger women are partly due to greater reporting of symptoms and use of medical care by women. Mortality rates are higher for the white population than the black population in the United States but the difference is becoming less among males. Between 1980 and 1985 COPD death rates (excluding asthma) increased by 12% in black males, by 7% in white males, by 43% in black females, and by 41% in white females.

Demographic, social, and economic factors were evaluated in a study of 1 million persons (Rogot et al., 1988). Standardized mortality ratios (SMR) for COPD in white males aged 25 and over were inversely related to education and income. The SMRs were 143 for family incomes under $5,000, 117 for incomes of $10,000–$14,000, and 42 for incomes of $25,000–$50,000.

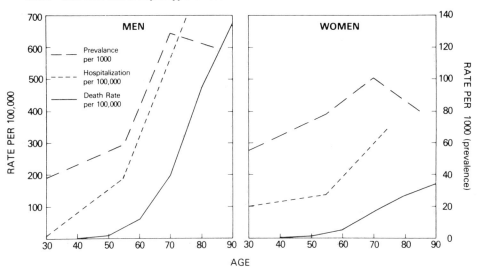

Figure 6 Prevalence, hospitalizations, and mortality from COPD by age and sex, United States, 1985.

IV. International Comparisons of COPD Mortality and Morbidity

Mortality statistics for selected causes of death in certain countries are published by WHO and additional information is available from the statistical office in Geneva (WHO, 1983–1986). Death rates for COPD and allied conditions for men and women aged 65–74 years are shown by country for the latest year available in Figure 7. Taken at face value, these data indicate substantial variation among countries for both sexes. The rates in men were highest in European countries, especially eastern European countries including Romania, East Germany, Poland, and Hungary and also in the British Isles. Death rates for COPD and allied conditions were lower among men in the United States and about the same as those among men in Italy, The Netherlands, Yugoslavia, Bulgaria, and Canada. Japanese men and men living in southern Europe (Spain, France, and Greece) had rates ranging from one-half to two-thirds of those in the United States and less than one-half of those for men in northern and eastern Europe. Death rates were lower among women than among men in every nation and the range of death rates was narrower. In general, rates were higher for women in those countries with high rates among men, but there were some exceptions. The COPD mortality was relatively low for women compared with men in East Germany, Poland, Belgium, and Finland.

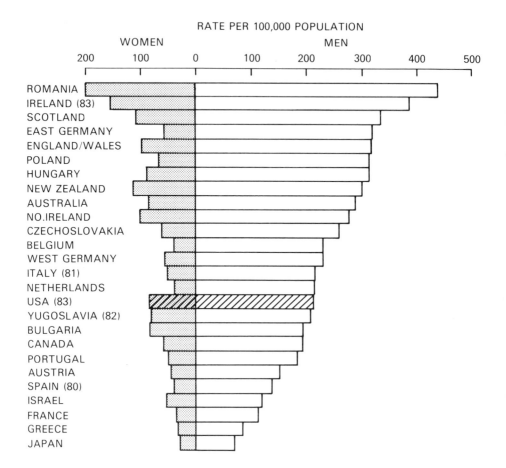

RATE PER 100,000 POPULATION

* ICD/9 codes 490-496

Source: World Health Organization, personal communication
October 31, 1986.

Figure 7 Death rates for COPD and allied conditions by sex, ages 65–74 years, by country, 1984.

Differences in COPD death rates among countries have attracted considerable attention for the last 30 years and have suggested a number of hypotheses including relationships between COPD death rates and smoking behaviors, type and processing of tobacco used in cigarettes, outdoor and indoor pollution, climate, frequency and management of respiratory infections, and genetic factors. Unfortunately, the ability to make inferences about these and other possible causative factors is severely curtailed by the lack of standardization of death certification and coding practices as well as by differences in education, diagnostic practices, and the availability and quality of medical care in different countries. To illustrate one of these problems, the proportion of COPD deaths attributed to the specific conditions bronchitis, emphysema, and asthma in 65–74-year-old men varies substantially (Thom, in press). Prior to about 1968 and the use of the 8th revision of the ICD, specific terminology was used extensively and WHO provided death rates for the combined conditions. During the 1970s, physicians in the United States and some other countries attributed an increasing proportion of these deaths to COPD or COLD, as discussed above. Since these deaths were not included in published data, international comparisons are not valid. Ability to make international comparisons has improved since the introduction of the 9th revision of the ICD, which includes deaths from COPD or chronic airways obstruction in the broad category of COPD and allied conditions (490–496). Comparisons for the restricted range of codes (490–492) or for the individual causes chronic bronchitis, emphysema, and asthma (490, 491, 492, 493) are misleading. For example Romania, with the highest mortality for the total COPD codes, ranks fourth when the restricted list is used and more than 40% of its deaths are omitted. Seventy percent of total COPD deaths in the United States are coded 496 and its rank would change from 16th to 24th among the 26 countries included in Figure 7 if these deaths were omitted. In contrast countries such as Poland, Czechoslovakia, and Italy make little use of the less specific category (COPD) and their death rates are not changed very much by including the newer category (496). While the emphasis here is on international comparisons in recent years, these data reinforce the need to consider diagnostic labels and death certificate coding practices in studies of trends over time within countries as well as between countries.

International differences in mortality rates stimulated studies of morbidity and mortality in residents of and migrants from selected countries. Migrants to the United States from Norway and Britain were compared with permanent residents of each country in an effort to determine the effect of the environment early and later on in life (Reid et al., 1966). Migrants from the United Kingdom to the United States had death rates for chronic nonspecific lung diseases similar to those of the US population but substantially lower than those of men who remained in their own country. Men who migrated from Norway, where death rates for chronic lung diseases are low, also had low death rates in the United States (Rogot, 1978). Cigarette smokers had higher death rates than nonsmokers regardless of their country of origin or residence at time of death.

Widespread use of the respiratory symptom questionnaire developed by the British Medical Research Council and increasing use of standardized methods to measure pulmonary function (Rogot, 1978), have provided morbidity information and improved the quality and comparability of data. But technical differences are greater than was appreciated earlier and, given the problems of making valid comparisons within a single large country such as the United States, information on morbidity in different countries must also be interpreted cautiously.

Prevalence rates in nonsmokers might be quite informative if the symptoms were ascertained and analyzed in the same way and reported singly and in combination for age-specific groups. Prevalence rates of airflow obstruction defined as a ratio of $FEV_{1.0}$ to FVC less than 60% are quite similar for populations of men in the United States, Canada, Finland, Yugoslavia, Poland, the Western Caroline Islands, and New Guinea and range from a low of 5-6% for East Boston to a high of 9% for New Guinea. Rates range from 2 to 5% in women (Department of Health and Human Services, 1984).

Results of the epidemiological studies currently available will be supplemented in the next few years by results from recent studies designed to make international comparisons more valid. Common protocols are being implemented in the United States and China, Poland, Italy, France, and elsewhere. Additional information may become available for some countries participating in collaborative studies for cardiovascular disease including the WHO-sponsored MONICA project, which is underway in 27 countries and over 40 different communities.

V. Trends in Prevalence of COPD and Cigarette Smoking

Cigarette smoking causes 80-90% of COPD in the United States and its influence on the frequency, distribution and trends in COPD morbidity and mortality is strong (Department of Health and Human Services, 1984). The history and current practice of cigarette smoking are different for men and women, for persons born at different times or in different places, and according to socioeconomic circumstances. In 1985, 33% of males and 28% of females 20 years and over smoked cigarettes but prevalence of smoking was higher in the past, especially among men. The percentage of former smokers is twice as high in men as in women over 45 years of age (Center for Disease Control, 1987). Men also smoke more heavily than women and they began smoking at younger ages.

Information on smoking habits for cohorts born between 1900 and 1960 suggests that the prevalence of smoking reached its peak in white men born between 1910 and 1930, in black men born between 1920 and 1950, and in white women born between 1930 and 1940 (Department of Health and Human Services, 1985). In addition to differences in the prevalence of smoking, there are also large differences in the numbers of cigarettes smoked by smokers. In 1980, the percentages of current smokers smoking 25 or more cigarettes per day ranged from 37 for white men and 25 for white women to 14 for black men and 9 for black women. There are socioeconomic differences in smoking habits in both sexes but they are greater among men. In 1983, the percentages of men who smoked were 24 for college graduates, 37 for high school graduates without college education, and 46 for men who did not finish high school. Comparable percentages among women were 18, 32, and 39 (Center for Disease Control, 1987).

Thus the differences between the sexes in exposure to cigarette smoke are compatible with higher morbidity and mortality from COPD among older men and with the earlier rise in COPD mortality in men. The decline in prevalence of smoking in men of all ages since 1965 is consistent with the leveling off or down-turn of mortality in middle-aged men. The more recent rise in COPD prevalence and mortality in women is also consistent with their having taken up smoking more recently. In the short term, COPD is likely to decrease among men but to increase in women over 65 years of age since the prevalence of current and former smokers is still rising in this age group of women. Reductions in smoking in all segments of the population can be expected to lead to less COPD in the future, if they are maintained.

Differences in exposure to tobacco smoke are also important as one explanation for international differences in COPD. Information on cigarette consumption is, unfortunately, not available for many of the countries included in Figure 7, but trends were reported for 18 countries at the Conference on the Decline in Coronary Heart Disease Mortality (Byington et al., 1979). In 1950, average cigarette consumption was high in the United States, Ireland, and the United Kingdom and substantially lower in Norway, Sweden, France, and Italy (Byington et al., 1979). Cigarette consumption increased in all 18 countries between 1950 and 1973, but the increase was particularly steep for Switzerland and Japan. Concordance between cigarette consumption and mortality rates for COPD is not as good among different countries as it is within subgroups of the United States population, but this is not surprising since per capita cigarette consumption is a very imprecise measure of exposure to tobacco smoke. However, ecological comparisons within and among different countries can be used as clues to stimulate the design of better studies and the collection of better data.

References

Byington, R., Dyer, A. R., Garside, D., Liu, K., Moss, D., Stamler, J., and Tsong, Y. (1979). Recent trends of major coronary risk factors and CHD mortality in the United States and other industrialized countries. Proceedings of the Conference on the Decline in Coronary Heart Disease, Mortality, U.S. DHEW, Public Health Service, NIH.

Centers for Disease Control (1987). *Smoking Tobacco and Health. A Fact Book*. DHHS Publication No. (CDC) 87-8397.

Department of Health and Human Services (1984). The Health Consequences of Smoking: Chronic Obstructive Lung Disease. A Report of the Surgeon General, DHHS (PHS), 84-50205.

Department of Health and Human Services (1985). The Health Consequences of Smoking. Cancer and Chronic Lung Disease in the Workplace. A Report of the Surgeon General. Office on Smoking and Health, DHHS (PHS) 85-50207.

Feinleib, M. (1987). Trends in COPD morbidity and mortality in the United States. Presented at the Workshop on the Rise of COPD Mortality, Bethesda, MD.

Kusserow, R. P. (1986). Inspection of DRG 88 Chronic Obstructive Pulmonary Disease. U.S. Department of Health and Human Services, Office of Analysis and Inspections, 1986.

National Center for Health Statistics (1974). Prevalence of Selected Chronic Respiratory Conditions, United States, 1970. Vital and Health Statistics, Series 10, No. 84. DHHS (HRA) 74-1511.

National Center for Health Statistics (1986a). Prevalence of Selected Chronic Respiratory Conditions, United States, 1979–81. Vital and Health Statistics, Series 10, No. 155. DHHS (PHS) 86-1583.

National Center for Health Statistics (C. S. Wilder) (1986b). Disability days, United States, 1983. Vital and Health Statistics. Series 10, No. 158. DHHS (PHS) 87-1586.

National Center for Health Statistics (1987). Current Estimates from the National Health Interview Survey, United States, 1986. Vital and Health Statistics, Series 10, No. 164. DHHS (PHS) 897-1592.

National Center for Health Statistics (1988a). Detailed Diagnosis and Procedures for Patients Discharged from Short-Stay Hospitals, United States, 1986. Vital and Health Statistics.

National Center for Health Statistics (1988b). Vital Statistics of the United States, Vol. II, Part A. Mortality, 1985.

Reid, D. D., Cornfield, J., Markush, R. E., Seigel, D., Pederson, E., and Haenszel, W. (1966). Studies of disease among migrants and native populations in Great Britain, Norway, and the United States. III.

Prevalence of cardiorespiratory symptoms among migrants and native born in the United States. In National Cancer Institute Monograph 19. *Epidemiological Approaches to the Study of Cancer and Other Chronic Disease.* Edited by W. Haenszel. Washington, D.C., U.S. Government Printing Office, USDHEW.

Rogot, E. (1978). Cardiorespiratory disease mortality among British and Norwegian migrants to the United States. *Am. J. Epidemiol.* **108**:181–191.

Rogot, E., Sorlie, P. D., Johnson, N. J., Glover, C. S., and Treasure, D. W. (1988). A Mortality Study of One Million Persons by Demographic, Social, and Economic Factors: 1979–1981 Follow-Up. U.S. Longitudinal Mortality Study. NIH 88-2896.

Thom, T. (in press). International comparisons of COPD mortality. *Am. Rev. Respir. Dis.*

World Health Organization (1983–1986). World Health Statistics Annual, 1983–1986.

3

Morbidity and Quality of Life in Patients with COPD

LOUIS LEVIN

University of New Mexico School of
  Medicine and
Pickard Presbyterian Convalescent
  Center
Albuquerque, New Mexico

DAVID C. LEVIN

University of Oklahoma Health
  Sciences Center and
Veterans Administration
  Medical Center
Oklahoma City, Oklahoma

This chapter assesses the morbidity of chronic obstructive pulmonary disease (COPD) as well as the effect that the disease has on the quality of life of the patient. Morbidity, including signs and symptoms, will be reviewed briefly, with particular attention to physical, emotional, and functional impairment. In the last decade, many important steps have been made toward the better evaluation of quality of life, as it is affected by COPD, using standard psychological and neuropsychological test instruments (Agle and Baum, 1977; Anthonisen, 1986; Calman, 1984; Cribb, 1985; Daughton et al., 1983; Grant and Heaton, 1985; Mahler et al., 1986; Make, 1986; Make and Paine, 1987; McSweeny et al., 1980, 1982; Prigatano et al., 1983, 1984). Increasing interest in this area has resulted in much discussion as to which variables to measure (Guyatt et al., 1985) and the recent development of a measure of quality of life specifically designed for use in patients with chronic lung disease (Guyatt et al., 1987). It is hoped that through a review of the large amount of psychological and clinical data on quality of life, a more logical approach can be achieved in evaluating and caring for patients with COPD.

I. Definition

Emphysema and chronic bronchitis are disabling disorders that frequently limit lifestyle and shorten life expectancy. COPD is second only to chronic cardiac disease as a cause of permanent and total disability (Krop et al., 1973). In 1981 COPD was the fifth leading cause of death in the United States, being responsible for at least 60,000 reported deaths (Higgins et al., 1982). The impact of the disease on the individual ranges from mild intermittent limitation of activity to severe chronic and recurrent illness. Ultimately many patients require extended hospital stay or chronic nursing care.

II. Risk Factors

Established risk factors for COPD include age, male sex, smoking, occupational exposures, air pollution, and familial and genetic factors including alpha-1-antitrypsin deficiency (Higgins et al., 1982; Petty, 1985; Tockman et al., 1981). There are frequent observations that the decline in lung function with age is significantly greater in smokers than in nonsmokers (Fletcher and Peto, 1977). In those who develop chronic airflow obstruction, the decrease in respiratory function is two or three times the expected change associated with aging. The person who stopped smoking at an earlier age will continue to experience age-related loss of function superimposed on the loss due to smoking. Patients are often unable to perform vigorous exertion once their FEV_1 falls much below 1.5 L (Burrows, 1985). When a patient's FEV_1 has decreased to the 1–1.5 L range, there will be continued loss of FEV_1 at a rate averaging 50 ml/year. On the basis of aging alone, life-long nonsmokers will lose about 30 ml, whereas continued heavy smokers will lose up to 80 ml/year (Paine and Make, 1986). However, Burrows (1980) makes three major suggestions: (1) it is unreasonable to assume that every mild ventilatory abnormality found on a routine survey represents an early stage of COPD; (2) one should be cautious in interpreting individual rates of decline in lung function, especially over periods less than 10 years; and (3) the precise preclinical course of most patients who develop severe disabling chronic airways obstruction is currently unknown (see chapter 6).

III. Morbidity

A. Dyspnea

The most bothersome and incapacitating symptom is dyspnea or pathological breathlessness, which becomes severe enough to interfere not only with the patient's ability to work and play but also with the activities of daily living. Exertional dyspnea is usually the first and most pronounced symptom in the emphysematous patient, who may otherwise be symptom-free. Vital capacity may be diminished, while residual volume and total lung capacity are increased, indicating air trapping and hyperinflation. As a result of anatomical destruction, both elastic recoil and diffusing capacity of the lung are often reduced. While these are fixed and lead to progressive deterioration, some of the physiological abnormalities, such as increased smooth muscle tone and mucus hypersecretion may be partially reversible (Make, 1986).

B. Recurrent Respiratory Infections

COPD patients have frequent acute viral and bacterial upper and lower respiratory infections, which often lead to worsening of their chronic bronchitis and airflow obstruction (Make, 1986). Though well-controlled studies supporting the use of broad-spectrum antibiotics are lacking, many authors suggest a decrease in hospitalizations in COPD patients who are given antibiotics early in the course of an exacerbation (Bates, 1982; Anthonisen et al., 1987). The role of respiratory infections in the initiation of COPD is not clearly delineated (Speizer and Tager, 1979), although a prior history of childhood "lung trouble" was associated with abnormal pulmonary function in the Tucson study (Burrows et al., 1977).

C. Lung Cancer

In a review of the COPD patients in the IPPB trial, Tockman and associates (1985) observed that 30 of 985 patients died of lung cancer during the 5 years of the study. Comparison of the incidence of lung cancer in the IPPB study with a group of men of similar age and smoking habits but without clinical evidence of COPD, demonstrated a significant association between COPD and lung cancer. In those patients of the same age and with similar smoking habits, airways obstruction increased the risk of lung cancer about fivefold. The presence of a decreased FEV_1 was a more important predictor of lung cancer risk than either age or smoking. While it is possible that increased airways obstruction predisposes a person to lung cancer, it is more likely that host factors are similar for the development of cancer and of COPD.

IV. Quality of Life

Major steps have been taken toward the better evaluation of the patient's quality of life, as it is affected by COPD. The greatest challenge facing investigators in their evaluation of "quality of life" is the development of a consistent meaning for the phrase. Calman (1984) states that the "quality of life is difficult to define and to measure." Moreover, such measurement may be of little importance from the patient's point of view, since action may be needed to modify the existing quality of life. Measurement and action need to be linked. Calman (1984) proposes the following definition: "A good quality of life can be said to be present when the hopes of the individual are matched and fulfilled by experience. To improve quality of life, therefore, it is necessary to narrow the gap between hopes and aspirations and what actually happens. The aim is to help people reach goals they have set for themselves." In a reply to Calman's hypothesis, Cribb (1985) states that in certain circumstances there is a need for a more systematic reminder of the factors relating to life quality, and a better means of taking those factors into account when making comparative policy judgments and selection of alternative treatments. Calman's formulation is to regard quality of life in terms of the patient's potential for improvement as seen by the patient. The greater the desired improvement, the lower the quality of life, and vice versa. Edlung and Tancredi (1985) agree that the exact meaning of the term "quality of life" is extremely difficult to define, since patients and health care providers often have different concepts of what to measure. As a concept "quality of life is open to a myriad of ideological uses, as well as potential abuses." It is obviously a useful term when used to justify health care services but raises a number of questions: Who is talking about quality of life? What sort of life is being specified and defined by whom?

V. Degree of Impairment

The problem is more difficult, when proceeding from a definition of "quality of life" to measurement of the degree of impairment or improvement (Anderson et al., 1986; Beattie, 1985; Daughton et al., 1983; Edlund and Tancredi, 1985; Gill, 1984; Tugwell et al., 1985). When treating a patient with COPD, one must ask the following questions: "To what extent is the life of the patient affected by his or her condition?" and "Would treatment improve the patient's quality of life?" (Gill, 1984). The complexity of the problem of the measurement of life quality is further emphasized when a review of the literature reveals a plethora of variables that have been studied by various workers (Anderson et al., 1986; Beattie, 1985; Daughton et al., 1983; Dudley et al., 1980; Edlund and Tancredi, 1985; Fishman and Petty, 1971; Gill, 1984; Guyatt et al., 1986; McSweeny et al., 1980; Pearlman and Jonsen, 1985; Prigatano et al., 1983; Prigatano et al., 1984; Tugwell et al., 1985).

McSweeny and co-workers (1980) tested their patients with three self-report evaluations concerned with four dimensions of life quality: emotional functioning, social role functioning, activities of daily living, and recreational pastimes. Further information was obtained from patients' spouses or relatives. Prigatano and associates (1983, 1984) studied mildly hypoxemic COPD patients and normal controls with tests similar to those used by the Nocturnal Oxygen Therapy Trial (NOTT) group (1980). Tests performed included sickness impact profile (SIP), profile of mood states (POMS), and Katz adjustment scale for relatives (KAS-R). Daughton and co-workers (1983) developed the additive daily activities profile test (ADAPT) and validated it against maximum oxygen consumption. Anderson and co-workers (1986) considered that the use of a quality of well being (QWB) scale was useful in overcoming a weakness of other tests, that of underreporting by the individual. They conclude that the interviewer-administered tests, using algorithms, are necessary if quality of life is to be measured with sufficient reliability and validity to evaluate major clinical trials and follow-up studies.

Daughton and associates (1983) validated the ADAPT scale against FEV_1 and found significant correlation between patients' FEV_1 and the two major scores in the total ADAPT score: maximal current activity (MCA) and the normative impairment index (NII). These findings suggested that the ADAPT could be useful in documenting activity level among pulmonary patients with mild to severe impairment. Burrows (1980) noted that after one had accounted for age, the postbronchodilator percentage predicted FEV_1 is the best predictor for survival.

In Prigatano's studies (1983, 1984) patients with COPD and mild hypoxemia reported significantly impaired function as measured by SIP compared to control subjects in all areas except (1) body care and movement and (2) eating. The POMS data demonstrated significant disturbances for five of the six subscores: tension–anxiety, depression–dejection, anger–hostility, fatigue, and vigor. KAS-R data completed by relatives showed that patients are distressed on three major dimensions of psychiatric disturbance: social obstreperousness, acute psychotism, and withdrawal depression. The composite study of the MMPI was characterized by significant elevations on hypochondriasis, depression, and hysteria, with slight elevations on psychasthenia and schizophrenia. The most common pattern was that of reactive depression. However, the authors point out that these patients might be identifying psychiatric problems that go beyond those expected in COPD. A very important finding was a highly significant difference in the average impairment rating (AIR), which indicated that there was a definite restriction in the higher cerebral problem-solving skills. This is of importance, since it may have been a major predictor of quality of life in these patients.

Sandhu (1986) points out that the psychological response to chronic pulmonary disease can be profound. Shortness of breath leads to fear and this, in turn, generates dyspnea. The fundamental changes in abilities and expectations lead to an arousal of negative emotions and attitudes, thus making it a problem for family, friends, and care givers to tolerate, understand, and cope with the patient. Isolation, denial, and repression are the classic defense of COPD patients (Sandhu, 1986).

Prigatano and co-workers (1984) found restrictions in quality of life functions in their patients with mild hypoxemia and COPD compared to an age-, sex- and education-matched control group. While the degree of physical limitation was minimal, the degree of psychosocial limitation was more marked. A greater percentage of the COPD patients were either not working or were working less. When compared with the COPD patients requiring home oxygen therapy in the NOTT, those with mild hypoxemia and COPD had much less physical limitation, but their psychosocial problems were similar in form and degree (Grant and Heaton, 1985). "This observation is of major importance and perhaps is the single most clinically relevant finding of this study" (Prigatano et al., 1984). The degree of physical limitation appears to be related to the degree of pulmonary disease. In contrast, the degree of psychosocial limitation does not appear to be so related, once chronic obstructive disease is present. Prigatano also focused on the identification of predictors of life quality in patients with COPD. Overall quality of life measures were clearly related to educational level, neuropsychological status, emotional or mood state, prebronchodilator FEV_1, and level of exercise completed. The last item correlated highly with severity of illness but not with psychosocial problems. It was noted that recent life changes were not greater than those found in control subjects, except on the health dimension. This suggests that changes in work, home life, marriage, social and personal life, and finances cannot account for the marked quality of life disturbances in patients with COPD. In this particular study of mildly hypoxic COPD patients ($FEV_1/FVC <$ 0.6 and $p_aO_2 > 55$ mmHg), it appeared that changes in health seem to be a very important predictor of life quality (Prigatano et al., 1984).

In a study of similar problems in a group of sicker, more hypoxic subjects, McSweeny and associates (1980) noted that patients with COPD experience negative changes in mood and social behavior that include depression, anxiety, irritability, and paranoia. These symptoms may arise from a multitude of disease-related factors such as breathlessness, sleep disturbance, hypoxia, and hypercapnia. These investigators concluded that patients with COPD experienced severe problems in almost all aspects of their lives. Depression seemed to be the most preponderant emotional disturbance noted. Fairly high levels of fatigue and anxiety were noted by patients and corroborated by their relatives. Also observed was impairment of psychological resiliency. In contrast to previous studies, patients did not report unusual degrees of suspicion and anger.

Dudley and co-workers (1980) observed a lack of overt hostility in COPD patients. The authors considered that this was a result of the patients having learned that expressions of anger required an excessive oxygen uptake. Home management activity and the general level of social interaction were particularly affected by the disease. Patients with COPD suffer from a deficit in basic behavioral function, particularly in ambulation, mobility, sleep, and rest. These patients reported a severe restriction in recreation and other leisure time activities. SIP studies suggested 40% to 50% reduction in pleasurable activities.

VI. Conclusion

Although many studies have been done to document the progressive deterioration in physiological and psychological functions of the COPD patient, much remains to be explained. Many studies have reported the benefits of a comprehensive rehabilitation program on the quality of life in patients with COPD. Not all program participants respond to such programs. Why not, and how can one identify these nonresponders in advance? Further studies need to be done in this area.

In an effort to decrease morbidity, a better understanding of the role of infection and the use of antibiotics should be helpful. Further data need to be collected on the possible benefits to quality, as well as quantity, of life, of oxygen therapy for COPD patients with a p_aO_2 between 55 and 60 mmHg.

With the dissemination of the recent documentation of the deleterious effects of COPD on the patient's quality of life, new psychological interventions to reverse this problem are to be encouraged.

Finally, future improvements in the quality of life of patients with COPD must include more successful methods to help control nicotine addiction associated with cigarette smoking, the primary risk factor for the development of COPD.

References

Agle, D. P., and Baum, G. L. (1977). Psychological aspects of obstructive pulmonary disease. *Med. Clin. North Am.* **61**:749–758.

Anderson, J. P., Bush, J. W., and Berry, C. C. (1986). Classifying function for health outcome and quality-of-life evaluation: self- versus interviewer modes. *Med. Care* **24**:454–470.

Anthonisen, N. R. (1986). Multi-institutional trials in treatment of patients with chronic obstructive pulmonary disease. *Semin. Respir. Med.* **8**:124–128.

Anthonisen, N. R., Manifreda, J., Warren, C. P. W., Hershfield, E. S., Harding, G. K. M., and Nelson, N. A. (1987). Antibiotic therapy in exacerbations of chronic obstructive pulmonary disease. *Ann. Intern. Med.* **106**:196–204.

Bates, J. H. (1982). The role of infection during exacerbations of chronic bronchitis. *Ann. Intern. Med.* **97**:130–131.

Beattie, R. R. (1985). Quality of life: the pursuit of health. *Aust. Fam. Physician* **14**:1291–1293.

Burrows, B. (1980). Course and prognosis of patients with chronic airways obstruction. *Chest* **77**(Suppl):250–251.

Burrows, B. (1985). Course and prognosis in advanced disease. In *Chronic Obstructive Pulmonary Disease: Second Edition, Revised and Expanded.* Edited by T. L. Petty. New York, Marcel Dekker, pp. 31–42.

Burrows, B., Knudson, R. J., and Lebowitz, M. D. (1977). The relationship of childhood respiratory illness to adult obstructive airway disease. *Am. Rev. Respir. Dis.* **115**:751–760.

Calman, K. C. (1984). Quality of life in cancer patients—an hypothesis. *J. Med. Ethics* **10**:124–127.

Cribb, A. (1985). Quality of life—a response to K C Calman. *J. Med. Ethics* **11**:142–145.

Daughton, D., Fix, A. J., Kass, I., McDonald, T., and Stevens, C. (1983). Relationship between a pulmonary function test (FEV$_1$) and the ADAPT Quality-of-Life Scale. *Percept Motor Skills* **57**:359–362.

Dudley, D. L., Glaser, E. M., Jorgenson, B. N., and Logan, D. L. (1980). Psychosocial concomitants to rehabilitation in chronic obstructive pulmonary disease: Part I. Psychosocial and psychological considerations. *Chest* **77**:413–420.

Edlund, M., and Tancredi, L. R. (1985). Quality of life: an ideological critique. *Perspect. Biol. Med.* **28**:591–607.

Fishman, D. B., and Petty, T. L. (1971). Physical, symptomatic and psychological improvement in patients receiving comprehensive care for chronic airway obstruction. *J. Chron. Dis.* **24**:775–785.

Fletcher, C. M., and Peto, R. (1977). The natural history of chronic airflow obstruction. *Br. Med. J.* **1**:1645–1648.

Gill, W. M. (1984). Measuring a patient's quality of life. *N. Z. Med. J.* **97**:329–30.

Grant, I., and Heaton, R. K. (1985). Neuropsychiatric abnormalities in advanced COPD. In *Chronic Obstructive Pulmonary Disease: Second Edition, Revised and Expanded.* Edited by T. L. Petty. New York, Marcel Dekker, pp. 355–373.

Guyatt, G. H., Bombardier, C., and Tugwell, P. X. (1986). Measuring disease-specific quality of life in clinical trials. *Can. Med. Assoc. J.* **134**:889–895.

Guyatt, G. H., Thompson, P. J., Berman, L. B., Sullivan, M. J., Townsend, M., Jones, N. L., and Pugsley, S. O. (1985). How should we measure function in patients with chronic heart and lung disease? *J. Chron. Dis.* **38**:517–724.

Guyatt, G. H., Berman, L. B., Townsend, M., Pugsley, S. O., and Chambers, L. W. (1987). A measure of quality of life for clinical trials in chronic lung disease. *Thorax* **42**:773–778.

Higgins, M. W., Keller, J. B., Becker, M., Howatt, W., Landin, J. R., Rotman, H., Weg, J. G., and Higgins, I. T. T. (1982). An index of risk for obstructive airways disease. *Am. Rev. Respir. Dis.* **125**:144–51.

Krop, H. D., Block, A. J., and Cohen, E. (1973). Neuropsychologic effects of continuous oxygen therapy in chronic obstructive pulmonary disease. *Chest* **64**:317–322.

Mahler, D. A., Barlow, P. B., and Matthay, R. A. (1986). Chronic obstructive pulmonary disease. *Clin. Geriatr. Med.* **2**:285–312.

Make, B. J. (1986). Pulmonary rehabilitation: myth or reality? *Clin. Chest Med.* **7**:519–540.

Make, B. J., and Paine, R. (1987). Pulmonary rehabilitation for COPD patients. *Hosp. Practice* **22**:26–34.

McSweeny, A. J., Heaton, R. K., Grant, I., Cugell, D., Solliday, N., and Timms, R. (1980). Chronic obstructive pulmonary disease: socioemotional adjustment and life quality. *Chest* **77**(Suppl):309–311.

McSweeny, A. J., Grant, I., Heaton, R. K., Adams, K. M., and Timms, R. M. (1982). Life quality of patients with chronic obstructive pulmonary disease. *Arch. Intern. Med.* **142**:473–478.

Nocturnal Oxygen Therapy Trial Group (1980). Continuous or nocturnal oxygen therapy in hypoxemic chronic obstructive lung disease. *Ann. Intern. Med.* **93**:391–398.

Paine, R., and Make, B. J. (1986). Pulmonary rehabilitation for the elderly. *Clin. Geriatr. Med.* **2**:313–335.

Pearlman, R. A., and Jonsen, A. (1985). The use of quality-of-life considerations in medical decision making. *J. Am. Geriatr. Soc.* **33**:344–352.

Petty, T. L. (1985). Definitions, clinical assessment, and risk factors. In *Chronic Obstructive Pulmonary Disease: Second Edition, Revised and Expanded*. Edited by T. L. Petty. New York, Marcel Dekker, pp. 1–30.

Prigatano, G. P., Parsons, O., Wright, E., Levin, D. C., and Hawryluk, G. (1983). Neuropsychological test performance in mildly hypoxemic patients with chronic obstructive pulmonary disease. *J. Consult. Clin. Psychol.* **51**:108–116.

Prigatano, G. P., Wright, E. C., and Levin, D. (1984). Quality of life and its predictors in patients with mild hypoxemia and chronic obstructive pulmonary disease. *Arch Intern. Med.* **144**:1613–1619.

Sandhu, H. S. (1986). Psychosocial issues in chronic obstructive pulmonary disease. *Clin. Chest Med.* **7**:629–642.

Speizer, F. E., and Tager, I. B. (1979). Epidemiology of chronic mucus hypersecretion and obstructive airways disease. *Epidemiol. Rev.* **1**:124–142.

Tockman, M. S., Anthonisen, R. N., and Wright, E. C. (1985). Airways obstruction and the risk of lung cancer. *Am. Rev. Respir. Dis.* **131**(Suppl):A64.

Tockman, M. S., Cohen, B. H., and Comstock, G. W. (1981). Risk factors for airways obstruction in a rural community. *Am. Rev. Respir. Dis.* **123**:139.

Tugwell, P., Bennett, K. J., Sackett, D. L., and Haynes, R. B. (1985). The measurement iterative loop: a framework for the critical appraisal of need, benefits and costs of health interventions. *J. Chron. Dis.* **38**:339–351.

4

Small Airway Disease: Structure and Function

JOANNE L. WRIGHT

University of British Columbia, Health Sciences Center Hospital
Vancouver, British Columbia, Canada

The small airways of the lung are presently defined, in general terms, as noncartilaginous airways less than 2 mm in internal diameter. Both the membranous and respiratory bronchioles are included in this definition, and extend from approximately Weibel generation 8 to 20 in the bronchial tree (Thurlbeck and Wang, 1974) or from generation 1 to 7 in the model by Horsfield and Cumming (1968), giving approximately 28×10^3 membranous bronchioles and 23.4×10^4 respiratory bronchioles. Much of the literature has grouped these airways as "terminal bronchioles," but in fact there are two distinct types: membranous bronchioles (conducting airways) have a complete fibromuscular wall, while the respiratory bronchioles (respiratory airways) are partially alveolated. The differences between the two airway types may be important since their differences in structure and location in the bronchial tree may alter pathological responses as well as affecting the amount of particulate or gaseous material to which they are exposed. The respiratory bronchiole has been largely ignored by physiologists and pathologists alike, and only recently have detailed analyses of its structure in subjects with airflow obstruction been carried out (see below).

The term small airway disease was coined by Hogg et al. in 1968 and reemphasized in 1971 by Macklem and co-workers. These workers were describing lesions in patients who had severe airflow obstruction, little emphysema, and a reticular pattern on chest radiograph. Since the catheters used in the study by Hogg et al. (1968) were wedged in airways 2-3 mm in diameter, the term "small airways" used by these workers probably included some small cartilaginous bronchi as well as the conducting airways. Respiratory bronchioles were not included in their concept. Since that time there have been numerous reports first describing and then quantifying the airway pathological changes. During these investigations, the concept of what constitutes "small airways" has changed to that described in the first paragraph. Even more importantly, the concept of the disease itself has evolved, and is now generally used to describe patients with mild to moderate chronic airflow obstruction.

Pulmonary physiology was in a stage of rapid development in the early 1960s. The airway partitioning technique used by Hogg et al. (1968) had been developed by Macklem and Mead (1967), ^{133}Xe was used to measure steady-state regional ventilation (Anthonisen et al., 1966), and the concept of airway closure had been introduced (Dollfuss et al., 1967). Numerous tests were therefore available for application, and they were suggested to be potentially useful in the identification of small airway disease. Many subsequent clinicopathological studies have shown definite correlations between some of these tests and the various components of airway disease, most often inflammation and fibrosis.

A potential conceptual problem is apparent in reviewing the literature regarding the correlations between airway disease and physiological tests. Closing volume and the nitrogen washout test, the helium flow tests, and the FEF_{25-75} were all thought to be able to detect airways pathological changes during a time when the usual spirometric tests were within normal limits. The term "early" was then applied. It is important to consider whether "early" represents mild disease that may be stable, or whether it represents a stage of disease that is gradually progressive, and, if arrested in its preliminary stages, will not progress to more severe disease. The difference between the two is important since the first option has no clinical significance, and all subsequent investigations have been based on the latter option. Throughout this paper, I will use the term "early" to indicate the preliminary stage of progressive airflow obstruction. Later sections discuss whether this concept is necessarily true.

In the following sections, I will first discuss some of the historical and other salient references that described the pathological appearance of the small airways. This will be followed by sections outlining the development of knowledge of small airway disease in the spheres of pathology, physiology, and clinicopathological relationships. A separate section will discuss whether we have indeed accomplished our intention of identifying airflow obstruction at an early stage. Final sections will be concerned with the relations of airway disease to emphysema, mineral dust exposure, and pulmonary hypertension.

I. Pathological Evidence for Small Airway Abnormalities

Although pathological alterations in the small airways have been recognized for a long time, the significance of these lesions has been largely ignored. Descriptive studies date back to Laennec, and Thurlbeck (1985) has a detailed list of historical developments in small airway disease. Descriptions of the lung in studies of chronic bronchitis (Reid, 1954) and emphysema (McLean, 1958) have documented airway inflammation and fibrosis. One of the better early descriptions of the pathological features of small airway disease was provided by Spain and Kaufman (1953), who described bronchioles with thick walls due to an inflammatory infiltrate, muscular hypertrophy, and a variable increase in fibrous tissue. They suggested that the airway lesions were the basic abnormality in emphysema, and that lung parenchymal destruction was secondary to airways obstruction. Leopold and Gough (1957) suggested that respiratory bronchiolar inflammation was very important in the causation of emphysema.

Two major advances in the pathological identification of disease of small airways were made by Bignon and colleagues, who were investigating the relationship of lung pathological conditions to right ventricular hypertrophy (Bignon et al., 1969, 1970; Depierre et al., 1972). First, they examined a large number of airways; although Anderson and Foraker (1962) had also measured airways, their complicated reconstructive technique was such that only a few airways could be examined per case. Second, they measured the internal diameter of membranous bronchioles, and expressed these data as a percentage of airways in different size values. This was an important new concept. The idea of a size-distribution histogram provided data superior to that of a single mean value, which could easily be skewed with a few very large or very small values. Using this technique, Bignon et al. (1969) initially showed a shift of bronchiolar size toward the narrower airways and, with measurements derived from both microscopic and casting techniques, were able to show that the bronchioles were narrowed throughout the lung and appeared to relate, at least in a gross fashion, to the severity of chronic respiratory failure.

Matsuba and Thurlbeck utilized the techniques of Bignon et al. in investigating airway size distribution changes in emphysema (1972) and chronic bronchitis (1973) from a group of "normal" (1971) lungs. They

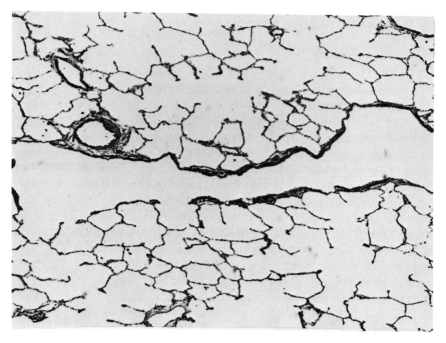

Figure 1 Grade 0 (normal) respiratory bronchiole. There is no inflammation or fibrosis (Masson trichrome X 64) (from Wright et al., 1985b).

found a shift toward the smaller-sized membranous bronchioles, with an excess of those airways less than 0.4 mm internal diameter, and a deficit of those in the size range 0.4–0.6 mm. They interpreted these findings as indicating airway lumen narrowing. This group of studies was important in that it reiterated and extended the value of airway size histograms. They emphasized proper morphometric technique discussing inflation, random sampling, and corrections for histological shrinkage. They also showed that airways sectioned in an elliptical plane could be examined, thus increasing the data base.

Linhartova and Anderson (1979) suggested that the airway narrowing could be related to increasing thickness of the wall, and showed that airways of lungs with emphysema were thicker than those without. They speculated, using a modeling technique, that such an alteration would result in earlier airway closure. Other workers, using a variety of methods (Linhartova et al., 1974, Wang and Ying, 1977) also found tortuosity, stenoses and dilatations, lesions that theoretically could alter flow properties within the airways, in groups of smokers.

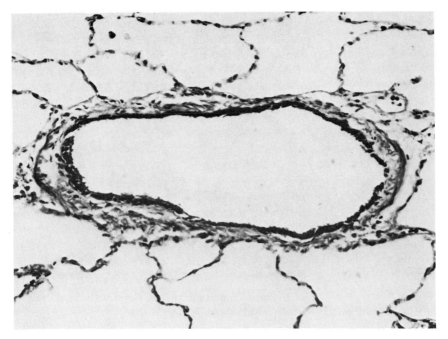

Figure 2 Grade 0 (normal) membranous bronchiole. No inflammation or fibrosis is present (Masson trichrome X 160) (from Wright et al., 1988).

The next major milestone in the investigation of small airways disease was the development of a grading scheme to quantitate pathological abnormalities. Niewoehner et al. (1974b) formulated a quantitative method based on the presence or absence of various pathological parameters (inflammation, fibrosis, goblet cell metaplasia, pigment deposition, and luminal mucus) in a given airway. Their report was also valuable in that it once again suggested the importance of the respiratory bronchiole in airways disease due to cigarette smoking. Cosio et al. (1977) improved the grading technique of Niewoehner by assigning numerical equivalents for the severity of each pathological parameter. The technique proved useful for the quantification of abnormalities in both the membranous and respiratory bronchioles (Wright et al., 1985b) (Figs 1–4). Subsequent studies by Cosio et al. (1980) and Hale and co-workers (1984) have shown that airways from cigarette smokers are narrowed, and there is inflammation of both the membranous bronchioles and respiratory bronchioles when compared to a group of lifetime nonsmokers.

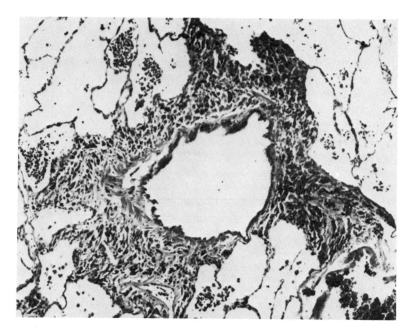

Figure 3 Grade 2 fibrosis of a membranous bronchiole. Note the thickened wall as a result of increased fibrous tissue (Masson trichrome X 64).

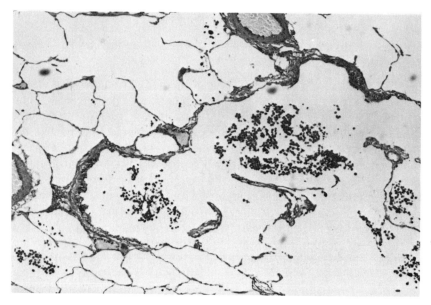

Figure 4 Grade 3 intraluminal inflammation in a respiratory bronchiole. Note the predominance of macrophages (Masson trichrome X 64) (from Wright et al., 1985b).

The grading technique markedly simplified estimation of airway pathology, and since it had a numerical equivalent, it could be used for correlations with physiological changes. In the initial report by Cosio et al. (1977), the airway inflammation and fibrosis seen in the lungs of young cigarette smokers (Niewoehner et al., 1974b) was confirmed as a major feature in small airways disease, and appeared to relate to abnormalities in the nitrogen washout curve and expiratory flow–volume curve as well as in the FEV_1.

II. Physiological Evidence Suggesting a Role for the Small Airways in Airflow Obstruction

Slightly predating, and advancing at the same time as, the descriptions and morphometric analyses of what we now know as small airways disease, experiments documenting airway resistance and airflow mechanics were being conducted. Macklem and Mead (1967) partitioned airways resistance, providing the technique that would be used by Hogg et al. (1968). Anthonisen and co-workers (1966) described a method to measure steady-state regional ventilation–perfusion ratios, and used this technique to show inequalities of ventilation in patients with emphysema and chronic bronchitis (Anthonisen et al., 1968). Dolfuss and colleagues (1967) introduced the concept of "closing volume," indicating the point at which the small airways closed. McCarthy et al. (1972) utilized this concept in investigating lung function in cigarette smokers. In a group of 32 smokers who had spirometry results within normal limits, 26 had a closing volume beyond the normal limit. The authors suggested that closing volume could detect airway abnormalities earlier than the conventional lung function tests. In 1968, Hogg and colleagues conducted a study that has become a physiological landmark. They measured total lung resistance and partitioned airways resistance and found that, in patients with obstructive lung disease, the peripheral airways accounted for the majority of lung resistance (Fig. 5), while in patients without COPD, they contributed only a small proportion of the total lung resistance. Although their values for peripheral resistance in normal lungs have been challenged (Van Brabandt et al., 1983), the data regarding COPD have not been disputed. Hogg et al. (1968) suggested that their data could be explained by narrowing and obliteration of the small airways. As Poiseuille's law would indicate, narrowing is of greater importance than obliteration, since resistance increases to the fourth power of the degree of narrowing, but only in direct proportion to the loss of airways.

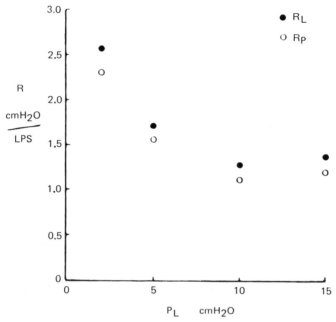

Figure 5   In this subject with severe airflow obstruction, peripheral resistance (R_p) accounts for the majority of the total lung resistance (R_1). Resistance is expressed in cm H_2O/L/sec. Pleural pressure is expressed in cm H_2O (Hogg et al., 1968).

The idea was then developed that the peripheral airways were a "quiet zone" (Mead, 1970), because a mild to moderate increase in their resistance would not be identified by the standard tests of pulmonary function, such as the FEV_1. This idea gained rapid acceptance, and soon a multitude of tests was developed specifically to detect small airway pathological change on the basis of the theory that such changes were "early" and might predict the development of clinically significant airflow obstruction. An excellent discussion of the physiology behind these tests can be found in the article by Dosman and Macklem (1976). Some tests such as frequency dependence of compliance, although very sensitive, require sophistication from equipment, technicians, and patients, and are generally unsuitable in the usual clinical setting (Woolcock et al., 1969). Others such as FEF_{25-75} and flow volume cuves on air and helium have a large normal range and a high variability. The single-breath N_2 test suffers from poor reproducibility and a large degree of intersubject variation (Buist, 1984). However, even when these caveats are borne in mind, many clinicopathological studies were able to find correlations between small airways pathological changes and abnormalities in the "tests for small airways."

III. Pathophysiological Correlations

After the descriptions of airways pathology and physiology, a variety of attempts were made to correlate pathological lesions with functional changes. These involved measurements of airway dimensions and/or the scores for the total or individual pathological parameters. Table 1 summarizes these studies and their findings. Niewoehner and colleagues (1974a) found a good correlation between frequency dependence of compliance and the mean internal diameter of the membranous bronchioles. Berend and co-workers (1979), using the relationship of internal bronchiolar diameter of the membranous bronchiole to the diameter of the adjacent small artery as an index of airway size, found that this value correlated with abnormalities of FEF_{25-75}, N_2 test, and difference in flow between air and helium at 50% vital capacity ($\Delta Vmax$ 50). In a subsequent study, Berend et al. (1981) found that the inflammatory score in the membranous bronchioles related to perturbations of the N_2 test, FEF_{25-75}, and the FEV_1 and, using postmortem lungs (Berend and Thurlbeck, 1982), found that flow at a transpleural pressure of 5 cmH_2O related to airway inflammation and fibrosis as well as grade of emphysema. These studies showed that airway pathological change could be correlated with a number of the specialized tests.

Petty et al. (1980, 1982) performed excised lung mechanics on postmortem lungs, classified the subjects into groups based on the value of the closing capacity, and examined membranous bronchiolar airway size distribution and inflammatory scores. They found that the group with the increased closing capacity had an increased number of airways less than 0.4 mm internal diameter signifying airway narrowing, and this group had an increased score for inflammation. Using both groups, they showed that mean internal bronchiolar diameter was correlated in a negative fashion with closing capacity as a percent predicted, and in a positive fashion with FEF_{25-75}. The mean inflammatory score also correlated with slope of phase III of the N_2 test (percent predicted) (Fig. 6). These studies suggested that the nitrogen washout test may be valuable in detecting airway pathological change in cigarette smokers.

Wright and colleagues (1983a) examined the relationships of pulmonary function tests, including N_2 washout, flow rates on air and helium, FEF_{25-75}, and FEV_1 to pathological conditions of both the membranous and respiratory

Table 1 Summary of Studies Carried Out to Correlate Airway Pathology and Physiology

Reference	Comparisons	Differences	Correlations
Niewoehner et al. (1974b)	Smoking, nonsmoking Respiratory bronchiolitis	Mural inflammation Respiratory bronchiolitis	NA
Niewoehner et al. (1974a)	NA	NA	IB: frequency dependence of compliance
Mitchell et al. (1976)	NA	NA	Chronic airflow Obstruction to airway Inflammation, airway Narrowing
Cosio et al. (1977)	Airway pathology groups	Increasing inflammation, fibrosis; increasing squamous cell metaplasia; decreasing pulmonary function	NA
Berend et al. (1979)	NA	NA	$IB/EAA + FEF_{25-75}$, FEV_1, CV/VC % pred
Petty et al. (1980)	Low and high closing capacity	Inflammation	NA
Berend et al. (1981)	NA	NA	$IB + \dot{V}_{50}$ inflammation — FEV_1, FEF_{25-75}; inflammation + CV/VC, phase III N_2 test; total pathology score — FEF_{25-75}

Petty et al. (1982)	Low and high closing capacity	Internal bronchiolar diameter	$IB - CC/TLC M FEV_1 \%$ pred
Wright et al. (1983b)	Smoking status	Goblet cell metaplasia RB inflammation (mural, lumen) RB fibrosis, pigment	NA
Wright et al. (1984	Groups based on the # pulmonary function tests abnormal	RB inflammation (mural, lumen) RB fibrosis	NA
Petty et al. (1984)	Emphysema-present/absent	Fibrosis score Pigment score Total pathology score	IB-total pathology score, K; $IB + Pl_{50}, Pl_{70}, Pl_{90}$ % airways $< 0.4mm + Pl_{50}, Pl_{70}, Pl_{90}$ fibrosis score $- Pst_{70}$
Pare et al. (1985)	Groups based on FEV_1 and density dependence of flow	MB inflammation	Inflammation $- \Delta\dot{V}_{50}, \Delta\dot{V}_{25}, FEV_1 > 80\%$ Inflammation $+ \Delta\dot{V}_{50}, \Delta\dot{V}_{25} FEV_1 < 80\%$

CV/VC, ratio of closing volume to vital capacity (nitrogen washout); CC/TLC, ratio of closing capacity to total lung capacity (nitrogen washout); FEF_{25-75}, forced expiratory flow at 25–75% vital capacity; FEV_1, forced expiratory volume in 1 sec; IB, internal bronchiolar diameter; IB/EAA, ratio of IB to external elastic lamina of adjacent artery; PHASE III, slope of phase III in the nitrogen washout; PL (50, 70, 90), pleural pressure at 50, 70, 90% vital capacity; PST 70, static pressure at 70% vital capacity; $\Delta\dot{V}$ (25,50), difference in flow between air and helium at 25, 50% vital capacity; NA, not applicable/not performed.

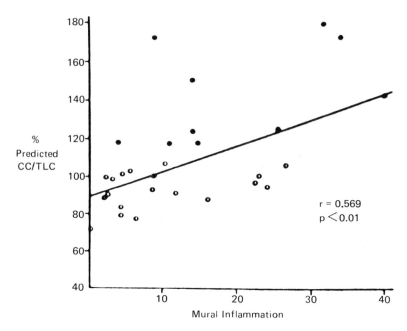

Figure 6 There is a positive relationship between intramural inflammation of membranous bronchioles and the closing capacity of the nitrogen washout test expressed as percent of total lung capacity (from Petty et al., 1980).

bronchioles. Inflammation and fibrosis of both airway types appeared to have the strongest associations with the individual tests. When the patients with FEV_1 greater than 80% predicted were classified into groups based on the number of tests that were abnormal, inflammation and fibrosis of the respiratory bronchioles were found to increase progressively with increased number of abnormal tests. It is interesting that nitrogen washout accounted for a single abnormal test in 8 of 12 cases, and 1 of 2 abnormal tests in 12 of 12 cases, the data again suggesting that the N_2 test was a predictor of airway pathological change, and became abnormal early in airflow obstruction. Some interesting data from Berend et al. (1984) provide a contrasting explanation of the alterations in the N_2 test in smokers. They found that in emphysema free lungs, the slope of phase III of the nitrogen washout curve significantly correlated with the measurement of K in the pressure volume curve when bronchiolar inflammation was held constant. They interpreted these data to suggest that the N_2 test reflects increasing inhomogeneity of elastic properties in the lung rather than bronchiolar disease per se, an explanation that provides ancillary support to the hypotheses of Saetta et al. (1985) (see section relating small airway disease to emphysema).

Pulmonary function, airways pathological conditions, and structural measurements have been examined in surgically excised lungs from nonsmokers, exsmokers, and current smokers. In an initial study (Wright et al., 1983b), respiratory bronchiolar inflammation and fibrosis was found to be a prominent feature differentiating nonsmokers from the two smoking groups. Both groups of smokers had a similar degree of airflow obstruction, but they also had a similar degree of emphysema. When wall structure was examined (Wright et al., 1987), the current and exsmokers had a similar increase in wall thickness compared to the nonsmokers. This increase in thickness was most prominent in the smaller airways, and did not have any obvious relationship to smoking intensity expressed in pack-years. A major finding in this paper was that if one classified the current and exsmokers into groups with and without emphysema, there was no difference in the wall thickness of either airway type between the groups with and without emphysema, nor was there any difference in the pulmonary function tests. These data strongly suggest that both the respiratory and membranous bronchioles are affected by the cigarette smoking habit, and that the fibrotic narrowing of these airways results in airflow obstruction that is independent of emphysema.

IV. Specialized Airway Tests: Are They Really Useful?

The three basic groups of small airway tests include the nitrogen washout, maximum flows breathing air and helium, and analysis of the expiratory flow–volume curve. Although there appears to be an overall relationship of airway pathological conditions to flow rates, Pare et al. (1985), unlike Cosio and colleagues (1977), found that density dependence of flow (measured by the differences in flow between air and helium) does not appear to be a good predictor of bronchiolar pathological conditions. The nitrogen washout test appears to have the most promise as a clinical tool in that it is simple, rapid, and is more frequently abnormal in cigarette smokers (McCarthy et al., 1972; Buist and Ross, 1973; Collins, 1973; Oxhaj, et al., 1977). As shown in the above clinicopathological studies, it also correlates with pathology abnormalities, primarily inflammation and fibrosis, of the respiratory and membranous bronchioles. These data are encouraging, but the cautions of Dosman and Macklem (1976) and of Buist (1984) must still be emphasized. It is not enough to simply have an abnormal test result; one must be able to use these tests to determine which subject will progress from mild airflow obstruction to more severe disease. To do this requires longitudinal studies, and until these data are available, the tests should be used in research settings.

Some intriguing data have been presented by Olofsson and co-workers (1986), who performed a longitudinal study in 460 men aged 50–60 years. The results showed that when the slope of phase III of the nitrogen washout test, corrected for age, smoking, and FEV_1, was steep at the start of the study, there was an enhanced rate of decline in the FEV_1 in the follow-up period. This was true when only the subjects who had a normal FEV_1 and an abnormal nitrogen washout test at the beginning of the study were considered.

In a North American study, Buist et al. (1984) examined the single-breath N_2 washout curve over a period of 7–11 years. When the subjects who had an abnormal final FEV_1 were examined, 114 of 151 had initially had an abnormality in the N_2 test, thus giving a sensitivity of 0.71. The specificity was calculated at 0.75 with 205 of 275 subjects having a normal N_2 test and a normal FEV_1; the significance of specificity in this setting is difficult to ascertain since the hypothesis states that FEV_1 could remain normal in the face of an abnormal N_2 test. These authors did not think that the N_2 washout test would be valuable as a predictor of significant airflow obstruction.

The two studies cited above are at variance. The data presented by Buist et al. (1984) would suggest that the small airway pathological changes reflected by the nitrogen washout test does not invariably progress to major airflow obstruction. The data of Olofsson and colleagues (1986), however, indicate that an abnormal slope of phase III of the nitrogen washout implies a steep rate of decline of the FEV_1. Further studies on this topic must obviously be performed before the nitrogen washout can be considered a test with definite predictive value.

V. Does Small Airways Disease Cause Emphysema?

Petty et al. (1984), investigating lungs with a wide range of emphysema, found that fibrosis of small airways was associated with airway narrowing, which in turn correlated with changes in both elastic recoil and the shape of the pressure volume curve (K). They suggested that the elastic recoil and the fibrotic reaction in the airway wall may both be due to an inflammatory process; several early investigators of emphysema had also suggested that there was a relationship between airway inflammation and development of alveolar destruction (Leopold and Gough, 1957; McLean, 1959; Bignon et al., 1970). Leopold and Gough (1957) blamed the respiratory bronchiole, while Anderson and Foraker (1962) proposed that inflammation in the membranous bronchioles resulted in adjacent alveolar destruction and loss of airway radial traction. Using a grading estimation of inflammation, Berend (1981) and Wright et al. (1984) failed to find a parallel between the severity of airway inflammation in the individual lobes of lung and the presence of gross emphysema in that lobe.

Linhartova and colleagues investigated the number (1971) and affixment pattern (Linhartova et al., 1982) of peribronchiolar alveoli in emphysema. They found that in nonemphysematous lungs, the distance between alveoli that could be found to attach to the bronchial wall was generally constant for bronchioles of all sizes. In emphysematous lungs, there were decreased numbers of attachments, and the affixment pattern was markedly altered. They suggested that these alterations may represent a causal relationship with airway deformities and therefore result in airflow alterations.

Petty et al. (1986) also examined alveolar attachments in lungs with and without emphysema. Unlike Linhartova's group, they did not find a difference between absolute numbers of attachments of the airways of emphysematous lungs compared to those without emphysema, but when the two groups were combined, they did find an overall negative relationship between number of attachments and increasing emphysema severity. These workers also found relationships between mean attachments and elastic recoil pressure at 70% total lung capacity, FEV_1, and closing capacity, but the significance of these associations is difficult to interpret because of the confounding presence of emphysema.

An elegant study by Saetta et al. (1985) has demonstrated a relationship between small airways inflammation and peribronchiolar alveolar destruction in smokers and nonsmokers. These workers did not estimate emphysema in the gross specimen, but measured mean interalveolar distance (Lm) as an index of airspace enlargement. Since the Lm was similar, and within the range considered normal in all groups examined, it is reasonably safe to assume that *significant* emphysema was not present, and the value of this study is in the choice of smoking as a discriminator. The study showed that there were marked differences between number of attachments, percentage abnormal attachments, and distance between attachments in the smoking groups compared to the nonsmoking group. Furthermore, when number of attachments was plotted against airway internal diameter, the slopes of the lines of nonsmokers and smokers were different, perhaps indicating that the larger membranous bronchioles (those between 1 and 2 mm internal bronchiolar diameter) were subject to greater alveolar destruction than the smaller airways (Fig. 7).

Saetta et al. (1985) showed that there was a greater degree of inflammation in the airways of smokers compared to nonsmokers, and that this

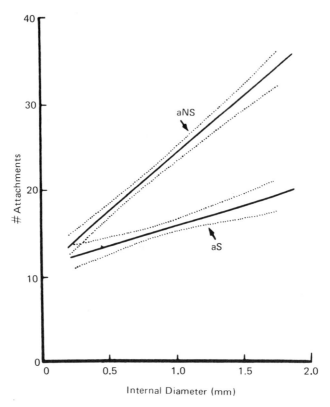

Figure 7 The number of alveolar attachments is related to the size of the airway. This relationship is different between nonsmokers and cigarette smokers (from Saetta et al., 1985).

inflammatory response, in the smoking groups, correlated strongly with degree of peribronchiolar alveolar destruction (Fig. 8). When the indices of peribronchiolar alveolar destruction were compared to function, there was no relationship to FEV_1, FEF_{25-75}, or lung volumes, but there were positive correlations with elastic recoil pressure at 90% total lung capacity and with K, indicating an association of peribronchiolar alveolar destruction with loss of elastic recoil. These data are interesting in relation to the work of Colebatch et al. (1985), who found alterations of K in smokers without airflow obstruction. A correlation can also be drawn with the data of Berend et al. (1984), who found that alteration of the nitrogen washout curve in emphysema-free lungs correlated best with K.

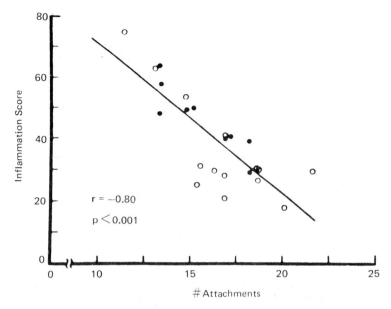

Figure 8 There is a negative relationship between airway inflammation and the number of alveolar attachments, suggesting that attachments are destroyed in inflamed airways (from Saetta et al., 1985).

The relationships identified by Saetta et al. (1985) are interesting when one considers the pathogenesis of airflow limitation. Increased resistance in the small airways and/or loss of elastic recoil have the potential to reduce airflow. The preceding sections have shown that inflammation and fibrosis of the small airways can produce obstruction to airflow, but loss of elastic recoil has always been considered to be due to emphysematous destruction. That this is not the sole cause has been shown by Berend et al. (1980) who found, in lungs with minimal emphysema, a loss of recoil greater than that expected; loss of alveolar attachments could provide an appropriate explanation for these results. The early loss of recoil in cigarette smokers identified by Corbin et al. (1979) may therefore have peribronchiolar alveolar attachment destruction as its morphological counterpart. Gross emphysema, however, appears to parallel rather than follow airways inflammation, as shown by the work of Greaves and Colebatch (1986) who recalculated the data of Mitchell et al. (1976). They interpreted the results to suggest that cumulative smoking history was a strong determinant of both emphysema and small airway disease, with no direct association between the two diseases.

The scheme of events in airflow obstruction may therefore be summarized in the following manner: an inflammatory and fibrotic response in the small airways results in airway wall thickening, lumen narrowing, and an increase in airflow resistance. Airway inflammation also results in destruction of peribronchiolar alveoli producing loss of elastic recoil, and loss of airway tethering with subsequent further distortion of airway lumen. Emphysematous destruction of alveolar parenchyma, at the present time, appears to be a pathological response separate from the airway disease, and the traditional notions of its physiological significance are now being challenged.

VI. Miscellaneous

A. Airway Disease and Dusts

If the small airways of the lung react to the materials of cigarette smoke by a relatively nonspecific process of inflammation and fibrosis, it should not be too surprising that other inhaled materials would produce a similar response. Indeed, one of the patients initially described by Bignon et al. (1970) was a miner, and an early article by Bates (1973) suggested that researchers look specifically for a relationship to dust exposure. A recent review by Becklake (1985) has discussed the physiological evidence and suggested that dust exposure of various kinds is associated with chronic airflow obstruction. There is also pathological evidence that the airways respond to many kinds of mineral dusts with a similar reaction, and that this reaction appears to be related to abnormal pulmonary function (Churg and Wright, 1983; Churg et al., 1985).

A large proportion of the experimental work in the relationships between abnormalities of airflow and pathological alterations of the airways in mineral-dust-exposed subjects has been concentrated on asbestos. Examination of the lungs of patients exposed to asbestos, and experimental instillation of asbestos into the lungs of animals, have shown abnormalities of the small airways, particularly the respiratory bronchioles (Begin et al., 1982; Glassroth et al., 1984; Wright et al., 1986; Wright and Churg, 1985a) (Fig. 9). Although a controversial issue, it is thought that workers exposed to asbestos mineral dusts may develop airflow obstruction (Begin et al., 1983; Cohen et al., 1984; Becklake, 1985), and the animal data suggest that the airway response to instilled asbestos dusts is indeed associated with obstruction to airflow and alteration of the lung volumes.

B. Airway Disease and Pulmonary Hypertension

Although there is abundant literature describing the pathological and physiological abnormalities of the pulmonary vasculature in emphysema,

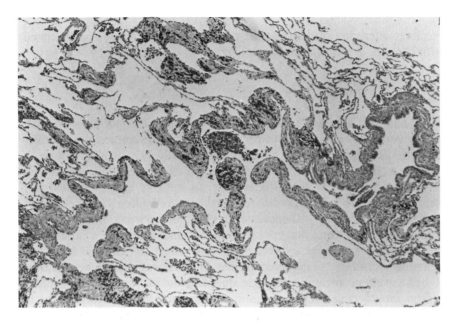

Figure 9 Membranous and subtending respiratory bronchiole in the lung of a hard rock miner. Note the thickened wall of the bronchiole because of the marked increase in fibrous tissue (Masson trichrome X 64) (from Cheng et al., 1985).

there has been very little written assessing the relationship between small airway disease and pulmonary vascular dysfunction. Bignon and co-workers (1969, 1970), investigating the association between right ventricular hypertrophy and emphysema, first suggested that there was a relationship between the presence of airway disease and pulmonary hypertension. Hale and colleagues (1984) quantitated the structure of both the small airways and the arteries in the lungs of nonsmokers and of smokers with and without chronic airflow obstruction. They found significant differences between the vessel structure of these groups, with increased proportion of intima and media in the vessels of the two smoking groups. They noted correlations between artery medial or intimal thickness and airway narrowing, inflammation, fibrosis, and muscular hyperplasia. Wright et al. (1983a) also found differences in vessel structure between nonsmokers and subjects with airflow obstruction and, in addition, showed that these abnormalities appeared to correlate with the pulmonary hemodynamic response to exercise and oxygen. These studies suggest that the inflammatory and fibrotic response of the airways to cigarette smoke results in alteration of the structure of the vasculature, which is associated with changes in vasculature physiology.

VII. Summary

There has been a great deal of controversy about the importance of small airway pathology in airflow obstruction. There are several reasons for this: First, the concept of small airway disease is relatively new, and, second, it is very difficult to divorce small airway disease completely from emphysema since they are often coexistent. In a highly intuitive statement, Bignon et al. (1969) remarked that "further investigations [are necessary] to determine whether inflammatory and fibrous narrowing of multiple bronchioles with minimal or no emphysema constitutes a clinico-pathologic entity, or an evolutionary stage in several chronic broncho-pulmonary diseases." Only recently has small airway disease been shown to be an event occurring in cigarette smokers, and may occur independently from emphysema. Finally, it is still the popular belief that emphysema is the most common association with COPD (Buist, 1984; Menkes et al., 1985; Nagai, et al., 1985a; Greaves and Colebatch, 1986). Certainly there is a strong association between emphysema and airflow obstruction in patients with severe disease (Mitchell et al., 1976; Nagai et al., 1985b; Hale et al., 1984), but also, when mild airflow obstruction is considered, there is good evidence to suggest that small airway disease is likely the prevalent association (Wright et al., 1983b, 1985b). In the study by Mitchell and colleagues (1976), inflammation of the membranous bronchioles was also correlated with the severity of chronic airflow obstruction.

Adequate methods of investigation are still a problem. Clinicopathological studies, by definition, must be performed on excised or autopsy specimens. It would be advantageous to be able to conduct these studies in vivo, but emphysema is difficult to quantify in vivo, either by pulmonary function tests or by the standard radiograph. It is also important not to go to the other extreme; an abnormal pulmonary function test cannot be conclusively attributed to small airway disease, and the cautionary notes of Dosman and Macklem (1976) and Buist (1984) must be reiterated.

It is frequently stated in regard to small airway disease that small airway disease is the major site of airflow obstruction and that small airway disease is an important intermediate step in the pathogenesis of emphysema, which is then responsible for airflow obstruction. It is my belief that neither of these statements is completely correct, and small airway disease represents a distinct entity usually associated with cigarette smoking, which is an important but not the only causative factor in airflow obstruction. The pathological and physiological data would suggest that inflammation and fibrosis in membranous and respiratory bronchioles occur as relatively early events in the cigarette smoking habit. Perhaps surprising is the relationship of physiological abnormalities to structural changes in the respiratory bronchiole. The cross-sectional area of this part of the bronchial tree is very large, and one would believe that abnormalities here would have very little effect. The relationships found in the various studies cited above would suggest that this belief should be reexamined.

There are fairly well documented correlations between airway pathological changes and perturbations in pulmonary function tests, but there does not appear to be a progressive deterioration in either the airway pathological parameters or the pulmonary function tests with continued exposure to cigarette smoke. The patient with an abnormality in FEF_{25-75}, nitrogen washout test, or density dependence of airflow must therefore be viewed as someone with abnormal airways who is at risk, but who may not invariably develop severe airflow obstruction. Until we can use the tests for small airway function to foresee destiny, the FEV_1 must remain the best indicator of airflow obstruction.

The data also indicate a relationship of airway disease with peribronchiolar alveolar destruction and loss of elastic recoil, but the question must be asked : "Does this represent emphysema?" The inflammatory reaction in the airway walls and lumens may act to alter the proteolysis–antiproteolysis balance and cause generalized lung destruction, but this is purely speculative and requires further investigation.

Small airway disease is an entity that, over the last 25 years, has gained widespread acceptance. Nonetheless, the concept that cigarette smoking causes three separate but interrelated conditons—mucus hypersecretion, emphysema, and small airway disease—is an important principle that is widely ignored. The understanding of the relationships between, and the exact physiological consequences of, these three diseases is crucial to an understanding of chronic obstructive pulmonary disease.

References

Anderson, A. E. and Foraker, A. G. (1962). Relative dimensions of bronchioles and parenchymal spaces in lungs from normal subjects and emphysematous patients. *Am. J. Med.* **32**:218–226.

Anthonisen, N. R., Dolovich, M. B., and Bates, D. V. (1966). Steady state measurement of regional ventilation to perfusion ratios in normal man. *J. Clin. Invest.* **45**:1349–1356.

Anthonisen, N. R., Bass, H., Oriol, A., Place, R. E., and Bates, D. V. (1968). Regional lung function in patients with chronic bronchitis. *Clin. Sci.* **25**:495–511.

Bates, D. V. (1973). The respiratory bronchiole as a target organ for the effects of dusts. *J. Occup. Med.* **15**:177–180.

Becklake, M. R. (1985). Chronic airflow limitation: its relationship to work in dusty occupations. *Chest* **88**:608–617.

Begin, R., Masse, S., and Bureau, M. A. (1982). Morphologic features and function of the airways in early asbestosis in the sheep model. *Am. Rev. Respir. Dis.* **126**:870–876.

Begin, R., Cantin, A., Berthiaume, Y., Boileau, R., Peloquin, S., and Masse, S. (1983). Airway function in lifetime-nonsmoking older asbestos workers. *Am. J. Med.* **75**:631–638.

Berend, N. (1981). Lobar distribution of bronchiolar inflammation in emphysema. *Am. Rev. Respir. Dis.* **124**:218–220.

Berend, N., Woolcock, A. J., and Marlin, G. E. (1979). Correlation between the function and structure of the lung in smokers. *Am. Rev. Respir. Dis.* **119**:695–705.

Berend, N., Skoog, C., and Thurlbeck, W. M. (1980). Pressure-volume characteristics of excised human lungs: effects of sex, age, and emphysema. *J. Appl. Physiol.* **49**:558–565.

Berend, N., Wright, J. L., Thurlbeck, W. M., Marlin, G. E., and Woolcock, A. J. (1981). Small airways disease: reproducibility of measurements and correlation with lung function. *Chest* **79**:263–268.

Berend, N. and Thurlbeck, W. M. (1982). Correlations of maximum expiratory flow with small airway dimensions and pathology. *J. Appl. Physiol.* **52**:346–351.

Berend, N., Glanville, A. R., and Grunstein, M. M. (1984). Determinants of the slope of phase III of the single breath nitrogen test. *Clin. Respir. Physiol.* **20**:521–527.

Bignon, J., Khoury, F., Even, P., Andre, J., and Brouet, G. (1969). Morphometric study in chronic obstructive bronchopulmonary disease. *Am. Rev. Respir. Dis.* **99**:669–695.

Bignon, J., Andre-Bougaran, J., and Brouet, G. (1970). Parenchymal, bronchiolar and bronchial measurements in centrilobular emphysema. *Thorax* **25**:556–567.

Buist, A. S. (1984). Current status of small airways disease. *Chest* **86**:100–105.

Buist, A. S., and Ross, B. B. (1973). Quantitative analysis of the alveolar plateau in the diagnosis of early airway obstruction. *Am. Rev. Respir. Dis.* **108**:1078–1087.

Buist, A. S., Vollmer, W., and Johnson, L. (1984). Does the single breath N_2 test identify the susceptible individual. *Chest* **85**:10S.

Churg, A., and Wright, J. L. (1983). Small airway lesions in patients with exposure to nonasbestos mineral dust. *Hum. Pathol.* **14**:688–693.

Churg, A., Wright, J. L., Wiggs, B., Pare, P. D., and Lazur, N. (1985). Small airway disease and mineral dust exposure: prevalence, structure and function. *Am. Rev. Respir. Dis.* **131**:139–143.

Cohen, B. M., Adasczik, A., and Cohen E. M. (1984). Small airways changes in workers exposed to asbestos. *Respiration* **45**:296–302.

Colebatch, H. J. H., Greaves, I. A., and Ng, C. K. Y. (1985). Pulmonary distensibility and ventilatory function in smokers. *Clin. Respir. Physiol.* **21**:439–447.

Collins, J. V. (1973). Closing volume—a test of small airway function? *Br. J. Dis. Chest* **67**:1–17.

Corbin, R. P., Loveland, M., Martin, R. R., and Macklem, P. T. (1979). A four-year follow-up study of lung mechanics in smokers. *Am. Rev. Respir. Dis.* **120**:293–304.

Cosio, M., Ghezzo, H., Hogg, J. C., Corbin, R., Loveland, M., Dosman, J., and Macklem, P. T. (1977). The relations between structural changes in small airways and pulmonary-function tests. *N. Engl. J. Med.* **298**:1277–1281.

Cosio, M. G., Hale, K. A., and Niewoehner, D. E. (1980). Morphologic and morphometric effects of prolonged cigarette smoking on the small airways. *Am. Rev. Respir. Dis.* **122**:265–271.

Depierre, A., Bignon, J., Lebeau, A., and Brouet, G. (1972). Quantitative study of parenchyma and small conductive airways in chronic nonspecific lung disease. *Chest* **62**:699–708.

Dollfuss, R. E., Milic-Emili, J., and Bates, D. V. (1967). Regional ventilation of the lung studied with boluses on Xe^{133}. *Respir. Physiol.* **2**:234–246.

Dosman, J. and Macklem, P. T. (1976). Disease of small airways. *Adv. Intern. Med.* **22**:355–376.

Glassroth, J. L., Bernardo, J., Lucey, E. C., Center, D. M., Jung-Legg, Y., and Snider, G. L. (1984). Interstitial pulmonary fibrosis induced in hamsters by intratracheally administered chrysotile asbestos. *Am. Rev. Respir. Dis.* **130**:242–248.

Greaves, I. A., and Colebatch, H. J. H. (1986). Observations on the pathogenesis of chronic airflow obstruction in smokers: implications for the detection of "early" lung disease. *Thorax* **41**:81–87.

Hale, K. A., Ewing, S. L., Gosnell, B. A., and Niewoehner, D. E. (1984). Lung disease in long-term cigarette smokers with and without chronic air-flow obstruction. *Am. Rev. Respir. Dis.* **130**:716–721.

Hogg, J. C., Macklem, P. T., and Thurlbeck, W. M. (1968). Site and nature of airway obstruction in chronic obstructive lung disease. *N. Engl. J. Med.* **278**:1355–1360.

Horsfield, K., and Cumming, G. (1968). Morphology of the bronchial tree in man. *J. Appl. Physiol.* **24**:373–383.

Leopold, J. G., and Gough, J. (1957). The centrilobular form of hypertrophic emphysema and its relation to chronic bronchitis. *Thorax* **12**:219–235.

Linhartova, A., and Anderson, A. E. (1979). Thickness and composition of nonrespiratory bronchiolar walls in normal and emphysematous lungs with some functional implications. *Bronchopneumologie* **29**:102–115.

Linhartova, A., Anderson, A. E., and Foraker, A. G. (1971). Radial traction and bronchiolar obstruction in pulmonary emphysema. *Arch. Pathol.* **92**:384–391.

Linhartova, A., Anderson, A. E., and Foraker, A. G. (1974). Topology of nonrespiratory bronchioles of normal and emphysematous lungs. *Hum. Pathol.* **5**:729–735.

Linhartova, A., Anderson, A. E., and Foraker, A. G. (1982). Affixment arrangements of peribronchiolar alveoli in normal and emphysematous lungs. *Arch. Pathol. Lab. Med.* **106**:499–502.

Macklem, P. T., and Mead, J. (1967). Resistance of central and peripheral airways measured by a retrograde catheter. *J. Appl. Physiol.* **22**:395–401.

Macklem, P. T., Thurlbeck, W. M., and Fraser, R. G. (1971). Chronic obstructive disease of small airways. *Ann. Intern. Med.* **74**:167–177.

Matsuba, K., and Thurlbeck, W. M. (1971). The number and dimensions of small airways in nonemphysematous lungs. *Am. Rev. Respir. Dis.* **104**:516–524.

Matsuba, K., and Thurlbeck, W. M. (1972). The number and dimensions of small airways in emphysematous lungs. *Am. J. Pathol.* **67**:265–276.

Matsuba, K., and Thurlbeck, W. M. (1973). Disease of the small airways in chronic bronchitis. *Am. Rev. Respir. Dis.* **107**:552–558.

McCarthy, D. S., Spencer, R., Greene, R., and Milic-Emili, J. (11972). Measurement of "closing volume" as a simple and sensitive test for early detection of small airway disease. *Am. J. Med.* **52**:747–753.

McLean, K. H. (1958). The pathology of emphysema. *Am. J. Med.* **25**:62–74.

McLean, K. H. (1959). The pathology of emphysema. *Am. Rev. Respir. Dis.* **80**:58–66.

Mead, J. (1970). The lung's "quiet zone." *N. Engl. J. Med.* **282**:1318–1319.

Menkes, H. A., Beaty, T. H., Cohen, B. H., and Weinmann, G. (1985). Nitrogen washout and mortality. *Am. Rev. Respir. Dis.* **132**:115–119.

Mitchell, R. S., Stanford, R. E., Johnson, J. M., Silvers, G. W., Dart, G., and George, M. S. (1976). The morphologic features of the bronchi, bronchioles, and alveoli in chronic airway obstruction: a clinicopathologic study. *Am. Rev. Respir. Dis.* **114**:137–145.

Nagai, A., West, W. W., Paul, J. L., and Thurlbeck, W. M. (1985a). The national institutes of health intermittent positive-pressure breathing trial: pathology studies. *Am. Rev. Respir. Dis.* **132**:937-945.

Nagai, A., West, W. W., Paul, J. L., and Thurlbeck, W. M. (1985b). The national institutes of health intermittent positive-pressure breathing trial: pathology studies. *Am. Rev. Respir. Dis.* **132**:946-953.

Niewoehner, D. E., and Kleinerman, J. (1974a). Morphologic basis of pulmonary resistance in the human lung and effects of aging. *J. Appl. Physiol.* **36**:412-418.

Niewoehner, D. E., Kleinerman, J., and Rice, D. (1974b). Pathologic changes in the peripheral airways of young cigarette smokers. *N. Engl. J. Med.* **291**:755-758.

Olofsson, J., Bake, B., Svardsudd, K., and Skoogh, B.-E. (1986). The single breath N_2-test predicts the rate of decline in FEV_1. *Eur. J. Respir. Dis.* **69**:46-56.

Oxhoj, H., Bake, B., and Wilhelmsen, L. (1977). Ability of spirometry, flow-volume curves and the nitrogen closing volume test to detect smokers. *Scand. J. Respir. Dis.* **58**:80-96.

Pare, P. D., Brooks, L. A., Coppin, C. A., Wright, J. L., Kennedy, S., Dahlby, R., Mink, S., and Hogg, J. C. (1985). Density dependence of maximum expiratory flow and its correlation with small airway pathology in smokers. *Am. Rev. Respir. Dis.* **109**:163-165.

Petty, T. L., Silvers, G. W., Stanford, R. E., Baird, M. D., and Mitchell, R. S. (1980). Small airway pathology is related to increased closing capacity and abnormal slope of phase III in excised human lungs. *Am. Rev. Respir. Dis.* **121**:449-456.

Petty, T. L., Silvers, G. W., and Stanford, R. E. (1982). Small airway dimension and size distribution in human lungs with an increased closing capacity. *Am. Rev. Respir. Dis.* **125**:535-539.

Petty, T. L., Silvers, G. W., and Stanford, R. E. (1984). Small airway disease is associated with elastic recoil changes in excised human lungs. *Am. Rev. Respir. Dis.* **130**:42-45.

Petty, T. L., Silvers, G. W., and Stanford, R. E. (1986). Radial traction and small airways disease in excised human lungs. *Am. Rev. Respir. Dis.* **133**:132-135.

Reid, L. (1954). Pathology of chronic bronchitis. *Lancet* **1**:275-278.

Saetta, M., Ghezzo, H., Kim, W. D., King, M., Angus, G. E., Wand, N.-S., and Cosio, M. G. (1985). Loss of alveolar attachments in smokers. *Am. Rev. Respir. Dis.* **132**:894-900.

Spain, D. M. and Kaufman, G. (1953). The basic lesion in chronic pulmonary emphysema. *Am. Rev. Respir. Dis.* **68**:24-30.

Thurlbeck, W. M. (1985). Chronic airflow obstruction. In *Chronic Obstructive Pulmonary Disease*. Edited by T. L. Petty. In *Lung Biology in*

Health and Disease, Vol. 28. Edited by C. Lenfant. New York, Marcel Dekker, pp. 129–203.

Thurlbeck, W. M. and Wang, N.-S. (1974). The structure of the lungs. In *Respiratory Physiology*. Edited by J. D. Widdicombe. London, Butterworth.

Van Brabandt, H., Cauberghs, M., Verbeken, E., Moerman, P., Lauweryns, J. M., and Van de Woestijne, K. P. (1983). Partitioning of pulmonary impedance in excised human and canine lungs. *J. Appl. Physiol.* **55**:1733–1742.

Wang, N.-S. and Ying, W.-L. (1977). The pattern of goblet cell hyperplasia in human airways. *Hum. Pathol.* **8**:301–311.

Woolcock, A. J., Vincent, N. J., and Macklem, P. T. (1969). Frequency dependence of compliance as a test for obstruction in the small airways. *J. Clin. Invest.* **48**:1097–1106.

Wright, J. L., Lawson, L. M., Pare, P. D., Hooper, R., Peretz, D., Nelems, J., Schulzter, M., and Hogg, J. C. (1983a). The structure and function of the pulmonary vasculature in mild COPD: the effect of oxygen and exercise. *Am. Rev. Respir. Dis.* **128**:702–707.

Wright, J. L., Lawson, L. M., Pare, P. D., Wiggs, B. J., Kennedy, S., and Hogg, J. C. (1983b). Morphology of peripheral airways in current smokers and ex-smokers. *Am. Rev. Respir. Dis.* **127**:474–477.

Wright, J. L., Lawson, L. M., Pare, P. D., Kennedy, S., Wiggs, B., and Hogg, J. C. (1984). The detection of small airways disease. *Am. Rev. Respir. Dis.* **129**:989–994.

Wright, J. L., Wiggs, B., and Hogg, J. C. (1984). Airway disease in upper and lower lobes in lungs of patients with and without emphysema. *Thorax* **39**:282–285.

Wright, J. L., and Churg, A. (1985a). Severe diffuse small airways abnormalities in long term chrysotile asbestos miners. *Br. J. Ind. Med.* **42**:556–559.

Wright, J. L., Cosio, M., Wiggs, B., and Hogg, J. C. (1985b). A morphologic grading scheme for membranous and respiratory bronchioles. *Arch. Pathol. Lab. Med.* **109**:163–165.

Wright, J. L., Filipenko, D., Dahlby, R., and Churg, A. (1986). Pathophysiologic correlations in asbestos-induced airway disease in the guinea pig. *Exp. Lung Res.* **11**:307–317.

Wright, J. L., Hobson, J., Wiggs, B. R., Pare, P. D., and Hogg, J. C. (1987). The effect of cigarette smoking on the structure of the small airways. *Lung* **165**:91–100.

5

Assessing the Effect of Exposure on Lung Function Loss Between Two Occasions: Issues of Confounding and Measurement Error

LES M. IRWIG

University of Sydney
Sydney, New South Wales, Australia

MARGARET R. BECKLAKE

National Centre for Occupational Health
University of the Witwatersrand
Johannesburg, South Africa
McGill University
Montreal, Quebec, Canada

HENNIE T. GROENEVELD

Institute for Biostatistics of the South
African Medical Research Council
Johannesburg, South Africa

I. Concepts of Confounding and Random Error of Measurement

Investigators often wish to explore the effect of exposure to airborne substances at work or in the general environment on respiratory health. One method is to examine lung function loss between two occasions in relationship to exposure. Longitudinal measurement allows greater certainty about causality and improves statistical power. However, appropriate analysis of longitudinal data requires due regard for (1) whether initial lung function is a confounder of the relationship between environmental factors and lung function loss; and, if so, (2) the consequences of random error of measurement in initial lung function. This chapter reviews the principles involved in these two points, examines how they are dealt with in the longitudinal lung function literature, and illustrates the importance of appropriate analytical techniques, especially the use of the reliability coefficient to correct for random error of measurement in initial lung function when it is considered a confounder. In this chapter, we explore these issues with regard to two-occasion longitudinal data only. However, the principles can be generalized to longitudinal data obtained on more numerous occasions.

A. Is Initial Lung Function a Potential Confounder of the Association between Environmental Exposure and Lung Function Loss?

A confounder is defined as a factor that distorts the apparent magnitude of the effect of exposure to a study factor on the risk of some outcome (Last, 1983). To be a confounder, a variable must be a risk factor for (cause or proxy thereof, or independent determinant of) the outcome; associated with exposure in the study population; and not an intermediate step in the causal path between the exposure and the outcome (Rothman, 1986). Which variables should be considered as confounders is a difficult decision in any analysis, and especially so in the case of longitudinal data (Fletcher et al., 1976; Weisberg, 1979; Hofman, 1983). Whether initial lung function should be considered a confounder of the association between exposure and lung function change is explored in the following two scenarios. In both scenarios, lung function is measured without error, initially at 40 and then at 50 years of age. The mean lung function loss between 40 and 50 years is greater in a group exposed to an environmental agent than in a group that is not exposed.

In the first scenario, the exposed group's exposure to the environmental agent only commences after the initial measurement of lung function at age 40. The exposed group was found to have a lower mean lung function at age 40 than that of the unexposed group. This could be due to a greater rate of loss from about 25 years of age (when their lung function was at its peak level) until 40 years of age. Continuation of this rate results in a greater loss of lung function in the exposed group, in the absence of any effect of the environmental exposure of interest (Fig. 1, line B). This phenomenon of lower lung function in middle age predicting subsequent loss is known as the horse-racing effect (Fletcher et al., 1976). It occurs because those with the lowest initial lung function are likely to have lost most since they reached their adult peak lung function in their 20s. Their subsequent loss represents no more than a continuation of their prior rate of loss. The rate of loss from the mid-20s to 40 years of age should be regarded in this example as a confounder; it is an independent determinant of lung function loss between the ages of 40 and 50 years and is associated with subsequent exposure. The confounder cannot be directly measured. However, based on the assumption that the exposed and unexposed groups had similar mean lung function in their mid-20s, we can use lung function at age 40 as a proxy measure of the loss from the mid-20s to 40 years of age. Note that analysis ignoring the confounder results in overestimation of the effect of exposure between 40 and 50 years of age. For example, in Figure 1, exposure would be found harmful when it had no effect (line B). Conversely if the exposed group had better lung function than the unexposed group at

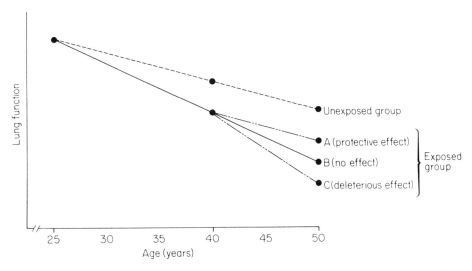

Figure 1 Lung function change with age in exposed and unexposed groups of men whose mean lung function differed at age 40. Exposure starts only after age 40.

40 years of age, the effects of exposure on lung function loss would be underestimated.

The second scenario differs from the first in that the exposed group commenced their exposure to the environmental agent in their mid-20s rather than only after the initial lung function measurement at age 40. In this case, a lower mean lung function in the exposed group at age 40 could be due entirely to their prior exposure. Adjusting loss for lung function at age 40 would essentially be adjusting for exposure. Therefore, while the unadjusted longitudinal data correctly show the effect of exposure, this would not be evident after adjustment for lung function at age 40. Clearly, lung function at age 40 should not be considered a confounder in this case because it is not an independent determinant of subsequent loss. It is a reflection of the effect of exposure on lung function change from the mid-20s to 40 years of age, which is the same effect of exposure that also causes the excessive loss from 40 to 50 years.

Obviously, many real-life scenarios fall between the two extremes presented, depending, for example, on when the exposure occurred, its variability over time, and exposure to several factors at different times. Whether initial lung function should be considered a potential confounder needs to be considered separately for every study.

B. When Initial Lung Function is Adjusted for, What are the Consequences if it is Measured with Random Error?

The consequences of random error of measurement in initial lung function when it is a confounder of the association between exposure and lung function loss are explained more fully in Appendix 1, but can be conceptualized as follows. It is easily shown that after adjustment for initial lung function, the regression coefficient of lung function loss on exposure is, with a change in sign, equivalent to the regression coefficient of the final lung function on exposure (Irwig, 1986) (Appendix 1). In the latter model, the effect of random measurement error in the confounder (initial lung function) is to attenuate the estimate of its correlation with both exposure and final lung function (Goldstein, 1979; Kupper, 1984). The partial regression coefficient of the final on initial lung function will be attenuated. This results in the regression of final lung function on exposure being underadjusted for initial lung function, even if the exposure and the final lung function are measured without error. This effect can be visualized by considering the analysis of covariance example shown in Figure 2 in which unexposed (u) and exposed (e) populations have different mean values for the confounder, initial lung function, which is represented on the x axis. The populations also have different mean values for the dependent

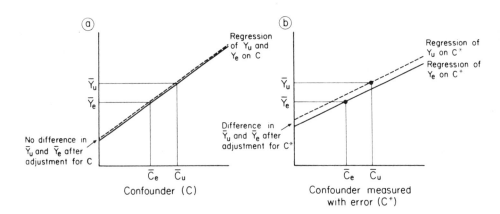

Figure 2 (a) No difference between the mean value of the dependent variable in exposed $(\bar{Y}_e)$ and unexposed $(\bar{Y}_u)$ groups after adjustment for a confounder (C). (b) Underadjustment occurs when C is measured with error so that the adjusted $\bar{Y}_e$ and $\bar{Y}_u$ are found to differ.

variable, final lung function (y axis). Consider first an analysis in which the confounder is measured *without* error (Fig. 2a). After one adjusts for the confounder using the unbiased regression coefficient, no effect of exposure is found, that is, the regression lines for the two exposure groups have the same intercept (Fig. 2a). The attenuated regression, as would be estimated if the confounder is measured with error, must still pass through the point defined by the mean for the dependent variable and the mean for the confounder in each exposure group. (Fig. 2b) The regression lines are still parallel but are "tilted" away from their true slopes around different pivots (the mean values) for the exposed and unexposed groups. Exposure is now estimated to have an effect on the dependent variable, final lung function, as shown by the differing intercepts of the regression lines for the exposed and unexposed groups (Fig. 2b).

II. How are Two-Occasion Longitudinal Lung Function Data Analyzed in the Literature?

We examined the pre-1985 literature on lung function loss (between two occasions) in relation to exposure to determine the major analytical methods used and whether any cognizance was taken of the issues discussed above. Common methods are listed below and illustrative references given.

A. Lung Function Loss Regressed Simultaneously on Exposure and Initial Lung Function

This method (Sparrow et al., 1982; Dontas et al., 1984; Beaty et al., 1984) assumes that initial lung function is a potential confounder. Most of the papers in which this method was used neither discuss the appropriateness of the model nor mention the problem arising because of random measurement error.

B. Lung Function Loss Related to Exposure

This method (Graham et al., 1981; Poukkula et al., 1982; Love and Miller, 1982; Siracusa et al., 1984) assumes that initial lung function is not a confounder. This assumption is justified if the initial lung function is not an independent determinant of loss or if the mean initial measurements do not differ between exposure groups. Few, if any, reports explicitly discussed whether initial lung function should be considered a determinant of loss. Several studies showed that initial measurements differed between exposure groups.

C. Lung Function Loss Regressed Simultaneously on Exposure and the Mean of the Initial and Final Measurement

Kauffman and co-workers (1982) considered initial lung function a confounder and regressed lung function loss on exposure and the mean of the initial and final height-adjusted lung function measurements. This follows the suggestion of Oldham (1964) that the mean value provides a lung function level against which to regress change without obtaining spurious negative regressions because of random error of measurement. However, this method can be shown to give biased estimates of the regression of change on initial lung function and exposure (Appendix 2). In some papers, the dependent variable was the ratio of lung function loss to the mean of the initial and final measurement (Jedrychowski, 1979; Krzyzanowski, 1980). Though not made explicit in any of the publications, the ratio model specifies that the absolute magnitude of loss is expected to be proportional to the initial level. In view of the horse-racing effect discussed earlier (Fletcher et al., 1976), this seems biologically unlikely.

D. Regression of Final Lung Function Measurement on Exposure after Adjusting for Initial Lung Function Measurement

Bosse and co-workers (1981) refer to a method suggested by Rosner (1979), who proposed a two-stage analytical procedure to control for confounding by initial lung function, by which the residuals of the final on the initial measurement are obtained and regressed on the exposure variable of interest. This method may be biased because the residuals are calculated from the regression coefficients of final on initial measurement rather than the corresponding partial regression coefficients (i.e., independent of exposure). In addition, no account is taken of the effect of random measurement error.

In summary, the literature contains a variety of methods used for analyzing longitudinal (two-occasion) data. Different methods may result in different conclusions because of different explicit or implicit assumptions about the relationship between loss and initial level. The conceptual issue of whether initial lung function was a potential confounder was usually not addressed. In most papers, exposure had commenced before the initial lung function measurement, although data were seldom given to quantify its duration. Information on differences in the distribution of initial lung function between exposure groups was often lacking. Only one method (regressing loss on the mean of initial and final measurements) attempts to take account of the effect of random error of measurement, and it can be shown to give biased results. We now present a method that can be used to obtain unbiased regressions of lung function change on exposure and initial lung function when it is measured with error.

III. Estimating Regression Coefficients Using Reliability Coefficients to Correct for Random Error of Measurement

If the true initial lung function values (L_1) are measured with random error (δ_1), resulting in a measurement M_1, then, if we assume that L_1 and δ_1 are independent and normally distributed:

$$\sigma_{M_1}^2 = \sigma_{L_1}^2 + \sigma_{\delta_1}^2$$

where σ = standard deviation

Regression coefficients are estimated with bias in the presence of random measurement error because $\sigma_{M_1}^2$ is used instead of $\sigma_{L_1}^2$ in the formulae for the calculation of the coefficients (see for example Eq. 5 in appendix 1). This effect is easily avoided if an estimate of $\sigma_{L_1}^2$ ($\hat{\sigma}_{L_1}^2$) is available for use in the regression formula. This can be obtained using the reliability or generalizability coefficient (G), defined as the ratio of the variance of true values ($\sigma_{L_1}^2$) to that of measurements ($\sigma_{M_1}^2$) (Goldstein, 1979; Shepard, 1981; Kupper, 1984):

$$G = \frac{\sigma_{L_1}^2}{\sigma_{M_1}^2} = \frac{\sigma_{M_1}^2 - \sigma_{\delta_1}^2}{\sigma_{M_1}^2} = 1 - \frac{\sigma_{\delta_1}^2}{\sigma_{M_1}^2}$$

The reliability coefficient is easily estimated as the correlation between repeat measurements of the same underlying level (Shepard, 1981). In the case of lung function measurements concerned with the detection of chronic airway obstruction, repeat measurements should be days or weeks apart so as to include both technical and short-term biological components of the random error variance. The $\sigma_{L_1}^2$ can be estimated as $G\sigma_{M_1}^2$, which can then be used in equations for the calculation of (partial) regression coefficients, such as that given in Eq. 5 in Appendix 1. Alternatively, the variance of each variable in a variance–covariance matrix can be corrected and the corrected matrix used to calculate regression coefficients (Warren et al., 1974). The variance of estimated regression coefficients are also obtainable (Warren et al., 1974) (Appendix 3).

Correction of regression coefficients using the reliability coefficient is based on the assumption that random measurement error is normally distributed and independent of the true level (Gardner and Heady, 1973; Warren et al., 1974; Shepard, 1981) of lung function. However, correction of regression coefficients is consistent if the error is not normally distributed, although the variance of the regression coefficient may be slightly biased (Warren et al., 1974).

In summary, the method presented is well established in the statistical literature as a technique to adjust regression analyses for random error of measurements. Its use requires an estimation of measurement reliability, the reliability coefficient, which is easily obtained. The method is easy to compute and generalizable to include several exposure variables. Despite its conceptual appeal and practical simplicity, it has not been widely used in analysis of longitudinal lung function data.

IV. Example

This illustrative example is concerned with loss of forced expiratory value in 1 sec (FEV$_1$) in relation to cigarette smoking in a data set chosen so that the initial FEV$_1$ and subsequent cigarette smoking were correlated. The source population consisted of white men aged between 18 and 22 years of age who began employment in South African mines in the mid 1960s and had spirometry performed at that time and again about 11 years later. Spirometry was performed using methods similar to those recommended by the American Thoracic Society (1979). Cigarette consumption was calculated as the average number of cigarettes smoked per day during the 11 years between initial and final spirometry. This was estimated from smoking histories reported annually at a medical examination. Details of the source population and study methods are given elsewhere (Irwig, 1986). From the source population of 433 men, a subset of 125 men was selected so that there was a moderate correlation (r = 0.45) between cigarette consumption and initial lung function. The data were analyzed using the methods commonly used in the literature, and that introduced in Section III. Results are shown in Table 1.

1. FEV$_1$ loss was regressed simultaneously on average cigarette consumption and the initial FEV$_1$ measurement without any correction for random error of measurement. Initial FEV$_1$ was a strong positive predictor of loss ($\hat{\beta} = 0.238$) whereas the regression coefficient for cigarette consumption was very small ($\hat{\beta} = 0.0032$, first column of Table 1).

2. FEV$_1$ loss was regressed on cigarette consumption without including initial FEV$_1$ in the model. Cigarette consumption was found to be a stronger predictor of FEV$_1$ loss than for method 1 ($\hat{\beta} = 0.0110$).

3. FEV$_1$ loss was regressed on average cigarette consumption and the mean of the initial and final FEV$_1$ measurements, that is (M$_1$ + M$_2$)/2. Initial FEV$_1$ showed a negative association with loss, whereas cigarette consumption predicted FEV$_1$ loss more strongly than in method 2.

Table 1 Regression Coefficients of FEV_1 Loss Over 11 Years on Initial FEV_1 and Cigarette Consumption by Different Methods

Independent variable	No correction for measurement error (Method 1)	Omitting initial FEV_1 from model (Method 2)	$(M_1 + M_2)/2$ as a proxy of M_1 (Method 3)	Regressing residuals (Method 4)	Correction using G (Method 5)
Initial FEV_1 (L)	$\hat{\beta}$ 0.238	NA	−0.193	0.258[a]	0.127
	SE 0.081		0.083	0.072	0.094
	p 0.004		0.02	0.0005	0.2
Cigarette consumption (average/day)	$\hat{\beta}$ 0.0032	0.0110	0.0162	0.0026	0.0068
	SE 0.0058	0.0054	0.0057	0.0052	0.0061
	p 0.6	0.04	0.005	0.6	0.3

[a]Coefficient of loss on initial FEV_1 without cigarette consumption in the model calculated from the regression of final on initial lung function (Appendix 1).

$\hat{\beta}$, Regression coefficient estimate; SE, standard error; NA, not applicable.

4. The residuals of final on initial FEV_1 were regressed on average cigarette consumption. The results were similar to method 1.

5. Corrected regression coefficients were obtained using the reliability coefficient as described in Section III. The reliability coefficient used for FEV_1 was 0.899, derived from repeat measurement on a sample of 331 men (Irwig, 1986). The regression coefficient for initial FEV_1 had a smaller absolute value than for any of the other methods, whereas the coefficient for cigarette smoking was between that of methods 1 and 2.

Different methods therefore result in widely differing estimates of the effect of smoking on FEV_1 loss, making the choice of method crucial. As suggested in the introduction, which method is appropriate depends on answers to the following three questions.

1. Could exposure have determined initial FEV_1? Men may certainly have started smoking before their initial FEV_1 measurement. However, they were on average 20 years old at the initial examination, and cigarette smoking could only be a small contributor to variability in initial FEV_1 measurements. It therefore would be appropriate to consider adjusting for initial lung function.

2. Does initial FEV_1 fulfil conventional criteria for potential confounding? In older men, initial FEV_1 is well established as an independent predictor of subsequent FEV_1 loss and there are good conceptual reasons (the "horse-racing" effect described in the introduction) for expecting those with the lowest initial FEV_1 to lose more over subsequent years (Fletcher et al., 1976). In the example chosen here, men were at or near their adult peak lung function, prior to their loss of FEV_1 with aging. There are no conceptual grounds for expecting "horse-racing" to occur in this age group: the race is yet to start. The literature on whether initial lung function is an independent determinant of loss in young men may be considered insufficient to decide that the coefficient should be regarded as zero (Irwig et al., 1988) (in which case initial lung function should be omitted from the analysis, as was done in method 2). If prior evidence is regarded as insufficient, the decision on whether initial lung function should be considered a potential confounder in young men may need to be made using the data from the same study in which the effect of exposure is being examined. Unbiased estimation of the coefficient is therefore crucial.

3. Does the method take into account the effect of random error of measurement? We have outlined the reason why random error in the measurement of initial lung function causes bias in the estimate of effect (partial regression coefficient) for both initial lung function itself and, more importantly, the exposure variable. Use of the reliability coefficient is

theoretically a sound way of reversing the consequences of random measurement error and method 5 in Table 1 must therefore be the analysis of choice. In fact, of those methods in which initial FEV_1 has been entered, method 5 is the one for which the absolute value of the regression coefficient for initial FEV_1 is closest to zero, and statistically not significant. If the decision about potential confounding is made on the basis of this study alone, method 5 could justifiably be followed in this example by an analysis omitting initial FEV_1 from the model (method 2).

Correction procedures using the reliability coefficient are very sensitive to the value of the reliability coefficient used. This is shown in Table 2, where analyses have been repeated using values of 0.85 and 0.95. Attention must therefore be paid to the details of the study designed to generate unbiased estimates of the reliability coefficient, and estimates must be based on large samples. The sample size on which the reliability coefficient is estimated is one of the determinants of the standard error of the corrected regression coefficients for all the independent variables in the model (Appendix 3). Those standard errors will always be larger than for uncorrected coefficients, as is evident from Table 1.

There may also be error in the measurement of the exposure variable, which can be corrected for simultaneously. Results of such an analysis, assuming a generalizability coefficient for smoking of 0.90, are shown in Table 3. The corrected estimate of the regression coefficient for cigarette smoking has a larger absolute value than when random measurement error in this variable is not corrected for, as expected from our knowledge of the attenuating effect of random measurement error in the exposure variable

Table 2 Sensitivity of Correction of Regression Analyses using Different Values of the Reliability Coefficient (G)

Independent variable		Correction using G of		
		0.85	0.899 (from Table 1)	0.95
Initial FEV_1	$\hat{\beta}$	0.060	0.127	0.185
	SE	0.105	0.094	0.087
	p	0.6	0.2	0.03
Cigarette consumption (average/day)	$\hat{\beta}$	0.0090	0.0068	0.0049
	SE	0.0063	0.0061	0.0059
	p	0.2	0.3	0.4

See Table 1 for abbreviations.

Table 3 Consequences of Random Error in Both Predictors

| | | Correction using G^a of 0.899 for FEV and | |
| | | Smoking Assumed Error-free (from Table 2) | Smoking G assumed to be 0.9 |
Independent variable			
Initial FEV$_1$	$\hat{\beta}$	0.127	0.120
	SE	0.094	0.098
	p	0.2	0.2
Cigarette consumption	$\hat{\beta}$	0.0068	0.0078
(average/day)	SE	0.0061	0.0070
	p	0.3	0.3

[a]G, Reliability coefficient.
See Table 1 for abbreviations.

of interest (Kupper, 1986). On the other hand, random error of measurement in the confounder may bias the estimate of the effect of exposure in either direction (Appendix 1). It is therefore more important to adjust for random measurement error in the confounders than in the exposure of interest (Kupper, 1984).

V. Conclusion

Whether initial lung function should be regarded as a confounder in longitudinal lung function studies of the effects of exposure is a conceptual issue that has been too frequently ignored. It should be addressed in each paper. If initial lung function is regarded as a confounder and included in the regression model, corrections should be made for its random error of measurement. This requires estimation of the reliability coefficient from short-term repeat measurements. These principles are generalizable to more complex situations, for example, where there are multiple types of exposure, or where the estimate of each individual's lung function loss is based on more than two lung function measurements.

Appendix 1: The Relationship between Exposure and Lung Function Change when Lung Function is Measured with Random Error

The general linear additive model, when initial lung function is considered a potential confounder of the relationship between environmental exposure and lung function loss, can be represented as:

$$L_2 - L_1 = \alpha + \beta_L L_1 + \beta_X X + \epsilon \tag{1}$$

where: L_1 = the *true* value or "level" (i.e., measured without random error) on the first occasion; L_2 = the true value on a second occasion, for example, 10 years later; α = a constant; X = the measurement of exposure (without error) to an environmental agent between the first and second occasion; β = the regression coefficient for each of the independent variables as indicated by its subscript; ϵ = the residual term, that is, a random deviation from the linear model.

Note that in this appendix, change is measured as the second minus the first lung function measurement. A negative value therefore indicates lung function loss. The model can be used to examine the relationship between change $(L_2 - L_1)$ and an environmental agent (X), after one takes into account any dependence of change on initial level (L_1). If there is exposure to more than one environmental agent, this can be represented by the inclusion of further terms (i.e., $X_1, X_2, X_3 \ldots X_n$). The model can also be expressed as (Werts and Linn, 1970):

$$L_2 = \alpha + (1 + \beta_L)L_1 + \beta_X X + \epsilon \tag{2}$$

Lung function L_i (i = 1 or 2) is usually observed with random error (δ_i) resulting in a measurement M_i, where:

$$M_i = L_i + \delta_i$$

The model from Eq. 1 then becomes (Goldstein, 1979):

$$M_2 - M_1 = \alpha + \beta_L M_1 + \beta_X X + \epsilon - \delta_1 + \delta_2 - \beta_L \delta_1 \tag{3}$$

alternatively expressed as:

$$M_2 = \alpha + (1 + \beta_L)M_1 + \beta_X X + \epsilon + \delta_2 - (1 + \beta_L)\delta_1 \tag{4}$$

The error terms now include δ_1 and $\beta_L \delta_1$, which are not independent of M_1 and therefore violate the necessary assumptions of regression analysis (Snedecor and Cochran, 1967). To explore this further, we use Eq. 4 as the preferred representation because it reduces longitudinal data analysis to a simple example of the errors-in-variables regression model (Warren et al., 1974).

The true (partial) regression coefficient for $X(\beta_{X|L_1})$, that is, the regression coefficient adjusted for L_1 is (Werts and Linn, 1970):

$$\beta_{X|L_1} = \frac{\sigma_{L_1}^2 \sigma_{XL_2} - \sigma_{XL_1} \sigma_{L_1 L_2}}{\sigma_x^2 \sigma_{L_1}^2 - \sigma_{XL_1}^2} \tag{5}$$

If L_1 is measured with random error, the expected covariance value of the terms (σ_{XL_1}, $\sigma_{L_1L_2}$) are unaltered because of the absence of association between measurement error and true values (Kupper, 1984). However, the variance of L_1 is overestimated. A simple illustration of how this may bias the estimate of $\beta_{X|L_1}$ is evident if one remembers that the sign of the regression coefficient is determined by the numerator of Eq. 5. This may truly be negative, but found to be positive if $\sigma_{L_1} \sigma_{XL_1}$ is inflated because $\sigma_{L_1}^2$ is replaced by $\sigma_{M_1}^2$. This is an example of underadjustment for a confounder because it is measured with error.

In summary, the partial regression of change on initial lung function is biased if the initial lung function is measured with random error. Note that the effect of random error is opposite in direction to the horse-racing effect (Fletcher et al., 1976). Because of the incorrect partial regression of change on initial measurement, adjustment for the confounding effect of initial lung function results in a biased regression coefficient of lung function change on environmental exposure.

Appendix 2: Bias in the Regression of Loss on Exposure if the Mean of Initial and Final Lung Function Measurements is a Covariate

With use of the same notation as in Appendix 1, the model is:

$$M_2 - M_1 = \alpha + \beta_L\left(\frac{M_1 + M_2}{2}\right) + \beta_X X + \epsilon - \delta_1 + \delta_2 - \beta_L\left(\frac{\delta_1 + \delta_2}{2}\right)$$

(6)

The method partly takes account of the association between the predictor and the residual because the variance of the $\beta_L\left(\dfrac{\delta_1 + \delta_2}{2}\right)$ term will be less than that $\beta_L\delta_1$ alone. The predictor is also less associated with δ_1 but is now associated with δ_2. However, the most important defect of the model is that it is biologically incorrect. It incorporates a component of change in the $(M_1 + M_2)/2$ term on which β_L is estimated (Blomqvist and Svardsudd, 1978). This results in overestimation of β_L and the possibility of showing a spurious positive association between lung function change and initial level. β_X may then also be incorrectly estimated. For example, if X is not associated with M_1 but is truly associated with change, it will be associated with M_2 and therefore with $(M_1 + M_2)/2$. The β_L estimate using the model in equation 6 will include part of the effect of X. Therefore β_X will be underestimated. This is easily demonstrated by analysis of the hypothetical data in the following table. The data are free of random error of measurement and not intended to represent lung function data.

Hypothetical data for X, M_1, and M_2
(all measured without error)

X	M_1	M_2
0	40	40
1	40	45
0	40	60
1	40	65
0	40	80
1	40	85
0	100	100
1	100	105
0	100	120
1	100	125
0	100	140
1	100	145

The least-squares regression equations calculated from this data set are:

$M_2 - M_1 = 20 + 5.00X + 0.00L_1$
        (using the error-free M_1 as the measure of L_1)
$M_2 - M_1 = 8.97 + 4.66X + 0.14L_1$
        (using $(M_1 + M_2)/2$ as the proxy of L_1).

Appendix 3: Example of Formulae for Variance Estimation of Regression Coefficients Corrected for the Consequences of Random Error of Measurement

When there is only one exposure variable (assumed free of random measurement error) and L_1 is measured with error, approximate formulae for the variance of regression coefficients (Warren et al., 1974) are:

$$\hat{\sigma}_{\hat{\beta}_L}^2 = \hat{\sigma}_{1+\beta_L}^2 = \frac{\hat{\sigma}_v^2}{n\hat{\sigma}_{L_1}^2\hat{G}_{M1}} + \left(\frac{1-\hat{G}_{M1}}{\hat{G}_{M1}}\right)^2 (1+\hat{\beta}_L)^2 \left(\frac{1}{n} + \frac{2}{n_1-1}\right)$$

$$\hat{\sigma}_{\hat{\beta}_X}^2 = \frac{\hat{\sigma}_v^2}{n\hat{\sigma}_X^2}$$

where terms are defined as in Appendix 1, and $\hat{\sigma}_v^2$ = the variance of the residuals around the corrected regression line; $\hat{G}_{M_1}$ = the reliability coefficient for M_1 (equivalent to G in Section III); n = sample size for estimation of the regression coefficients; n_1 = number of pairs of measurements for estimation of G_{M_1}.

This formula assumes that the reliability coefficient is estimated on a subset of the sample used for estimating the other parameters. Alternative formulae when the reliability coefficient is estimated on a totally independent data set give slightly smaller values of $\hat{\sigma}_{\beta_L}^2$ (Fuller and Hidiroglou, 1978).

References

American Thoracic Society. (1979). ATS Statement–Snowbird workshop on standardization of spirometry. *Am. Rev. Respir. Dis.* **119**:831–838.

Beaty, T. H., Menkes, H. A., Cohen, B. H., and Newill , C. A. (1984). Risk factors associated with longitudinal change in pulmonary function. *Am. Rev. Respir. Dis.* **129**:660–667.

Blomqvist, N., and Svardsudd, K. (1978). A new method for investigating the relation between change and initial value in longitudinal blood pressure data. II. Comparison with other methods. *Scand. J. Soc. Med.* **6**:125–129.

Bosse, R., Sparrow, D., Rose, C. L., and Weiss, S. T. (1981). Longitudinal effect of age and smoking cessation on pulmonary function. *Am. Rev. Respir. Dis.* **123**:378–381.

Dontas, A. S., Jacobs, D. R. Jr., Corcondilas, A., Keys, A., and Hannan, P. (1984). Longitudinal versus cross-sectional vital capacity changes and affecting factors. *J. Gerontol.* **39**:430–438.

Fletcher, C., Peto, R., Tinker, C., and Speizer, F. E. (1976). *The Natural History of Chronic Bronchitis and Emphysema—An Eight-Year Study of Early Chronic Obstructive Lung Disease in Working Men in London.* Oxford, Oxford University Press, pp. 195–208.

Fuller, W. A., and Hidiroglou, M. A. (1978). Regression estimation after correcting for attenuation. *J. Am. Stat. Assoc.* **73**:99–104.

Gardner, M. J., and Heady, J. A. (1973). Some effects of within-person variability in epidemiological studies. *J. Chron. Dis.* **26**:781–795.

Goldstein, H. (1979). Some models for analysing longitudinal data on education attainment. *J. R. Stat. Soc.* [A] **142**:407–442.

Graham, W. G. B., O'Grady, R. V., and Dubuc, B. (1981). Pulmonary function loss in Vermont granite workers. A long-term follow-up and critical reappraisal. *Am. Rev. Respir. Dis.* **123**:25–28.

Hofman, A. (1983). Change viewed on the level. *Int. J. Epidemiol.* **12**: 391–392.

Irwig, L. M. (1986). Correcting for the effect of measurement error on the association between environmental exposure and respiratory impairment. Johannesburg, Institute for Biostatistics of the South African Medical Research Council, Research Report No. 1.

Irwig, L. M., Groeneveld, H. T., and Becklake, M. R. (1988). Relationship of lung function loss to initial level: correcting for measurement error using the reliability coefficient. *J. Epidemiol. Commun. Health*, **42**:383–389

Jedrychowski, W. (1979). A consideration of risk factors and development of chronic bronchitis in a five-year follow-up study of an industrial population. *J. Epidemiol. Commun. Health* **33**:210–214.

Kauffman, F., Drouet, D., Lellouch, J., and Brille, D. (1982). Occupational exposure and 12-year spirometric changes among Paris area workers. *Br. J. Ind. Med.* **39**:221–232.

Krzyzanowski, M. (1980). Changes of ventilatory capacity in an adult population during a five-year period. *Bull. Eur. J. Physiopathol. Respir.* **16**:155–170.

Kupper, L. L. (1984). Effects of the use of unreliable surrogate variables on the validity of epidemiologic research studies. *Am. J. Epidemiol.* **120**:643–648.

Last, J. M. (Ed.) (1983). *A Dictionary of Epidemiology*. New York, Oxford University Press (for the International Epidemiological Association).

Love, R. G., and Miller, B. G. (1982). Longitudinal study of lung function in coal-miners. *Thorax* **37**:193–197.

Oldham, P. D. (1964). A note on the analysis of repeated measurements of the same subjects. *J. Chron. Dis.* **15**:969–977.

Poukkula, A., Huhti, E., and Makarainen, M. (1982). Chronic respiratory disease among workers in a pulp mill. A ten-year follow-up study. *Chest* **81**:285–289.

Rosner, B. (1979). The analysis of longitudinal data in epidemiologic studies. *J. Chron. Dis.* **32**:163–173.

Rothman, K. (1986). *Modern Epidemiology*. Boston, Little Brown, pp. 89–94.

Shepard, D. S. (1981). Reliability of blood pressure measurements: implications for designing and evaluating programs to control hypertension. *J. Chron. Dis.* **34**:191–209.

Siracusa, A., Cicioni, C., Volpi, R., et al. (1984). Lung function among asbestos cement factory workers: cross-sectional and longitudinal study. *Am. J. Ind. Med.* **5**:315–325.

Snedecor, G. W., and Cochran, W. G. (1967). *Statistical Methods*, 6th Ed. Iowa, The Iowa State University Press, pp. 164–166.

Sparrow, D., Bosse, R., Rosner, B., and Weiss, S. T. (1982). The effect of occupational exposure on pulmonary function: a longitudinal evaluation of fire fighters and non-firefighters. *Am. Rev. Respir. Dis.* **125**:319–323.

Warren, R. D., White, J. K., and Fuller, W. A. (1974). An errors-in-variables analysis of managerial role performance. *J. Am. Stat. Assoc.* **69**:886–893.

Weisberg, H. I. (1979). Statistical adjustments and uncontrolled studies. *Psychol. Bull.* **86**:1149–1164.

Werts, C. W., and Linn, R. L. (1970). A general linear model for studying growth. *Psychol. Bull.* **73**:17–22.

6

Natural History of Chronic Airflow Obstruction

BENJAMIN BURROWS

University of Arizona College of Medicine
Tucson, Arizona

The generally accepted concept of the evolution of clinically significant chronic airflow obstruction (CAO) is that it results from many years of a moderately excessive decline in lung function that occurs in those smokers especially "sensitive" to the effects of cigarettes. This course was first suggested by the relatively modest increase in rates of decline in FEV_1 observed in patients who were clinically ill with "chronic obstructive lung (or pulmonary) disease" (COPD). These rates would need to have been present for many years to explain the severity of the functional impairment (Burrows and Earle, 1969). More direct evidence about the early natural history of CAO came from the classic study by Fletcher and co-workers (1976), which showed a relationship between the mean "level" of the FEV_1 and its rate of decline with time ("slope"). This has been interpreted to mean that a lower FEV_1 in later adult life is due to more rapid reduction in FEV_1 during adult life, the so-called "horse-racing effect," rather than being the result of starting adult life with a lower FEV_1, which declines at the same rate as the rest of the population. This relationship of "slope" and "level" of FEV_1 has often been considered definitive evidence that mild ventilatory impairment is present for many years prior to the development of clinical illness and that the slow evolution of the disease should allow its

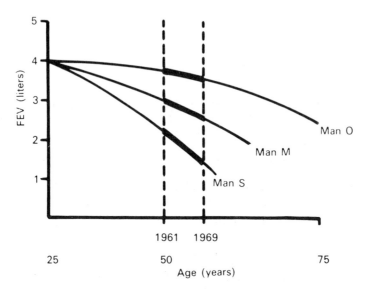

Figure 1   Rapid loss causing low FEV_1 and steep FEV_1 slope. Graphs of FEV_1 against age for three hypothetical men, all born in 1911 and all with an FEV_1 of 4 L at age 25. Man S develops severe airflow obstruction, man O develops very little, and man M moderate obstruction. The heavy lines indicate the FEV_1 regression lines that Fletcher et al. (1976) found during their study.

detection at a preclinical stage. This model of the evolution of clinically significant CAO is shown in Figure 1.

I. The London Study

Despite its wide acceptance, the London study of Fletcher and co-workers has important limitations, and concerns have been expressed about its conclusions concerning early detection of those likely to progress to clinically significant CAO. These concerns may be summarized as follows.

1. The "level" of FEV_1 used was a weighted mean of the FEV_1 values obtained over the course of the study (adjusted for body size by dividing by height[3]). The "level" therefore included some of the observed decline in FEV_1. There is an inherent mathematical relationship between "slope" and "level" when the latter is calculated in this manner. No positive correlation between *initial* FEV_1 impairment and subsequent decline could be shown, presumably because

of "regression toward the mean" (see chapter by Irwig in this volume).

2. The analyses included both smokers and nonsmokers. It is unclear how much of the correlation of "slope" and "level" resulted from smokers having both low levels of function and high rates of decline. Thus, it is uncertain that the "horse-racing effect" was present within the smoking group alone, even though the basic premise of the authors is that one can differentiate rapid-declining "susceptible smokers" from "nonsusceptible smokers" by their FEV_1 level.

3. Despite a demonstrated relationship of both "slope" and "level" to age, this was not controlled in the analyses.

4. The group studied included only working males aged 30–60 years of age, most of whom were very heavy smokers and all of whom lived in London during a period of heavy air pollution.

5. "Asthmatic" patients were excluded from most of the analyses although they did tend to show high rates of decline in FEV_1.

6. Despite the possible biases noted above, which might tend to increase their correlation, "slope" versus "level" showed a correlation coefficient of only 0.35. Thus, the mean level of the FEV_1 explained only 12% of the variance in its rate of change, even when a quartic function of FEV_1 was used to maximize the relationship.

II. The Tucson Study

A recent report (Burrows et al., 1987a) addresses some of these issues. The correlation of mean FEV_1 level (expressed as FEV_1/Ht^3) with FEV^1 change in 30–60-year-old men was almost identical to that noted by Fletcher et al. (1976), but after age was controlled for, this was significant only in smokers. Even in them, however, the relationship was dependent on inclusion of part of the decline in FEV_1 in the calculation of its mean value; neither the actual initial FEV_1/Ht^3 nor an initial FEV_1/Ht^3 estimated from the regression of FEV_1 over time predicted subsequent course. As in Fletcher's data, there appeared to be significant regression toward the mean, which confounded any predictive usefulness for the initial FEV_1, whether it was expressed as FEV_1/Ht^3 or as a percentage predicted value. However, the initial FEV_1/FVC ratio did prove to be a useful predictor of subsequent decline in FEV_1 in male smokers. When both age and initial FEV_1/FVC ratio were used to predict the rate of change in FEV_1, the multiple correlation coefficient was 0.48. It reached 0.58 when the percentage change in

FEV_1 per year rather than the actual rate of change in milliliters/year was used as the dependent variable.

The superiority of the FEV_1/FVC ratio to the FEV_1 itself as a predictor variable was ascribed to the following: the FEV_1/FVC ratio is more specific for early airways disease than the actual FEV_1 level; a poor initial effort will usually have less effect on the FEV_1/FVC ratio than on the actual FEV_1, minimizing regression toward the mean; the physiological intersubject variability in FEV_1 which is not accounted for by age and body size is reduced by dividing by the FVC; and regression to the mean is less marked when a different variable indicative of the disease under study is used to predict change than the one used to measure the subsequent rate of decline.

Most of the relationships noted above appeared to result from an almost uniformly elevated rate of decline in those male smokers who entered the study with an FEV_1/FVC ratio of $< 70\%$. In them, screening spirometry did appear to predict accurately the development of clinically significant COPD during the next decade. However, the observed rates of decline in these subjects were often very rapid, as they were also in many subjects in the study of Fletcher et al. (1976) and in reports of others (Howard and Astin, 1969; Bates, 1973). This raised a question about the "window of time" available for early detection of COPD. It appears possible that the transition from the mild functional decrease seen in most smokers to clinically significant impairment occurs over a relatively short time in late middle age. If so, early detection would require regular spirometric screening of smokers at 3–5-year intervals after the age of 40.

In all studies, rapid functional decline appears to terminate with smoking cessation and is not seen in exsmokers (Fletcher et al., 1976; Burrows et al., 1987a; Wilhelmsen et al., 1969; Comstock et al., 1970; Bosse et al., 1980; Kauffman et al., 1979; Camilli et al., 1987). Indeed, evidence for the above concept of the evolution of COPD has been demonstrated only in men who continue to smoke, a point that requires emphasis. It remains possible that this type of early natural history is seen in only one form of CAO, the type that appears to be directly dependent on persistent bronchial irritation (usually by cigarette smoking), which is generally associated with emphysema, and that may depend, at least in part, on the protease–antiprotease systems within the lung. It has been suggested that there may be another form of chronic airflow obstruction with a different pathogenetic mechanism (Burrows, 1984) and a different preclinical course (Burrows, 1981).

III. The Role of Asthma and Bronchial Hyperreactivity

There has been considerable interest in the possibility that asthma, even in a subclinical form, represents an important risk factor for persistent airways obstructive disease (AOD) in later life. A history of childhood asthma or bronchitis has been associated with reduced ventilatory function in adults and an apparent increased susceptibility to cigarettes in at least one cross-sectional study (Burrows et al., 1977). Because of the likelihood of preferential recall of childhood illnesses by functionally impaired adults, these data do little more than provide an interesting hypothesis regarding the pathogenesis of some forms of adult AOD. However, a variety of other observations would seem compatible with this hypothesis.

Certain features suggesting an asthmatic type of disorder, such as eosinophilia (Burrows et al., 1980; Van de Lende, 1969) and a high serum IgE level (Burrows et al., 1982) have been associated with ventilatory impairment in middle-aged and elderly adults. There appears to be important smoking–IgE interactions, and the relationships of IgE to airways obstruction were demonstrable only in subjects in whom there were asthmatic or bronchitic symptoms in association with the functional abnormality (Burrows et al., 1983). The insidious development of ventilatory impairment described earlier and most evident in older male smokers shows no obvious relationship to immunological factors or to stigmata of asthma. However, a more "asthmatic–bronchitic" type of diseases also appears to be occurring, and the data suggest that an asthmatic predisposition may be important in the pathogenesis of this type of disorder. This would be compatible with the "Dutch hypothesis" suggested by the group in Groningen many years ago (Orie et al., 1961), in which an "asthmatic predisposition" was considered essential to the development of persistent AOD.

A variety of other evidence is compatible with this theory. Rapid declines in FEV_1 have been associated with bronchial hyperreactivity (Barter and Campbell, 1976; Tabona et al., 1984; Taylor et al., 1985) and with increased responsiveness to bronchodilators (Barter and Campbell, 1976; Vollmer et al., 1985). Unfortunately, studies of bronchial reactivity or responsiveness have generally been carried out following the functional decline, making it difficult to determine whether bronchial lability is a risk factor or simply a feature of the disease. In either case, the observations suggest that a rapid decline in lung function in adult life may be associated with some of the cardinal features of asthma. Furthermore, despite the expected variability in function that might confound the data, an excessive decline in ventilatory function has been reported in adults with known asthma (Vollmer et al., 1985; Schacter et al., 1984; Brown et al., 1984), suggesting that there may be a chronic and a progressive form of the disease.

The course of clinically established disease may also differ in different forms of COPD. In series in which persistent asthmatics have been systematically excluded, the course of the disease is generally one of steady decline in function with a relatively high mortality. Longevity in these patients appears closely related to the initial level of functional impairment. The literature relating to this area has been reviewed recently (Burrows, 1985). However, it is unclear whether these data are applicable to patients whose disease has a major asthmatic component.

Data from The Netherlands suggest that the more asthmatic, or at least more bronchodilator- and steroid-responsive, forms of chronic airflow obstruction may have a more benign course and a lower mortality than other types of chronic AOD (Postma et al., 1979, 1985); these findings are also compatible with the clinical impressions of many chest physicians. In these studies, survival appeared more closely related to the degree of reversibility of the disease than to the actual level of FEV_1 (Postma et al., 1979), and steroid-responsive patients showed less progressive deterioration of function than others being evaluated (Postma, 1985). Nevertheless, even this type of disease can be a serious and disabling disorder.

A more recent report (Burrows et al., 1987b) would appear to confirm that there are two different forms of persistent airflow obstruction and that even after the development of clinically significant ventilatory impairment, they have quite different clinical courses. Subjects with features most suggestive of a "chronic asthmatic bronchitis" showed a low mortality and remarkable stability of function over a 10 year follow-up period. Those with more typical COPD (presumably with a more emphysematous type of disease) showed a much higher mortality rate and a decline in FEV_1 in the range of 70 ml/year. The latter subjects closely resembled those in earlier reports on the course and prognosis of COPD (Burrows and Earle, 1969). It was thought likely that the better course of the more asthmatic subjects reflected their responsiveness to therapy.

IV. Conclusion

In summary, it appears that there are at least two different types of chronic airflow obstruction. One ("chronic asthmatic bronchitis") may well depend on an "asthmatic predisposition." It is likely to be manifested by variable lung function and bronchial hyperreactivity in its preclinical stages. It probably represents the type of disease that conforms to the so-called "Dutch hypothesis." On the other hand, a more insidiously developing progressive form of disease, probably associated with emphysematous obstruction of the lung, appears to follow a more predictable course (the "horse-racing effect"). It appears directly related to smoking and has no relationship to any of the classic features of asthma. It has a relatively rapid progression and poor prognosis once a clinically significant degree of ventilatory impairment has occurred.

Acknowledgments

This work was supported by Specialized Center of Research Grant No. HL 14136 from the National Heart, Lung and Blood Institute.

References

Barter, C. E., and Campbell, A. H. (1976). Relationship of constitutional factors and cigarette smoking to decrease in 1-second forced expiratory volume. *Am. Rev. Respir. Dis.* **113**:305–314.

Bates, D. V. (1973). The fate of the chronic bronchitic: a report of the ten-year follow-up in the Canadian Department of Veterans Affairs coordinated study of chronic bronchitis. *Am. Rev. Respir. Dis.* **108**:1043–1077.

Bosse, R., Sparrow, B., Garvey, A. J., Costa, P. T. Jr, Weiss, S. T., and Rowe, J. W. (1980). Cigarette smoking, aging, and decline in pulmonary function: a longitudinal study. *Arch. Environ. Health* **35**:247–252.

Brown, P. J., Greville, H. W., and Finucane, K. E. (1984). Asthma and irreversible airflow obstruction. *Arch. Environ. Health* **35**:247–252.

Burrows, B. (1981). An overview of obstructive lung diseases. *Med. Clin. North Am.* **65**:455–471.

Burrows, B. (1984). Possible pathogenetic mechanisms in chronic airflow obstruction. *Chest* 85(Supplement): 12S–15S.

Burrows, B. (1985). Course and prognosis in advanced disease. In *Chronic Obstructive Pulmonary Disease.* Edited by T. L. Petty. Vol 28, *Lung Biology in Health and Disease.* New York, Marcel Dekker, pp. 31–42.

Burrows, B., and Earle, R. H. (1969). Course and prognosis of chronic obstructive lung disease. *N. Engl. J. Med.* **280**:397–404.

Burrows, B., Knudson, R. J., and Lebowitz, M. D. (1977). The relationship of childhood respiratory illness to adult obstructive airway disease. *Am. Rev. Respir. Dis.* **115**:751–760.

Burrows, B., Hasan, F. M., Barbee, R. A., Halonen, M., and Lebowitz, M. D. (1980). Epidemiologic observations on eosinophilia and its relationship to respiratory disorders. *Am. Rev. Respir. Dis.* **122**:709–719.

Burrows, B., Halonen, M., Lebowitz, M. D., Knudson, R. J., and Barbee, R. A. (1982). The relationship of serum immunoglobulin E, allergy skin tests, and smoking to respiratory disorders. *J. Allergy Clin. Immunol.* **70**:199–204.

Burrows, B., Lebowitz, M. D., Barbee, R. A., Knudson, R. J., and Halonen, M. (1983). Interactions of smoking and immunologic factors in relation to airways obstruction. *Chest.* **84**:657–661.

Burrows, B., Knudson, R. J., Camilli, A. E., Lyle, S. K., and Lebowitz, M. D. (1987a). The "horse-racing effect" and predicting decline in forced expiratory volume in one second from screening spirometry. *Am. Rev. Respir. Dis.* **135**:788–793.

Burrows, B., Bloom, J. W., Traver, G. A., and Cline, M. G. (1987b). The course and prognosis of different forms of chronic airways obstruction in a sample from the general population. *N. Engl. J. Med.* **317**:1309–1314.

Camilli, A. E., Burrows, B., Knudson, R. J., Lyle, S. K., and Lebowitz, M. D. (1987). Longitudinal changes in forced expiratory volume in one second in adults. Effects of smoking and smoking cessation. *Am. Rev. Respir. Dis.* **135**:794–799.

Comstock, G. W., Brownlow, W. J., Stone, R. W., and Sartwell, P. E. (1970). Cigarette smoking and changes in respiratory findings. *Arch. Environ. Health.* **21**:50–57.

Fletcher, C. M., Peto, R., Tinker, C. M., and Speizer, F. E. (1976). *The Natural History of Chronic Bronchitis and Emphysema: An Eight Year Study of Early Chronic Obstructive Lung Disease in Working Men in London.* Oxford, Oxford University Press, 1976.

Howard, P., and Astin, T. W. (1969). Precipitous fall of the forced expiratory volume. *Thorax* **24**:492–495.

Kauffman, F., Querleux, E., Drouet, D., Lellouch, J., and Brille, D. (1979). Twelve year FEV_1 changes and smoking habits among 556 workers in the Paris area. *Bull. Eur. Physiopathol. Respir.* **15**:723–737.

Orie, N. G. M., Sluiter, H. J., deVries, K., Tammeling, G. J., and Withop, J. (1961). The host factor in bronchitis. In *Bronchitis, an International Symposium.* Edited by N. G. M. Orie and H. J. Sluiter. Assen, Royal Vangorcum, pp. 43–59.

Postma, D. S., Burema, J., Gimeno, F., May, J. F., Smit, J. M., Steinhuis, E. J., van de Weele, L. Th., and Sluiter, H. J. (1979). Prognosis in severe chronic obstructive pulmonary disease. *Am. Rev. Respir. Dis.* **119**:357–367.

Postma, D. S., Steinhuis, E. J., Van de Weele, L. T., and Sluiter, H. J. (1985). Severe chronic airflow obstruction: can corticosteroids slow down progression? *Eur. J. Respir. Dis.* **67**:56–64.

Shachter, E. N., Doyle, C. A., and Beck, G. J. (1984). A prospective study of asthma in a rural community. *Chest* **85**:623–630.

Tabona, M., Chan-Yeung, M., Enarson, D., MacLean, L., Dorken, E., and Schulzer, M. (1984). Host factors affecting longitudinal decline in lung spirometry among grain elevator workers. *Chest* **85**:782–786.

Taylor, R. G., Joyce, H., Gross, E., Holland, F., and Pride, N. B. (1985). Bronchial reactivity to inhaled histamine and annual rate of decline in FEV_1 in male smokers and ex-smokers. *Thorax* **40**:9–16.

Van de Lende, R. (1969). In *Epidemiology of Chronic Nonspecific Lung Disease (Chronic Bronchitis)*. Vol. 1. *A Critical Analysis of Three Field Surveys of CNSLD Carried Out in the Netherlands*. Assen, Royal Vangorcum, pp. 140–146.

Vollmer, W. M., Johnson, L. R., and Buist, A. S. (1985). Relationship of response to a bronchodilator and decline in forced expiratory volume in one second in population studies. *Am. Rev. Respir. Dis.* **132**:1186–1193.

Wilhelmsen, L., Orha, I., and Tibbling, G. (1969). Decrease in ventilatory capacity between ages 50 and 54 in a representative sample of Swedish men. *Br. Med. J.* **3**:553–556.

7

Cigarette Smoking

DAVID B. COULTAS and JONATHAN M. SAMET

University of New Mexico School of Medicine
Albuquerque, New Mexico

Until the early 1900s, cigarette consumption was a relatively uncommon mode of tobacco consumption throughout the world, and chronic obstructive pulmonary disease (COPD) was also uncommon. By midcentury, increasing occurrence of chronic respiratory diseases had become evident through both clinical observation and review of trends of mortality (Stuart-Harris, 1954, 1968a,b). For example, in the United States in 1950, 3,157 deaths were attributed to "bronchitis unqualified," "chronic bronchitis," or "emphysema," codes compatible with clinically diagnosed COPD. Over the next 30 years, the number of deaths in categories related to COPD increased to 52,348. By 1964, the evidence was sufficiently compelling to support the conclusion by the Advisory Committee to the Surgeon General that "cigarette smoking is the most important of the causes of chronic bronchitis in the United States, and increases the risk of dying from chronic bronchitis and emphysema" (U.S. Dept. H.E.W., 1964). The 1964 report did not consider the evidence as sufficient for classifying the relationship between smoking and COPD as causal. However, reports published during the 1970s firmly linked reduced lung function and increased mortality from chronic bronchitis and emphysema with cigarette smoking. In

1984, the Surgeon General (U.S. Dept. H.H.S., 1984) concluded that cigarette smoking accounts for 80–90% of cases of COPD.

The evidence that cigarette smoking causes COPD comes from diverse and complementary lines of investigation, including in vitro studies, animal experiments, laboratory observations in humans, pathophysiological observations in humans, and epidemiological studies. In vitro experiments have shown the toxic effects of cigarette smoke on cellular and biochemical systems and provided insights into the mechanisms by which smoking contributes to the development of COPD. Animal models of emphysema and cigarette smoke provide an approach for assessing cellular, biochemical, and morphological changes in the lungs after injury. Investigations of disease mechanisms in humans have been based on measurements of markers of injury in blood or bronchoalveolar lavage fluid of smokers and nonsmokers. In another human approach, the pulmonary pathological findings from surgical or autopsy findings on smokers and nonsmokers have been correlated with physiological parameters and risk factors. Cross-sectional and longitudinal surveys of populations have been conducted worldwide to compare disease frequency in smokers and nonsmokers. The results of these different approaches to investigating smoking and COPD will be discussed in this chapter with the goal of demonstrating the causal association between smoking and COPD.

This chapter highlights the voluminous evidence showing that cigarette smoking causes COPD. While it is now widely accepted that cigarette smoking causes COPD, the evidence merits review in this volume because research on mechanisms, determinants of susceptibility, and other environmental risk factors must be conducted in the context of the extensive information available on cigarette smoking (Snider, 1986; Janoff et al., 1987). Furthermore, the epidemiological data can be used by clinicians to improve the accuracy of diagnoses of COPD. The evidence will be reviewed using criteria for causality originally described by Hill (1965) and subsequently modified by others (Tugwell et al., 1985). These criteria are not simply a checklist for establishing causation (Rothman, 1986) but provide an approach for summarizing a large amount of data and facilitating interpretation and a decision on causality. The criteria include evidence from human experiments, strength of association, consistency of association, temporal relationship, dose–response gradient, biological plausibility, epidemiological plausibility, specificity, and analogy (Tugwell et al., 1985). Representative data are reviewed for each of these criteria.

I. Human Experiments

A human experiment to determine if cigarette smoking causes COPD would require the random allocation of subjects to be smokers or nonsmokers, and follow-up of the two groups for the development of COPD. Because this experiment is neither ethical nor feasible, it has not been conducted. However, through epidemiological investigation, data can be obtained from the natural experiment offered by the decision of some persons to become smokers.

II. Strength of Association

The strength of an association is measured by the relative frequency of disease occurrence or mortality in an exposed group, for example, smokers, compared to an unexposed group, for example, nonsmokers. In a cohort or follow-up study, the usual measures of association are incidence or mortality ratios; in cross-sectional and case–control studies, the odds ratio, the ratio of the odds of exposure in affected and unaffected subjects, is generally calculated (Rothman, 1986). A greater degree of association, as asssessed by these measures, strengthens the causal explanation for an association, although weaker associations may be as biologically plausible as stronger associations. Stronger associations, however, are less likely to result from uncontrolled bias (Hill, 1965). This section reviews studies of morbidity and mortality from COPD to document the strength of association between COPD and cigarette smoking.

With regard to morbidity, epidemiological criteria for COPD are generally based on level of FEV_1, often in combination with level of the FEV_1 to FVC ratio. Surprisingly few reports provide data on the prevalence of COPD in smokers and nonsmokers in population samples (U.S. Dept. H.H.S., 1984). However, the published studies document a strong association between cigarette smoking and the prevalence of reduced lung function on spirometry, indicative of COPD. For example, Knudson and co-workers (1976) found that among 2,735 subjects from Tucson, Arizona, ages 8–90 years of age, 8.3% of asymptomatic nonsmokers and 13.3% of asymptomatic smokers had a FEV_1 and/or FEV_1/FVC in the lowest fifth percentile predicted for that population. In a sample of over 8,000 men and women, 18 years of age or older, from three southern California communities, Detels and co-workers (Detels et al., 1979; Rokaw et al. 1980) showed that the prevalence of a FEV_1 less than 75% predicted was nearly twice as great among current smokers compared to those who had never smoked. (Fig. 1). Using multiple logistic regression, Tager et al. (1978) found that lifetime cigarette consumption was the only significant predictor of a FEV_1 less than 65% predicted (odds ratio = 9.3) among 1,251 men and women from East Boston, Massachusetts. Age, respiratory symptoms, relation to a subject with chronic bronchitis or chronic airways obstruction, and current smoking were not important predictors. Other

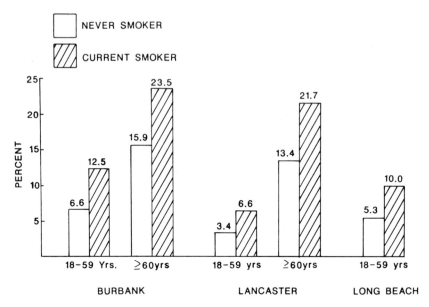

Figure 1 Prevalence of FEV_1 less than 75% predicted in three southern California communities by age group and smoking status (prevalence age and sex adjusted using 1970 white population of the United States as standard population) (from Detels et al., 1979; Rokaw et al., 1980).

cross-sectional studies have also shown a higher prevalence of airflow obstruction among smokers than nonsmokers (Ferris et al., 1979; Beck et al., 1981).

The Tecumseh study, a large population-based investigation of risk factors for many chronic diseases in residents of Tecumseh, Michigan, provides information on the incidence of COPD and smoking. Higgins and associates (1982) obtained lung function measurements in 1962, and again in 1979, from 2,954 men and women, 16–64 years of age at the first measurement. During follow-up, 5.3% of males and 3.1% of females developed obstructive airways disease, defined as a FEV_1 less than 65% of predicted and a FEV_1/FVC ratio 80% or less. For subjects who smoked throughout the period of follow-up compared with nonsmokers, relative risks for developing airways obstruction were 5.5 and 7.7 for males and females, respectively.

Mortality from COPD is also increased in cigarette smokers compared to nonsmokers (U.S. Dept. H.H.S., 1984). In the longitudinal study of British doctors (Doll and Peto, 1976; Doll et al., 1980), over 40,000 male and female physicians were followed for approximately 20 years. Increased mortality ratios for emphysema and/or chronic bronchitis were found among smokers

Table 1 Mortality Ratios[a] for COPD in Smokers from Selected Populations

Study Population	Emphysema	Bronchitis	Both
34,000 male British physicians			24.7
68,000 males from California in various occupations	12.3		
78,000 male Canadian veterans	5.9	11.4	
440,500 males[b]	45–64 yr		
562,700 females[b]	6.6		
	4.9		
290,000 male U.S. veterans	14.8	5.1	12.1

[a]Reference group is nonsmokers with a mortality ratio of one.
[b]From 25 states in the United States; age range 45–64 years.
Source: U.S. Dept. H.H.S., 1984.

compared to nonsmokers; the mortality ratios ranged from 10.5 to 38.0 among categories of gender and number of cigarettes smoked per day. Similar results were obtained by Hammond (1966) from the American Cancer Society 25-State Study that included over 1 million men and women. Among men and women 45–64 years of age, the mortality ratios for emphysema in smokers compared with nonsmokers were 6.6 and 4.9, respectively. The ratios were even higher in men over 64 years of age. Numerous other prospective studies have documented increased mortality ratios from COPD among smokers (Table 1) (U.S. Dept. H.H.S., 1984).

These and other data document a strong association between cigarette smoking and COPD. In nearly every population examined, smokers have substantially greater occurence of COPD than nonsmokers (U.S. Dept. H.H.S., 1984). In fact, the only other strong risk factor for COPD is alpha$_1$-antitrypsin deficiency.

III. Consistency of Association

To meet the criterion of consistency, a similar conclusion on the association between smoking and COPD must be reached from studies of different design among different populations. Numerous populations have been studied worldwide using different measures of COPD. Regardless of the outcome measure, prevalence or incidence of airflow obstruction, mortality, doctor-diagnosed COPD, mean level of FEV_1, or rate of decline of lung function, smokers have a greater frequency of abnormalities than nonsmokers (U.S. Dept. H.H.S, 1984). Lower levels of lung function among smokers than nonsmokers were documented in over 45 reports from cross-sectional and longitudinal investigations involving over 130,000 subjects summarized in the 1984 report of the U.S. Surgeon General (U.S. Dept. H.H.S., 1984). Eight major prospective studies of about 2 million subjects document marked increases in mortality from COPD in smokers compared to nonsmokers (U.S. Dept. H.H.S., 1984).

IV. Temporal Relationship

This criterion implies that exposure to cigarette smoke must precede the development of COPD. In the conceptual model that is commonly accepted for the development of COPD (Fig. 2), clinically evident disease develops after sustained cigarette smoking has resulted in sufficient loss of ventilatory function to produce impairment. Observations made on children and adults document an appropriate temporal sequence between smoking and the development of COPD. In nonsmokers without respiratory disease, ventilatory function begins to decline at approximately 25–35 years of age. The FEV_1 drops by about 25 ml annually in nonsmokers (U.S. Dept. H.H.S., 1984). In cigarette smokers, the average rate of loss of ventilatory function is much greater; some smokers may lose 100 ml or more annually (Fletcher et al., 1976; U.S. Dept. H.H.S., 1984). However, not all cigarette smokers develop COPD, and it is the susceptible minority with higher rates of decline who are at greatest risk for the disease. Smoking during childhood could predispose to the development of COPD if the level of lung function achieved during lung growth was reduced by smoking.

Data from several study designs, including longitudinal studies of lung function during growth, studies of lung histopathological appearance in younger and older smokers and nonsmokers, and longitudinal studies during the period of lung function decline are consistent with an appropriate temporal relationship between cigarette smoking and COPD. The results of these three categories of investigation are reviewed in this section.

During childhood and adolescence, cigarette smokers have a decreased rate of lung growth and a lower mean level of lung function compared to nonsmokers. To examine childhood risk factors for the development of COPD, Tager et al. (1985) obtained questionnaire data and spirometry measurements annually, from 1975 to 1982, on 669 subjects who were 5–19 years of age in 1975. For males and females the rates of growth of FEV_1 and FEF_{25-75} were lower for current smokers compared to those not smoking. A mathematical model projected that on average, children who start smoking

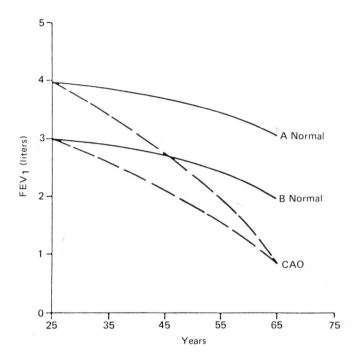

Figure 2 Conceptual model of decline of FEV$_1$ in persons achieving full lung growth (A) and not achieving full lung growth (B). Excessive decline results in the development of chronic air flow obstruction (CAO) (from Samet et al., 1983).

at age 15 years will only achieve 92% and 90% of their expected FEV$_1$ and FEF$_{25-75}$, respectively, at age 20 years. In three southern California communities, Tashkin et al. (1983) obtained pulmonary function measurements from 198 subjects, 13–23 years of age between 1973 and 1974, and repeated the studies on 183 subjects 5 years later. Eighteen males started smoking during the 5-year interval. At the first test, mean FEV$_1$, FVC, and flow rates were higher for these 18 subjects compared to those who remained nonsmokers, but after 5 years the function of the smokers and nonsmokers was similar except that flow at 75% of the FVC was lower in smokers than nonsmokers. Similar effects of smoking on lung function were not observed among females. The attainment of a lower level of lung function during childhood, because of smoking or other injuries to the lung, may increase the risk for the subsequent development of COPD, although longitudinal data directly testing this hypothesis are unavailable.

Abundant data have documented that cigarette smoking by adults reduces lung function level and predisposes to the development of COPD. In the Tecumseh study (Higgins et al., 1982) a lower percentage predicted FEV_1 at the initial examination in 1962 was associated with an increased risk for developing chronic airways obstruction in 1979. Using data from this population, a multiple logistic model was developed to predict the risk of developing COPD within 10 years in men and women between 25 and 64 years of age. The model was then applied to data collected in other epidemiological investigations in Baltimore, Boston, Framingham, Louisiana, Stavely, and Tucson (Higgins et al., 1984). The probability of developing COPD within 10 years was predicted from a summary score, which increased with age, number of cigarettes smoked per day, and lower levels of FEV_1. In addition, the change over a 10-year period in the number of cigarettes smoked per day resulted in an increased score with increased consumption, or a decreased score with decreased consumption. In each population, the relative risk for developing COPD increased among subjects with a high score, predictive of a 10% or greater incidence of COPD over 10 years, compared to subjects with a predicted incidence of less than 10% (Table 2). Other investigators, using longitudinal data, have also found an association between a low initial level of lung function, and an increased risk for the development of COPD (Lebowitz et al., 1984; Peach et al., 1986; Burrows et al., 1987).

Histopathological studies confirm that smoking affects the lung in smokers before the development of frank COPD. Histopathological abnormalities develop in young smokers and these abnormalities worsen in older smokers. Changes in the small airways (2 mm in diameter and less) are among the earliest manifestations of cigarette smoking. Niewoehner and co-workers (1974) examined the lungs of 20 smokers and 19 non-smokers who died suddenly at a mean age of 25 years. A pattern of small airways injury in smokers, termed respiratory bronchiolitis, was readily identified. Clusters of brown pigmented macrophages were found in the respiratory bronchioles, which also displayed increased numbers of inflammatory cells and denuded epithelium. To assess the pathological effects of longer durations of smoking Cosio and co-workers (1980) compared the airway morphology in 25 smokers and 14 lifelong nonsmokers over the age of 40 years who had died suddenly. They found alterations similar to those reported by Niewoehner et al. (1974) but also demonstrated changes that suggested more severe damage with an increased number of goblet cells, increased amounts of smooth muscle, and an excess of narrowed small airways less than 400 mm in diameter among the smokers.

The attainment of a lower level of lung function because of active or passive smoking at a young age combined with an accelerated decline from smoking as an adult may increase the risk for COPD (Fig. 2). Numerous longitudinal investigations in adults have documented an increased loss of

Table 2 Relative Risks for Developing COPD Over a 10-Year Period in Different Study Populations Using the Tecumseh Index of Risk[a]

Study Population	Relative Risk[b]	
	Men	Women
958 men and 1,159 women, Tecumseh	12.8	11.3
700 men and 558 women, Baltimore	8.0	6.8
97 men and 231 women, Boston	—	2.2
309 men and 48 women, Louisiana	7.2	8.6
502 men, Stavely	6.9	—
377 men and 493 women, Tucson	13.2	17.1
1,088 men and 1,549 women, Framingham[c]	3.6	6.5

[a]See text for description of the Tecumseh Index of Risk.
[b]Relative risk = /incidence of COPD with risk $\geq 10\%$ incidence of COPD with risk $< 10\%$.
[c]Based on index of risk within 15 years.
Source: Higgins et al., 1984

lung function among cigarette smokers compared to nonsmokers (U.S. Dept. H.H.S., 1984); sufficient loss leads to COPD in susceptible smokers (Fletcher et al., 1976). Fletcher and colleagues (1976) conducted one of the first large longitudinal investigations of the effect of cigarette smoking on lung function. Between 1961 and 1969, these investigators obtained questionnaire data and pulmonary function measurements every 6 months from 792 men, 30–59 years of age, who were working in West London. For men between 50 and 59 years of age, the rates of decline for nonsmokers, light smokers (less than 15 cigarettes/day), and heavy smokers (15 or more cigarettes/day) were -42 ml/year, -47 ml/year, and -66 ml/year, respectively (Fletcher and Peto, 1977). Clement and Van de Woestijne (1982) evaluated 2,406 male members of the Belgian Air Force for 3–15 years and found excess mean declines in FEV_1 in smokers compared to nonsmokers. After adjustment for age, height, and weight, excess mean changes in FEV_1 were 1.5 ml/year for nonsmokers, -2.8 ml/year for ex-smokers, -3.4 ml/year for smokers of less than 20 cigarettes/day, and -12.6 ml/year for smokers of more than 20 cigarettes/day. Also, subjects with a reduced FEV_1, regardless of their smoking habits, had an increased mean rate of decline compared to the group of subjects with a normal

FEV_1. Between 1971 and 1981, Beaty and co-workers (1984) evaluated 1,912 men and women from Baltimore for an average of 4.7 years in a longitudinal investigation of risk factors for COPD. For both sexes, only advancing age and smoking were associated with increased decline in FEV_1. In three communities in the Los Angeles, California area, Tashkin and associates (1984) obtained questionnaire and pulmonary function data from 2,401 subjects between 1973 and 1975 and again 5 years later. The mean differences in FEV_1 from the two observations were greatest in current smokers and lowest for those who had never smoked.

Evidence from a wide variety of study designs strongly supports an appropriate temporal relationship between cigarette smoking and the development of COPD. Although longitudinal data on the effects of cigarette smoking are not available from childhood through adulthood, cigarette smoking does impair lung growth in children and accelerates lung function decline in adults. These effects of cigarette smoking precede clinically apparent COPD, and are consistent with the conceptual model for the development of COPD proposed in Figure 2.

V. Dose-Response Gradient

Demonstration of increased risk of COPD with an increasing dose of cigarette smoke would meet the dose–response criterion. However, dose–response relationships have not been directly described because the specific causative agent or agents have not been identified among the thousands of substances in tobacco smoke (U.S. Dept. H.H.S., 1984). However, exposure–response relationships have been readily demonstrated between the occurrence of COPD and exposure estimates based on questionnaire measures of smoking. The usual estimates of exposure to cigarette smoke in active smokers are the pack-years of consumption and the average number of cigarettes smoked daily. Other aspects of smoking, such as type of cigarette and pattern of inhalation, may also influence the dose in active smokers.

In active smokers, numerous investigations have shown increased risks for developing COPD, and for mortality from COPD, as the number of cigarettes smoked and the duration of smoking increase. During lung growth, among 669 subjects 5–19 years of age, Tager et al. (1985) found that the percentage predicted values for FEV_1 and FEF_{25-75} decreased with an increasing number of cigarettes smoked. The effects of the cumulative number of cigarettes on lower lung function values were observed despite a median total consumption of only 7,300 cigarettes. In adult participants in the Framingham Heart Study, Ashley and co-workers (1975) found a progressive decline in the FEV_1/FVC ratio with increasing pack-years of cigarettes (Table 3). Using FEV_1 or deviation of FEV_1 from predicted value as the outcome measure, results from New Hampshire (Ferris et al., 1973), Tucson (Burrows et al., 1977), and six other United States cities (Ferris et al., 1979; Dockery et al., 1988) have all demonstrated an increasing decline in FEV_1 with increasing consumption of cigarettes (Table 3, Fig. 3). To estimate the risk for COPD associated with cigarette consumption, Higgins et al. (1982) defined obstructive airways disease as a FEV_1 less than 65% of predicted and a FEV_1/FVC ratio 80% or less, and found that risk for COPD increased among men and women with the number of cigarettes smoked per day (Table 3). In studies of mortality from COPD, mortality ratios of smokers compared to nonsmokers uniformly increase with an increasing number of cigarettes smoked daily (U.S. Dept. H.H.S., 1984).

Although reduction in the number of cigarettes smoked probably decreases risk for cigarette-related diseases, the magnitude of the reduction in risk may not be as great as anticipated because of compensatory changes in smoking patterns. Benowitz and associates (1986) measured urinary mutagenicity, an indicator of tar exposure, and blood concentrations of nicotine and carbon monoxide in 13 volunteer cigarette smokers after decreasing their average number of cigarettes from 37/day to 5/day for 3–4 days. Despite an 86% reduction in the number of cigarettes smoked, the subjects' exposure to tar and nicotine only decreased 50%.

Because complete elimination of cigarette smoking is unlikely, the development and promotion of less hazardous cigarettes, low in tar and nicotine, has been suggested as one approach to decreasing exposure and thus decreasing cigarette-related diseases (Hammond, 1980). Over the last 30 years, declines in tar and nicotine yields have been documented with measurements made by smoking machine (U.S. Dept. H.H.S., 1981). However, it is not certain that the inhaled dose of cigarette smoke has declined in parallel; compensatory alterations in smoking pattern may result in increased inhaled doses of smoke components above those predicted by machine yields (Benowitz et al., 1983).

Little information is available regarding the risk of COPD and the types of cigarettes smoked. The tar content of cigarettes smoked, as measured by smoking machine, does not have a strong association with level of pulmonary function (Sparrow et al., 1983; Higenbottam et al., 1980; Paoletti et al., 1985; Peach et al., 1986). The conflicting results among the available studies of cigarette tar content and lung function may result from difficulties in accurately quantifying exposure to tar. While methodological problems limit the epidemiological approach to evaluating potential benefits of lower-yield cigarettes (Samet, 1985), the preponderance of the evidence to date weighs against a strong effect of the lower yield products in protection against COPD.

Table 3 Results of Dose–Response Effects of Cigarette Smoking on Lung Function from Selected Investigations

Study Population (ref)	Findings

1,238 men and women, 37–69 years of age from Framingham, MA (Ashley et al., 1975)	Decline in FEV_1/FVC ratios with each pack-year of cigarettes
	
	37–49 years
	  Males −0.084
	  Females −0.039
	
	50–59 years
	  Males −0.090
	  Females −0.098
	
	60–64 years
	  Males −0.098
	  Females −0.043

848 men and women, 30–80 years of age from Berlin, NH (Ferris et al., 1973)	By multiple linear regression, FEV_1 drops by 0.01 L for each cigarette smoked per day
2,369 men and women, above 14 years of age from Tucson AZ (Burrows et al., 1977)	By multiple regression analysis, FEV_1 drops by 0.31 and 0.24% of predicted value per pack-year of smoking in men and women, respectively

8,480 men and women 25–74 years of age from six U.S. communities (Ferris et al., 1979)

Mean residual FEV$_1$ (L) after correction for height and age

Lifetime packs	Male	Female
None	0.25	0.06
<3,000	0.21	0.04
3,000–8,999	0.01	−0.05
9,000–17,999	−0.19	−0.20
≥18,000	−0.45	−0.28

2,955 men and women, 30–80 years of age from Tecumseh, MI (Higgins et al., 1982)

Relative risks for obstructive airways disease

Number of cigarettes/day	Male	Female
None	1.0	1.0
1–19	1.9	4.8
≥20	4.7	8.3

8,191 men and women 25–74 years of age from six U.S. communities (Dockery et al., 1988)

By multiple regression analysis, male and female smokers of average height lose 7.4 ml on average for each pack-year and 4.4 ml per year, respectively.

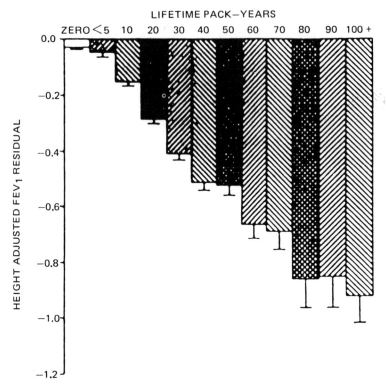

Figure 3 Mean difference (residual) of height adjusted FEV₁ from expected values for healthy never smokers from six U.S. cities versus lifetime pack-years (from Dockery et al., 1988).

Patterns of smoking cigarettes, including inhalation, puff volume, duration of holding smoke in the mouth before inhalation, and depth and duration of inhalation may all affect the dose of cigarette smoke deposited in the lungs. The available epidemiological data, based on questionnaire responses about the depth of inhalation and decline in lung function, provide conflicting results on these aspects of smoking behavior (U.S. Dept. H.H.S., 1984). The inconsistencies may result from inaccuracies in assessment of smoking pattern and from the small degree of effect that may be associated with smoking pattern. For example, Dockery and co-workers (1988) found a difference of only -39 ml in the mean residual FEV₁, which was lower among subjects who reported that they inhaled slightly or not at all compared to those subjects who inhaled moderately or deeply.

More refined measurement of smoking behavior has not provided additional insight. To assess smoking patterns more accurately, Medici and associates (1985) measured smoke-flow and chest movements during cigarette smoking in 91 smokers with different types of respiratory disease and degrees of lung function abnormalities. For all smokers, the only difference was a short puff-inhalation time—a measure of the duration of smoke retention in the mouth—among those subjects with emphysema. Whether the association reflects cause, resulting from a greater delivery of smoke components to the lung, or a consequence of the disease remains to be determined.

Few investigations have examined the effects of cigarette type and smoking patterns on mortality. Mortality from all causes and from COPD may be reduced among those who smoke low tar and nicotine cigarettes (Hammond et al., 1976; Lee and Garfinkel, 1981). In the study of British doctors (Doll and Peto, 1976), the mortality ratio from COPD among men who reported inhaling cigarette smoke compared to those who did not was 1.53, an excess possibly reflecting the increased dose of cigarette smoke associated with inhalation.

Reduction of exposure, through smoking cessation, also reduces risk for COPD. Smoking cessation has been shown to reduce the risk of developing COPD in several epidemiological investigations. In the 8-year follow-up of 792 British men, Fletcher and colleagues (1976; Fletcher and Peto, 1977) found that the slopes of FEV_1 decline were similar for nonsmokers and exsmokers. For those subjects who stopped smoking during the 15-year follow-up in the Tecumseh study, the relative risk (RR) of developing a FEV_1 less than 65% predicted was 3.5 for males and 7.6 for females; the relative risks were 5.5 and 7.7 for male and female smokers, respectively. Over a 5-year interval Tashkin et al. (1984) evaluated 2,401 subjects and found that exsmokers at the beginning of the study and subjects who quit smoking during the follow-up period had smaller mean losses of FEV_1 compared to those who continued to smoke. Among males, the mean differences were 0.28 L for nonsmokers, 0.26 L for exsmokers, and 0.31 L for those who quit during the study. Among women the mean differences were similar in the three groups. The findings for men suggest that either a period of greater than 5 years is needed before the accelerated decline in FEV_1 returns to normal, or the results may be due to a lower cumulative consumption of cigarettes by the exsmokers. Camilli et al. (1987) examined the effects of smoking and smoking cessation on change in FEV_1 during a mean duration of follow-up of 9.4 years in 1,705 adults from Tucson. In general, smoking cessation reduced rate of decline to that of nonsmokers, but the benefits were greatest in males 50–69 years of age (Fig. 4).

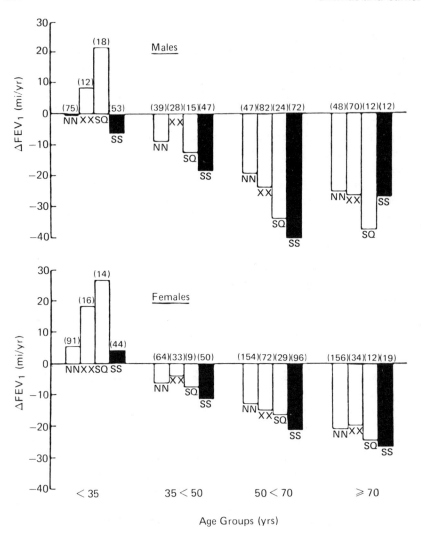

Figure 4 Mean change in FEV_1 (ΔFEV_1) values in nonsmokers (NN), consistent exsmokers (XX), subjects who quit smoking during the follow-up period (SQ), and consistent smokers (SS) in four age groups by sex from Tucson, Arizona. Numbers of subjects in each category are shown in parentheses (from Camilli et al., 1987).

Smoking cessation also reduces mortality from COPD, but mortality among former smokers probably never returns to that of those who have never smoked (U.S. Dept. H.H.S., 1984). In a prospective study of 294,000 United States veterans, the mortality ratio for bronchitis and emphysema was 12.1 for current smokers and decreased to 2.6 among exsmokers, but only after more than 20 years of cessation (Rogot and Murray, 1980).

In summary, the available evidence strongly supports increasing risk for COPD as exposure to cigarette smoke increases; the exposure measures used are undoubtedly surrogates for the doses of the many toxic components of cigarette smoke. Risk may be lowered by decreasing the number of cigarettes smoked or by smoking low tar and nicotine cigarettes, but the degree of protection is small because exposure is not greatly altered. Finally, smoking cessation offers a definite reduction in risk, but the risk may not return to that of the lifelong nonsmoker because of irreversible injury.

VI. Biological Plausibility

Several lines of evidence support the biological plausibility of the association between cigarette smoking and COPD. The evidence includes the cellular and biochemical changes found in the lungs of cigarette smokers, the pathophysiological changes observed in young asymptomatic smokers and older cigarette smokers with COPD, and the experimental data from animal models and in vitro systems (Janoff et al., 1987). In this section these various types of data are considered in relation to effects on the airways and the lung parenchyma.

The pattern of lung injury associated with cigarette smoking has been comprehensively described elsewhere (U.S. Dept. H.H.S., 1984) (Table 4). In the large airways, cigarette smoke causes an increase in mucous gland size and in goblet cell number. These changes result in increased mucus production and the associated symptom of chronic bronchitis. Large airway injury may contribute to airflow obstruction, but the predominant sites for the increased airflow resistance in COPD are the peripheral airways and lung parenchyma (U.S. Dept. H.H.S., 1984).

As described previously, changes in the small airways are one of the earliest manifestations of cigarette smoking's effects on the lung. To characterize the physiological consequences of small airways injury associated with smoking cigarettes, Cosio and associates (1978) correlated small airways morphology with lung function in 36 patients donating lung tissue at thoracotomy for a localized lesion. With increasing cumulative consumption of cigarettes, both inflammation and fibrosis of the

Table 4 Pathological Changes and Physiological Manifestations of Lung Injury by Cigarette Smoke

	Large Airways	Small Airways	Parenchyma
Pathological changes	Mucous gland hyperplasia, inflammation and edema, bronchial smooth muscle	Goblet cell metaplasia, inflammation, and fibrosis of the respiratory bronchiole	Emphysema, minimal interstitial fibrosis
Functional consequences	? $\downarrow FEV_1$	$\downarrow FEV_1$, $\downarrow FEV_1\%$ $\uparrow TLC$, $\uparrow RV$, $\downarrow DLCO$ Accelerated annual decline of FEV_1	$\downarrow FEV_1$, $\downarrow FEV_1\%$ $\uparrow TLC$, $\uparrow RV$, $\downarrow DLCO$ Accelerated annual decline of FEV_1

Source: U.S. Dept. H.H.S., 1985.

respiratory bronchioles increased. Furthermore, the FEV_1/FVC ratio and the maximum midexpiratory flow rate (FEF_{25-75}), which are measures of airflow obstruction, progressively decreased with the amount smoked. Physiological measures of airflow obstruction also correlated with the severity of small airways abnormalities. Similar results were reported by Berend and co-workers (1979) from 21 smokers and 1 nonsmoker who had lobectomies for peripheral lung tumors. The correlations between bronchiolar narrowing and the FEV_1 and FEF_{25-75} were 0.44 and 0.45, respectively.

Since the discovery, about 20 years ago, that alpha$_1$-antitrypsin deficiency is associated with familial panlobular emphysema (Laurell and Eriksson, 1963), the role of proteases and antiproteases in the development of emphysema in cigarette smokers has been intensively investigated (Janoff, 1985). Current concepts of the development of emphysema emphasize lung inflammation and an imbalance between proteolytic enzymes and their inhibitors (Janoff, 1985; Niewoehner, 1988). Observations that smokers, in comparison with nonsmokers, have an increased number of neutrophils in peripheral blood (Yeung and Bunico, 1984), in bronchoalveolar lavage fluid, and in lung biopsy specimens (Hunninghake and Crystal, 1983) provide indirect evidence for an increased elastase burden in lungs of cigarette smokers, since neutrophils are the primary source of elastase (Janoff, 1985). Further indirect evidence for the role of neutrophils in the development of COPD was provided by Martin and co-workers (1985) who performed bronchoalveolar lavage in 48 men who were current or exsmokers with variable degrees of airflow obstruction. Those subjects with a FEV_1 percentage predicted less than 60% had a higher proportion of neutrophils in bronchoalveolar lavage fluid compared to subjects with FEV_1 levels 60% or greater. To evaluate changes in elastase levels with smoking, Fera and associates (1986) measured neutrophil elastase levels in bronchoalveolar fluid from five smokers, before and immediately after smoking four cigarettes, and five other smokers, before and 1 hr after smoking. Increased neutrophil elastase levels were measured among the smokers lavaged immediately after smoking but not among those lavaged 1 hr after smoking. The findings of increased neutrophils and elastase levels in lungs of cigarette smokers support lung injury by elastase as a mechanism that may result in COPD. Other biochemical alterations from cigarette smoking may also mediate lung injury: Decreased levels or activity of antiproteases (Janoff, 1985), increased oxidant activity of neutrophils (Anderson et al., 1987), impaired antioxidant mechanisms (Toth et al., 1986; Taylor et al., 1986; Galdston, et al., 1987), and reduced efficacy of elastin repair (Janoff, 1985).

The major parenchymal injury associated with cigarette smoking is emphysema, defined as "abnormal dilation of air spaces distal to the terminal bronchioles accompanied by destruction of air space walls" (U.S. Dept. H.H.S., 1984). To quantitate the destructive changes in lung parenchyma from cigarette smoke, Saetta and co-workers (1985) examined the lungs of eight lifelong nonsmokers who died suddenly at a mean age of 70 years, and of 23 smokers with a mean age of 66 years. Of the cigarette smokers, 22 underwent a surgical resection of a localized lesion and 1 was examined as an autopsy case. Disruption of alveolar and duct spaces was found about three times as often in the smokers as in the nonsmokers and these destructive changes were inversely correlated with level of FEV_1 among the smokers.

Emphysema and small airways injury contribute to the physiological impairment found in COPD; in individual patients with COPD, either type of injury may be predominant, but both are probably important (U.S. Dept. H.H.S., 1984). However, not all cigarette smokers develop COPD. To characterize the morphological changes that appear with smoking and overt COPD, Hale and co-workers (1984) examined 14 lungs from non-smokers, 25 lungs from smokers without severe lung disease who died suddenly, and 18 lungs from smokers with chronic airflow obstruction from an autopsy service. The mean ages of the subjects were 72 years, 58 years, and 64 years. Among the smokers with chronic airflow obstruction, mean bronchiolar diameter, percent of bronchioles less than 400 μm in diameter, and severity of emphysema correlated with FEV_1, $r = 0.54$, $r = 0.51$, and $r = 0.74$, respectively. The severity of emphysema was highest among the smokers with chronic airflow obstruction compared to the nonsmokers and smokers without airflow obstruction. Other pathological changes, bronchiolar inflammation, fibrosis, and amount of smooth muscle, showed a progressive increase in severity from the nonsmokers to smokers with chronic airflow obstruction, although none of these features were important for predicting level of FEV_1 independent of emphysema. Nagai and associates (1985) examined lungs from 48 patients with a mean age of 64 years, a mean FEV_1 of 31%, and an arterial partial pressure of oxygen of 55 mmHg or greater. All 48 patients died during the National Institutes of Health Intermittent Positive Pressure Breathing trial. Bronchiolar lesions, including the proportion of bronchioles less than 400 μm in diameter, goblet cell metaplasia, and increased pigmentation of bronchioles were inversely correlated with percentage predicted FEV_1, with correlations of -0.46, -0.32, and -0.40, respectively. The average interalveolar diameter, a morphological measurement of emphysema, was also inversely correlated with percentage predicted FEV_1, $r = -0.33$.

Animal models of emphysema provide further evidence for possible pathogenic mechanisms by which cigarette smoke causes COPD. In a recent review, Janoff (1985) categorizes animal experiments into five models:

elastase-induced emphysema, augmentation of elastase-induced emphysema, progression of elastase-induced emphysema, spontaneously occurring emphysema, and emphysema produced by agents other than proteases. The intrapulmonary instillation of proteases produces emphysematous changes, and exposure of animals to cigarette smoke after protease-induced lung injury results in impairment of the normal repair mechanisms, which may play a role in progression of emphysema. Other data suggest that retention of active proteases in alveolar macrophages and on lung proteins may result in a sustained release of proteases that causes progression of lung destruction. Further evidence that proteases may play a major role in the development of emphysema can be found in studies of mice with spontaneously occurring enlarged lungs and bullae, as found in human emphysema (Szapiel et al., 1981). Investigation of these mice shows increased numbers of alveolar macrophages and neutrophils, sources of proteases, and partial inactivation of an antiprotease found in lung lavage fluid (Rossi et al., 1984; Chan and Matulionis, 1984). Although most animal studies have used protease-induced injury to study mechanisms that produce emphysema, in two recent investigations in rats, prolonged exposure to tobacco smoke resulted in emphysema.

Diverse but complementary forms of data support the biological plausibility of the association between cigarette smoking and COPD. In young, asymptomatic cigarette smokers, an increased number of inflammatory cells may initiate alveolar damage and the small airways are injured. Furthermore, protective mechanisms against inflammatory cell injury are probably impaired by cigarette smoke. The progressive destruction of the small airways and of the parenchyma is ultimately manifest as COPD.

VII. Epidemiological Plausibility

The application of this criterion requires that available data not conflict with current knowledge on the natural history and biology of the disease. Findings among cigarette smokers and nonsmokers, reviewed in the sections on temporal relationship and biological plausibility, provide abundant evidence to support the epidemiological plausibility of cigarette smoking as the major cause of COPD.

VIII. Specificity

The criterion of specificity requires that smoking cause only COPD. However, cigarette smoke is a complex mixture that has numerous toxic components with a multiplicity of effects. The association of smoking with many adverse health outcomes other than COPD is well documented (U.S. Dept. H.E.W., 1979). Unique exposure–disease connections are rare and specificity cannot be used as a major determinant for evaluating causation (Rothman, 1986).

IX. Analogy

The rationale for this criterion suggests that if one exposure can cause disease, other exposures that act similarly are potential causes. Fulfillment of the analogy criterion for smoking and COPD requires an established relationship between another exposure and the development of COPD. Although other environmental agents alone have not been shown to cause COPD, a host factor, $alpha_1$-antitrypsin deficiency, is an established cause of emphysema and provides an analogous relationship. Unchecked proteolytic activity in patients with $alpha_1$-antitrypsin deficiency results in panlobular emphysema (Laurell and Eriksson, 1963). Available data likewise suggest an imbalance between protease and antiprotease activity in cigarette smokers (Janoff, 1985). The similarities between an established cause of emphysema, $alpha_1$-antitrypsin deficiency, and cigarette smoking meet the criterion of analogy.

X. Conclusions

The association of cigarette smoking with morbidity and mortality from COPD may result from chance, bias, or cause. Chance can be dismissed in view of the numerous investigations with statistically significant results and bias is an implausible explanation for the voluminous evidence of association between smoking and COPD. However, the determination that the relationship between cigarette smoking and COPD is causal requires careful scrutiny of the available data.

The nine criteria for causation proposed by Hill (1965) are largely met by the evidence on smoking and COPD. Data from human experimentation are not available for obvious reasons, and cigarette smoking does not invariably predict the occurrence of COPD. However, the epidemiological data obviate the need for experimental data and few diseases have single causes. Despite these shortcomings with reference to the nine criteria, cigarette smoking can be judged as the major cause of COPD; from a public health standpoint, COPD would be a rare disease in the absence of cigarette smoking.

The available clinical and epidemiological data do show a strong and consistent association between cigarette smoking and COPD. The repeated demonstration worldwide of pulmonary function and structural abnormalities among smokers that are uncommon in nonsmokers provides powerful evidence for a causal link between cigarette smoking and COPD. Results from longitudinal investigations in children show that cigarette smoking causes lower lung function levels among those who actively and passively smoke, and as adults, children affected by smoking may be at increased risk for developing COPD. In adults who smoke, progressive decline in lung function in susceptible smokers leads to clinically evident COPD. Regardless of study design, the prevalence and incidence of COPD, and mortality from COPD are increased with the amount smoked. Also, with smoking cessation the rate of decline of lung function decreases, resulting in a lower risk of developing, and dying from, COPD. Pathological findings of small airways inflammation and parenchymal destruction from smoking cigarettes, coupled with laboratory evidence of an increased inflammatory cell population in lungs of cigarette smokers, provide biological plausibility.

Because all cigarette smokers do not develop COPD, individual susceptibility factors, as yet unidentified, probably determine risk from smoking (Snider, 1986). The major unanswered research question regarding smoking and COPD is identification of the factors determining individual susceptibility to cigarette smoke. The genetic characteristics and environmental factors that may act during childhood or adulthood to influence susceptibility are discussed in other chapters. Factors that may help identify the high-risk smoker include a low level of lung function (Burrows et al., 1987) and a high cumulative cigarette consumption (Dockery et al., 1988). The use of sophisticated physiological measurements has been suggested as a method for determining which smoker is at risk for development of COPD, but these tests have not been highly predictive in prospective studies (Stanescu et al., 1987; Habib et al., 1987; Buist et al., 1988).

Cigarette smoking is causally associated with the development of COPD, and most cases in the United States can be attributed to this addictive behavior. The strong association of cigarette smoking with COPD has both clinical and public health implications. Clinicians should be cautious in making the diagnosis of COPD in nonsmokers, particularly if the level of alpha$_1$-antitrypsin is within normal limits. Conversely, a history of cigarette smoking, particularly if the daily level of consumption has been high, increases the likelihood of COPD. However, only a minority of smokers develop COPD, so the disease should not be diagnosed on the basis of smoking history alone.

Acknowledgments

Dr. Coultas is a recipient of an Edward Livingston Trudeau Scholar Award from the American Lung Association.

References

Anderson, R., Theron, A. J., and Ras, G. J. (1987). Regulation by the anti-oxidants ascorbate, cysteine, and dapsone of the increased extracellular and intracellular generation of reactive oxidants by activated phagocytes from cigarette smokers. *Am. Rev. Respir. Dis.* **135**:1027-1032.

Ashley, F., Kannel, W. B., Sorlie, P. D., and Masson, R. (1975). Pulmonary function: relation to aging, cigarette habit, and mortality. The Framingham Study. *Ann. Intern. Med.* **82**:739-745.

Beaty, T. H., Menkes, H. A., Cohen, B. H., and Newill, C. A. (1984). Risk factors associated with longitudinal change in pulmonary function. *Am. Rev. Respir. Dis.* **129**:660-667.

Beck, G. J., Doyle, C. A., and Schachter, E. N. (1981). Smoking and lung function. *Am. Rev. Respir. Dis.* **123**:149-155.

Benowitz, N. L., Hall, S. M., Herning, R. I., Jacob, P., Jones, R. T., and Osman, A.-L. (1983). Smokers of low-yield cigarettes do not consume less nicotine. *N. Engl. J. Med.* **309**:139-142.

Benowitz, N. L., Payton, J., Kozlowski, L. T., and Yu, L. (1986). Influence of smoking fewer cigarettes on exposure to tar, nicotine, and carbon monoxide. *N. Engl. J. Med.* **315**:1310-1313.

Berend, N., Woolcock, A. J., and Marlin, G. E. (1979). Correlation between the function and structure of the lung in smokers. *Am. Rev. Respir. Dis.* **119**:695-705.

Buist, A. S., Vollmer, W. M., Johnson, L. R., and McCamant, L. E. (1988). Does the single-breath N_2 test identify the smoker who will develop airflow limitation? *Am. Rev. Respir. Dis.* **137**:293-301.

Burrows, B., Knudson, R. J., Cline, M. G., and Lebowitz, M. D. (1977). Quantitative relationships between cigarette smoking and ventilatory function. *Am. Rev. Respir. Dis.* **115**:195-205.

Burrows, B., Knudson, R. J., Camilli, A. E., Lyle, S. K., and Lebowitz, M. D. (1987). The "horse-racing effect" and predicting decline in forced expiratory volume in one second from screening spirometry. *Am. Rev. Respir. Dis.* **135**:788-793.

Camilli, A. E., Burrows, B., Knudson, R. J., Lyle, S. K., and Lebowitz, M. D. (1987). Longitudinal changes in forced expiratory volume in one second in adults. *Am. Rev. Respir. Dis.* **135**:794-799.

Chan, S.-K., and Matulionis, D. (1984). The relationship between the inactivation of alpha$_1$-protease inhibitor and the predisposition to emphysema in the tight-skin mouse (abstract). *Am. Rev. Respir. Dis.* **129**(2):300.

Clement, J., and Van de Woestijne, K. P. (1982). Rapidly decreasing forced expiratory volume in one second or vital capacity and development of chronic airflow obstruction. *Am. Rev. Respir. Dis.* **125**:553-558.

Cosio, M., Ghezzo, H., Hogg, J. C., Corbin, R., Loveland, M., Dosman, J., and Macklem, P. T. (1978). The relations between structural changes in small airways and pulmonary-function tests. *N. Engl. J. Med.* **298**:1277–1281.

Cosio, M. G., Hale, K. A., and Niewoehner, D. E. (1980). Morphologic and morphometric effects of prolonged cigarette smoking on the small airways. *Am. Rev. Respir. Dis.* **122**:265–271.

Detels, R., Rokow, S. N., Coulson, A. H., Tashkin, D. P., Sayre, J. W., and Massey, F. J. (1979). The UCLA population studies of chronic obstructive respiratory disease. I. Methodology and comparison of lung function in areas of high and low pollution. *Am. J. Epidemiol.* **109**:33–58.

Dockery, D. W., Speizer, F. E., Ferris, R. G., Jr., Ware, J. H., Louis, T. A., and Spiro, A. III (1988). Cumulative and reversible effects of lifetime smoking on simple tests of lung function in adults. *Am. Rev. Respir. Dis.* **137**:286–292.

Doll, R., and Peto, R. (1976). Mortality in relation to smoking: 20 years' observations on male British doctors. *Br. Med. J.* **2**(6051):1525–1536.

Doll, R., Gray, R., Hafner, B., and Peto, R. (1980). Mortality in relation to smoking: 22 years' observations on female British doctors. *Br. Med. J.* **280**(6219):967–971.

Fera, T., Abboud, R. T., Richter, A., and Johal, S. S. (1986). Acute effect of smoking on elastaselike esterase activity and immunologic neutrophil elastase levels in bronchoalveolar lavage fluid. *Am. Rev. Respir. Dis.* **133**:568–573.

Ferris, B. G., Higgins, I. T. T., Higgins, M. W., and Peters, J. M. (1973). Chronic nonspecific respiratory disease in Berlin, New Hampshire, 1961 to 1967. A follow-up study. *Am. Rev. Respir. Dis.* **107**:110–122.

Ferris, B. G. Jr., Speizer, F. E., Spengler, J. D., Dockery, D., Bishop, Y. M. M., Wolfson, M., and Humble, C. (1979). Effects of sulfer oxides and respirable particles on human health. Methodology and demography of populations in study. *Am. Rev. Respir. Dis.* **120**:767–779.

Fletcher, C. M., Peto, R., Tinker, C., and Speizer, F. E. (1976). *The Natural History of Chronic Bronchitis and Emphysema. An Eight-Year Study of Early Chronic Obstructive Lung Disease in Working Men in London.* New York, Oxford University Press.

Fletcher, C., and Peto, R. (1977). The natural history of chronic airflow obstruction. *Br. Med. J.* **1**:1645–1648.

Galdston, M., Feldman, J. G., Levytska, V., and Magnusson, B. (1987). Antioxidant activity of serum ceruloplasmin and transferrin available iron-binding capacity in smokers and nonsmokers. *Am. Rev. Respir. Dis.* **135**:783–787.

Habib, M. P., Klink, M. E., Knudson, D. E., Bloom, J. W., Kaltenborn, W. T., Knudson, R. J. (1987). Physiologic characteristics of subjects exhibiting accelerated deterioration of ventilatory function. *Am. Rev. Respir. Dis.* **136**:638–645.

Hale, K. A., Ewing, S. L., Gosnell, B. A., and Niewoehner, D. E. (1984). Lung disease in long-term cigarette smokers with and without chronic air-flow obstruction. *Am. Rev. Respir. Dis.* **130**:716–721.

Hammond, E. C. (1966). Smoking in relation to the death rates in one million men and women. In *Epidemiological Approaches to the Study of Cancer and Other Chronic Diseases.* National Cancer Institute Monograph No. 19, edited by W. Haenszel. U.S. Department of Health, Education, and Welfare, Public Health Service, National Institutes of Health, National Cancer Institute, pp. 127–204.

Hammond, E. C. (1980). The long-term benefits of reducing tar and nicotine in cigarettes. In *Banbury Report 3, A Safe Cigarette?* Edited by G. B. Gori and F. G. Bock. Cold Spring Harbor, Cold Spring Harbor Press, pp. 13–18.

Hammond, E. C., Garfinkel, L., Seidman, H., and Lew, E. A. (1976). "Tar" and nicotine content of cigarette smoke in relation to death rates. *Environ. Res.* **12**:263–274.

Higenbottam, T., Shipley, M. J., Clark, T. J. H., Rose, G. (1980). Lung function and symptoms of cigarette smokers related to tar yield and number of cigarettes smoked. *Lancet* **1**:409–412.

Higgins, M. W., Keller, J. B., Becker, M., Howatt, W., Landis, J. R., Rotman, H., Weg, J. G., and Higgins, I. (1982). An index of risk for obstructive airways disease. *Am. Rev. Respir. Dis.* **125**:144–151.

Higgins, M. W., Keller, J. B., Landis, J. R., Beaty, T. H., Burrows, B., Demets, D., Diem, J. E., Higgins, I. T. T., Lakatos, E., Lebowitz, M. D., Menkes, H., Speizer, F. E., Tager, I. B., and Weill, H. (1984). Risk of obstructive pulmonary disease. Collaborative assessment of the validity of the Tecumseh index of risk. *Am. Rev. Respir. Dis.* **130**:380–385.

Hill, A. B. (1965). The environment and disease: association or causation? *Proc. R. Soc. Med.* **58**:295–300.

Hunninghake, G. W., and Crystal, R. G. (1983). Cigarette smoking and lung destruction. Accumulation of neutrophils in the lungs of cigarette smokers. *Am. Rev. Respir. Dis.* **128**:833–838.

Janoff, A. (1985). Elastases and emphysema. Current assessment of the protease-antiprotease hypothesis. *Am. Rev. Respir. Dis.* **132**:417–433.

Janoff, A., Pryor, W. A., and Bengali, Z. H. (1987). Effects of tobacco smoke components on cellular and biochemical processes in the lung. *Am. Rev. Respir. Dis.* **136**:1058–1064.

Knudson, R. J., Burrows, B., and Lebowitz, M. D. (1976). The maximal expiratory flow-volume curve: its use in detection of ventilatory abnormalites in a population study. *Am. Rev. Respir. Dis.* **114**:871–879.

Laurell, C. B., and Eriksson, S. (1963). The electrophoretic alpha 1-globulin pattern of serum in alpha 1-antitrypsin deficiency. *Scand. J. Clin. Invest.* **15**:132–140.

Lebowitz, M. D., Knudson, R. J., and Burrows, B. (1984). Risk factors for airways obstructive diseases: a multiple logistics approach. *Chest* **85**:11–12s.

Lee, P. N., and Garfinkel, L. (1981). Mortality and type of cigarette smoked. *J. Epidemiol. Commun. Health.* **35**:16–22.

Martin, T. R., Raghu, G., Maunder, R. J., and Springmeyer, S. C. (1985). The effects of chronic bronchitis and chronic airflow obstruction on lung cell populations recovered by bronchoalveolar lavage. *Am. Rev. Respir. Dis.* **132**:254–260.

Medici, T. C., Unger, S., and Ruegger, M. (1985). Smoking pattern of smokers with and without tobacco-smoke-related lung diseases. *Am. Rev. Respir. Dis.* **131**:385–388.

Nagai, A., West, W. W., and Thurlbeck, W. M. (1985). The National Institutes of Health Intermittent Positive Pressure Breathing Trial: Pathology studies II. Correlation between morphologic findings, clinical findings, and evidence of expiratory air-flow obstruction. *Am. Rev. Respir. Dis.* **132**:946–953.

Niewoehner, D. E. (1988). Cigarette smoking, lung inflammation, and the development of emphysema. *J. Lab. Clin. Med.* **111**(1):15–27.

Niewoehner, D. E., Kleinerman, J., and Rice, B. (1974). Pathologic changes in the peripheral airways of young cigarette smokers. *N. Engl. J. Med.* **291**:755–758.

Paoletti, P., Camilli, A. E., Holberg, C. J., and Lebowitz, M. D. (1985). Respiratory effects in relation to estimated tar exposure from current and cumulative cigarette consumption. *Chest* **88**:849–855.

Peach, H., Hayward, D. M., Ellard, D. R., Morris, R. W., and Shah, D. (1986). Phlegm production and lung function among cigarette smokers changing tar groups during the 1970s. *J. Epidemiol. Commun. Health* **40**:110–116.

Rogot, E., and Murray, J. L. (1980). Smoking and causes of death among U.S. veterans: 16 years of observation. *Public Health Rep.* **95**:213–222.

Rokaw, S. N., Detels, R., Coulson, A. H., Sayre, J. W., Tashkin, D. P., Allwright, S. S., and Massey, F. J. Jr. (1980). The UCLA population studies of chronic obstructive respiratory disease 3. Comparison of pulmonary function in three communities exposed to photochemical oxidants, multiple primary pollutants, or minimal pollutants. *Chest* **78**:252–262.

Rossi, G. A., Hunninghake, G. W., Gadek, J. E., Szapiel, S. V., Kawanami, O., Ferrans, V. J., and Crystal, R. G. (1984). Pathogenesis of hereditary emphysema in the tight-skin mouse: evaluation of a potential source of proteases within the alveolar structures. *Am. Rev. Respir. Dis.* **129**:850–855.

Rothman, K. J. (1986). *Modern Epidemiology*. Boston/Toronto, Little, Brown, pp. 16–21, 35–40.

Saetta, M., Shiner, R. J., Angus, G. E., Kim, W. D., Wang, N.-S., King, M., Ghezzo, H., and Cosio, M. G. (1985). Destructive index: a measurement of lung parenchymal destruction in smokers. *Am. Rev. Respir. Dis.* **131**:764–769.

Samet, J. M., Tager, I. B., and Speizer, F. E. (1983). The relationship between respiratory illness in childhood and chronic airflow obstruction in adulthood. *Am. Rev. Respir. Dis.* **127**:508–523.

Samet, J. M. (1985). Less hazardous cigarettes and diseases of the lung. *Chest* **88**:802–803.

Snider, G. L. (1986). Chronic obstructive pulmonary disease—a continuing challenge. *Am. Rev. Respir. Dis.* **133**:942–944.

Sparrow, D., Stefos, T., Bosse, R., and Weiss, S. T. (1983). The relationship of tar content to decline in pulmonary function in cigarette smokers. *Am. Rev. Respir. Dis.* **127**:56–58.

Stanescu, D. C., Rodenstein, D. O., Hoeven, C., and Robert, A. (1987). Sensitive tests are poor predictors of the decline in forced expiratory volume in one second middle-aged smokers. *Am. Rev. Respir. Dis.* **135**:585–590.

Stuart-Harris, C. H. (1954). The epidemiology and evolution of chronic bronchitis. *Br. J. Tuber. Dis. Chest* **48**:169–178.

Stuart-Harris, C. H. (1968a). Chronic bronchitis, Part I. *Abst. World Med.* **42**:649–669.

Stuart-Harris, C. H. (1968b). Chronic bronchitis, Part II. *Abst. World Med.* **42**:737–751.

Szapiel, S., Fulmer, J. D., Hunninghake, G. W., Kawanami, O., Ferrans, V. J., and Crystal, R. G. (1981). Hereditary emphysema in the tight-skin mouse. *Am. Rev. Respir. Dis.* **123**:680–685.

Tager, I., Tishler, P. V., Rosner, B., Speizer, F. E., and Litt, M. (1978). Studies of the familial aggregation of chronic bronchitis and obstructive airways disease. *Int. J. Epidemiol.* **7**:55–62.

Tager, I. B., Munoz, A., Rosner, B., Weiss, S. T., Carey, V., and Speizer, F. E. (1985). Effect of cigarette smoking on the pulmonary function of children and adolescents. *Am. Rev. Respir. Dis.* **131**:752–759.

Tashkin, D. P., Clark, V. A., Coulson, A. H., Bourque, L. B., Simmons, M., Reems, C., Detels, R., and Rokaw, S. (1983). Comparison of lung function in young nonsmokers and smokers before and after initiation of the smoking habit. A prospective study. *Am. Rev. Respir. Dis.* **128**:12–16.

Tashkin, D. P., Clark, V. A., Coulson, A. H., Simmons, M., Bourque, L. B., Reems, C., Detels, R., Sayre, J. W., and Rokaw, S. N. (1984). The UCLA population studies of chronic obstructive respiratory disease VIII. Effects of smoking cessation on lung function: a prospective study of a free-living population. *Am. Rev. Respir. Dis.* **130**:707–715.

Taylor, J. C., Madison, R., and Kosinska, D. (1986). Is antioxidant deficiency related to chronic obstructive pulmonary disease? *Am. Rev. Respir. Dis.* **134**:285–289.

Toth, K. M., Berger, E. M., Beehler, C. J., and Repine, J. E. (1986). Erythrocytes from cigarette smokers contain more glutathione and catalase and protect endothelial cells from hydrogen peroxide better than do erythrocytes from nonsmokers. *Am. Rev. Respir. Dis.* **134**:281–284.

Tugwell, P., Bennett, K. J., Sackett, D. L., and Haynes, R. B. (1985). The measurement iterative loop: a framework for the critical appraisal of need, benefits and costs of health interventions. *J. Chron. Dis.* **38**:339–351.

U.S. Department of Health, Education, and Welfare (1964). Smoking and Health Report of the Advisory Committee to the Surgeon General of the Public Health Service. U.S. Department of Health, Education, and Welfare, Public Health Service, Washington, D.C. PHS Publication No. (PHS) No. 1103, pp. 45,277.

U.S. Department of Health, Education, and Welfare (1979). Smoking and Health. A Report of the Surgeon General. U.S. Department of Health, Education, and Welfare, Public Health Service, Office of the Assistant Secretary of Health, Office on Smoking and Health, Washington, D.C. DHEW Publication No. (PHS) 79-50066, pp. 4/1–4/77, 5/1–5/74, 6/1–6/52, 8/1–8/93.

U.S. Department of Health and Human Services (1981). The Health Consequences of Smoking. The Changing Cigarette. A report of the Surgeon General. U.S. Department of Health and Human Services, Public Health Service, Office on Smoking and Health, Rockville, Maryland. DHHS Publication No. (PHS) 81-50156, pp. 3–26, 48–59.

U.S. Department of Health and Human Services (1984). The Health Consequences of Smoking. Chronic Obstructive Lung Disease: A Report of the Surgeon General. U.S. Department of Health and Human Services, Public Health Service, Office on Smoking and Health, Rockville, Maryland. DHHS Publication No. (PHS) 84-50205, pp. 9, 75–118, 185–250, 348–352, 361–412.

U.S. Department of Health and Human Services (1985). The Health Consequences of Smoking. Cancer and Chronic Lung Disease in the Workplace. A Report of the Surgeon General. U.S. Department of Health and Human Services, Public Health Service, Office on Smoking and Health, Rockville, Maryland. DHHS Publication No. (PHS) 85-50207, p. 149.

Yeung, M. C., and Buncio, A. D. (1984). Leukocyte count, smoking, and lung function. *Am. J. Med.* **76**:31–37.

8

Genetic and Perinatal Risk Factors for the Development of Chronic Obstructive Pulmonary Disease

SUSAN REDLINE

Roger Williams General Hospital
Brown University Medical School
Providence, Rhode Island

SCOTT T. WEISS

Harvard Medical School
Brigham and Women's Hospital
Beth Israel Hospital
Boston, Massachusetts

Numerous studies have sought to identify a genetic basis for chronic obstructive pulmonary disease (COPD). COPD does not refer to a specific phenotype, however, but describes the presence of significant airflow obstruction with different degrees of incomplete reversibility, variably associated with mucus hypersecretion and emphysema (Fanta, 1981). It is generally recognized that COPD may be a heterogeneous entity, and that the pathophysiological roles played by host and environmental factors may vary among different subsets of the population with COPD. Furthermore, even identical phenotypes (e.g., FEV_1 levels each of 1.0 L) may be produced by different physiological mechanisms that influence the elastic recoil properties of the lung or the structure and function of the airways. Imprecise definitions of phenotype, and diversity in the pathogenetic determinants of the phenotype, limit the ability to identify modes of inheritance.

Given these limitations, we shall review the genetic–epidemiological evidence that suggests a genetic component for the development of COPD, and then review the available data regarding specific biological properties of the lungs that may be inherited. An attempt will be made to differentiate genetic causes from those that relate to prenatal factors and to environmental influences shared among family members. Potentially inherited properties that may increase susceptibility to cigarette smoke will be emphasized. These include airway responsiveness and the perhaps genetically related determinants of atopy and autonomic function; protease homeostasis; lung defense mechanisms possibly related to blood markers; lung growth characteristics; and smoking habits (Table 1). This list is not exhaustive, and we will not specifically discuss cystic fibrosis. The interested reader is referred to several other reviews for a consideration of factors not discussed here (Cohen, 1980; Kauffmann, 1984).

I. Familial Aggregation of Respiratory Symptoms, Disease, and Pulmonary Function

A familial basis for COPD, possibly genetic, is suggested by studies that have demonstrated the aggregation of respiratory symptoms, disease, and level of function among family members. In many studies, familial similarities in respiratory symptoms or in level of lung function are demonstrated (Higgins and Keller, 1975; Astemborski et al., 1985; Speizer et al., 1976; Leeder et al., 1976a; Tager et al., 1976). A familial association *between* different respiratory symptoms (e.g., wheeze and bronchitis) has also been described (Leeder et al., 1976b; Speizer et al., 1976). To what extent associations that relate different symptoms, or that relate symptoms with pulmonary function level, indicate the operation of similar pathogenetic mechanisms and are based on common genetic mechanisms is not well understood. However, some investigators have suggested that childhood respiratory symptoms (e.g., wheeze) may be causally related to conditions of chronic airflow obstruction.

A familial aggregation of respiratory *symptoms* was suggested by Leeder and associates (1976a) in a British study of 2000 children evaluated for 5 years. A greater prevalence of asthma and wheeze was demonstrated among children whose parents reported similar symptoms than among children of asymptomatic parents (5.4% versus 2.5%, and 27.7% versus 19.6%, for asthma and wheeze, respectively). These effects persisted following adjustment for parental smoking. Although a recall bias may have been operative in this study, symptomatic children demonstrated lower peak flow rates than did asymptomatic children. Sibbald and associates (1980) similarly demonstrated that asthma was reported more often by the first-degree relatives (siblings and parents) of children with asthma or wheezy bronchitis (prevalence rates of 13% and 11% for asthma and wheezy bronchitis, respectively) as compared with relatives of controls (4%). Thes findings could relate to the operation of nongenetic familial

Table 1 Factors that Could be
Inherited to Account for
Familial Aggregation of COPD

Lung dimensions
Pi genotype
Airway responsiveness
Atopy
Autonomic function
ABO blood group
Male sex

influences, such as smoking and infectious exposures, that may cause similar health effects in household members. Their results also may relate, as in the previous study, to a preferential reporting of disease by the relatives of asthmatics compared to relatives of controls.

Twin studies, which exploit the genetic differences between monozygotic (MZ) and dizygotic (DZ) twins, also have demonstrated a familial, perhaps genetic, basis for respiratory symptoms. These studies have demonstrated greater concordance rates for asthma for MZ twins (ranging from 15% to 59%) than for dizygotic (DZ) twins (4–19%) (Redline et al., 1987; Lubs, 1971; Konig and Godfrey, 1974). Similar concordance rates for the symptom "cough" and for the presence of dyspnea also have been demonstrated (Cederlof et al., 1967; Fabsitz et al., 1985). Such differences in concordance rates between groups that differ in their degree of genetic identity suggest the influence of genetic factors on phenotype. However, greater similarities in the phenotype of MZ than DZ twins may also relate to greater similarities in environmental exposures that occur in MZ than in DZ twinships.

Respiratory *disease*, defined as asthma, bronchitis, or emphysema, was shown to aggregate in 37,000 households surveyed in the United States (Speizer et al., 1976). In this study, the prevalence of asthma or bronchitis was 25% higher among the children from households with at least one parent with respiratory disease than it was in the children of asymptomatic parents. Similarly, in Tecumseh, Michigan, a greater prevalence of chronic bronchitis or asthma was demonstrated among children who had at least one parent with a history of respiratory disease than among the offspring of parents without such a history (Higgins and Keller, 1975). A sibship aggregation of disease additionally was suggested. In both of these studies, prevalence of disease was greater when both parents were affected than if only one parent was affected, which suggests a polygenic mode of inheritance.

A familial aggregation of chronic bronchitis also was demonstrated by Tager and associates (1978) in a population-based study of 1770 subjects from 430 randomly chosen households in East Boston. First-degree relatives of an affected propositus were found to have a relative risk of 1.4 for chronic bronchitis compared with relatives of unaffected kindred. The prevalence of chronic bronchitis progressively decreased in second- and third-degree relatives of affected propositi. A decreasing prevalence of disease in these subjects could be due to a lesser influence of shared environmental exposures among more distant relatives. However, such a relationship between genotypic and phenotypic similarities also suggests a polygenic mode of inheritance. In this study, as in the previously discussed studies, the possibility of reporting bias cannot be excluded.

Measurements of pulmonary function in randomly chosen household members may provide objective support for a familial basis for pulmonary disease that is free of recall bias, and may more specifically indicate conditions of chronic airflow obstruction than does information obtained from questionnaires. In numerous family studies, a familial aggregation of level of pulmonary function, expressed as either a continuous measurement or dichotomized as "normal" or "low," has been demonstrated.

In a matched-pair study of 1441 relatives of 114 index cases with COPD and of 114 control subjects, Kueppers and associates (1977) demonstrated a greater reported prevalence of chronic respiratory disease in the relatives of cases than in relatives of controls. Measurement of FEV_1 on a smaller sample of subjects revealed that although this concordance of symptoms was due in part to reporting bias, a greater number of relatives of cases than relatives of controls had levels of FEV_1 less than 70% of the predicted level (15.5% [9/58] versus 4.8% [3/63], respectively). However, smoking exposure was also greater in the relatives of cases. Similarly, in a family study of subjects identified through a pulmonary function laboratory, Larson and associates (1970) demonstrated a higher prevalence of reduced lung function among the siblings and children of 61 patients with COPD as contrasted with the prevalence among the (genetically unrelated) spouses of these patients (Larson et al., 1970). Furthermore, a disproportionately elevated prevalence of COPD among the smoking, as contrasted with the nonsmoking, relatives of cases of COPD suggested an interaction between smoking and genetic factors. In a more representative population-based sample of subjects, Higgins and Keller also demonstrated that reduced level of pulmonary function aggregated within families (Higgins and Keller, 1975). Approximately one-half of the children in this study whose age-, sex-, and height-adjusted levels of FEV_1 were within the lowest tertile of the population distribution were the offspring of adults who also had low levels of FEV_1.

In addition to a familial aggregation of respiratory disease defined as a critically low level of pulmonary function, there are familial similarities in continuously measured levels of lung function in healthy subjects. Correlations in age-, sex-, and height-adjusted levels of FEV_1 and FVC among generally healthy relatives have been found to vary according to their genetic identity (Redline et al., 1989; Higgins and Keller, 1975). Particularly important is the remarkable consistency in genetic estimates derived with the use of different statistical methods: path (Lewitter et al., 1984; Devor et al., 1984); variance component (Astemborski et al., 1985); or correlational analyses (Redline et al., 1986) and in studies of populations with different age ranges and representing different genotypic relationships. Parent–child correlations in FEV_1 have been found to range from 0.14 to 0.33, 0.18 to 0.25, and 0.20 to 0.29 in two population-based studies of nuclear families and in one study of adult twin families (Higgins et al., 1975; Tager et al., 1976; Redline et al., 1989). In these three studies, sibship correlations for FEV_1 ranged from 0.23 to 0.66, 0.26, and 0.17 to 0.28, respectively. Such correlations possibly could be produced by nongenetic familial influences, such as similarities in exposures to active and passive smoking, indoor and outdoor air pollution, and respiratory infections. However, both a variance analysis of pulmonary function, (Devor and Crawford, 1984) partitioning genetic and environmental contributions to phenotype among relatives drawn from a population-based sample, and an analysis of genotypic and phenotypic similarities among family members of MZ and DZ adult twins who differed in their degree of shared environment (Redline et al., 1987) have suggested that a common familial environment contributed little to these familial similarities in lung function.

II. Implications of Familial Aggregation Studies

The demonstration of a decreasing prevalence of disease (e.g., chronic bronchitis, asthma) and lesser degrees of similarity in level of lung function among relatives with decreasing genetic identity suggests that lung function/disease is determined by multifactorial genetic influences. The identification of more specific modes of inheritance would require the identification of differences in disease prevalence among different groups of relatives. For example, a recessive mode of inheritance is suggested by the demonstration of a sibship aggregation of a trait, and little vertical transmission. X-linked and dominant modes of inheritance require the demonstration of specific patterns of similarity in phenotype between parents and children, which in the former case (X-linked) varies according to gender. Such patterns of inheritance for the majority of cases of COPD have not been described. The genetic epidemiologist, however, may be unable to identify specific modes of inheritance for phenotypes that are produced by heterogeneous genetic mechanisms; such patterns of inheritance may only be evident in pedigree studies, and may not be observed when data on multiple families are combined. Furthermore, the familial clustering of disease may be influenced by a myriad of pre and postnatal environmental exposures that may influence phenotypic expression. Given these limitations, we will next attempt to examine evidence that may suggest a genetic basis for *specific* physiological properties and polymorphisms that could account for a familial aggregation of COPD.

III. What May Be Inherited?

A. Lung Dimensions

An appreciation of the longitudinal behavior of pulmonary function has increased our understanding of who may be at greatest risk of critically low levels of FEV_1 with cigarette exposure. Longitudinal studies of pulmonary function in nonsmoking adults suggest that FEV_1 decreases by approximately 20–40 ml/yr after age 35 years (Beaty et al., 1984; Dockery et al., 1985). Age- and size-corrected levels of pulmonary function, expressed in percentiles relative to the population distribution, appear to be constant over time in individual nonsmokers, a phenomenon described as "tracking" (Dockery et al., 1985) (Fig. 1). In smokers, however, adjusted levels of FEV_1 may cross percentiles over time. In such individuals (i.e., "rapid decliners") annual rates of decline in FEV_1 may be as much as 60–120 ml/yr (Fletcher et al., 1976). Figure 2 demonstrates patterns of pulmonary function change for two "rapid decliners," each of whom suffer a 120 ml/yr decline in FEV_1 between ages 35 and 60 years but in whom baseline level of lung function is low (3.5 L) or high (5.0 L). Although a maximum loss of 3.0 L in FEV_1 is expected for both subjects, only the subjects with a relatively low "starting" level of pulmonary function has reached a level of FEV_1 so critically low that "disease" is recognized. Therefore, at least theoretically, the maximum level of pulmonary function attained in early adulthood may determine, and be an important risk factor for, the subsequent development of COPD.

"Tracking" of FEV_1 growth also has been demonstrated in early childhood (Dockery et al., 1983) (Fig. 1). This suggests that level of FEV_1

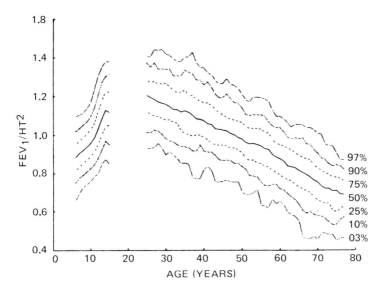

Percentiles of FEV_1/HT^2 vs. age for white females

Figure 1 Age-related change in FEV_1/HT^2 for white females for percentiles of FEV_1/HT^2.

measured at least as early as age 6 years determines subsequent level measured until puberty, and probably beyond. Therefore, level of pulmonary function measured in early childhood may predict the maximal level of pulmonary function in early adulthood.

Is "starting" level of pulmonary function genetically determined? The answer appears to be, at least in part, yes. Path analyses of the relationship of pulmonary function between family members, (Lewitter et al., 1984) and heritability estimates for pulmonary function in young and older twins (Redline et al., 1987) suggest an important genetic influence on the "native" level of pulmonary function. These relationships are most evident in children and may diminish in older individuals in whom environmental factors may become progressively more influential (Lewitter et al., 1984). In adult MZ twins, in whom genetic identity is absolute, there are, however, substantial intraclass correlations in levels of FEV_1 and FVC that are not substantially altered when one considers a number of environmental exposures potentially shared by both members of a twinship such as smoking, occupational exposure, and childhood respiratory illness. Functional similarity between twins also is supported by smaller studies demonstrating greater radiographic similarities in tracheal and chest wall

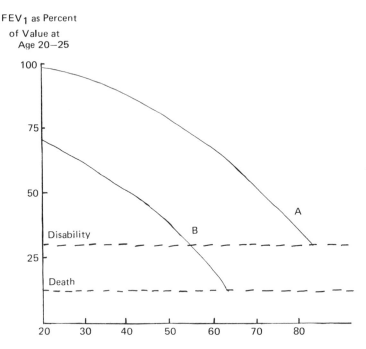

Figure 2   Demonstration of the importance of early adulthood lung function on the late adulthood lung function in circumstances of identically rapid annual decline in lung function.

dimensions in MZ than DZ twins (Kawakami, et al., 1986) that also suggest a genetic basis for "native" level of pulmonary function.

B. Protease Homeostasis

Early reports of emphysema occurring in families with severely deficient levels of the enzyme α_1-antiprotease (α_1 AP), (Eriksson, 1964) provided the first and, as of yet, only clearly genetic cause (other than cystic fibrosis) for COPD. Antiprotease phenotype is inherited in an autosomal codominant pattern. Severely deficient levels (less than 15% of normal) occur in only approximately 1% of the population who are homozygous for the Z allele (Fagerhol and Cox, 1981; Morse, 1978; Kauffmann, 1984), a proportion too small to explain susceptibility to cigarette smoke in the majority of subjects with COPD. However, heterozygosity for the Z or for other variant alleles (associated with 30–80% normal α_1AP levels) occurs in approximately 7% of the population and has been hypothesized to be an important risk factor for the development of COPD (Lieberman, 1971; Kueppers et al., 1969; Mittman et al., 1974).

Population studies that support heterozygosity as a genetic factor for COPD include comparisons of Pi phenotype in cases of COPD and controls, and in the relatives of such index cases (reviewed in detail by Kauffmann, 1984). Shigeoka and associates (1976), for example, found the prevalence of the PiMZ phenotype to be 1.5–4 times greater in patients with COPD than in controls (Shigeoka et al., 1976). However, subsequent, more representative, population studies in Tucson, AZ (Morse et al., 1977), and Baltimore, MD (Khoury et al., 1986), have failed to find a consistent association of heterozygosity with FEV_1 level or with rate of decline in FEV_1 despite careful characterization of phenotype. In particular, a collaborative study that examined pulmonary function in 143 cases with PiMZ phenotype and 143 normal subjects (PiM) matched for relevant covariates showed no significant differences in pulmonary function assessed with spirometry or with "more sensitive" tests of pulmonary dysfunction (DLCO, closing volume, and density dependence of expiratory flow) between these groups (Bruce et al., 1984). This study had a statistical power of 95% in detecting modest (200 ml) differences in lung function and strongly suggests that in the general population heterozygosity does not significantly increase susceptibility to COPD. Previously observed relationships between heterozygosity and pulmonary disease in the relatives of cases of COPD have been interpreted to be due to additional familial, genetic or environmental, factors that interacted with heterozygosity and predisposed to disease. Of considerable interest are preliminary findings that suggest that there may be a disease locus for emphysema close to the a_1-antiprotease gene. In this study, a significantly increased frequency of a specific restriction fragment length polymorphism of the a_1-antiprotease gene was demonstrated in patients with bronchiecstasis or with emphysema unassociated with antiprotease deficiency, as compared to controls (Kalsheker et al., 1987). If this finding is confirmed, it might explain the familial patterns of emphysema observed in some but not in all heterozygotes.

The failure to demonstrate an epidemiological association of the a_1 heterozygous phenotypes and respiratory disease furthermore should be interpreted within the context of laboratory studies that indicate a multiplicity of interactions that influence protease homeostasis. For example, the occurrence of emphysema in PiZ individuals, most probably a result of an inherited inability to inhibit sufficiently elastin degradation mediated by human leukocyte elastase, may represent a simpler case of protease–antiprotease imbalance compared to what may occur in the majority of smokers (Janoff, 1985). In smokers, protease imbalance may occur rather as a result of numerous mechanisms acting to increase elastin degradation and impair elastin repair. Laboratory studies suggest that smoking may cause a diversity of effects: augmented release of human leukocyte elastase as well as at least one elastase (a metalloenzyme resistent to α_1AP) from macrophages (Hinman et al., 1980); functional inactivation of normally secreted α_1AP by oxidants that are directly in cigarette smoke and oxidants that are secondarily released during the inflammatory cell reaction to smoking (Johnson and Travis, 1979); and impaired elastin repair due to the defective function of the elastin-related cross-linking enzyme, lysyl oxidase (Laurent et al., 1983), also due to inactivation by smoking-related oxidants. Therefore, if susceptibility to cigarette smoke is related to complex interactions among a number of host characteristics that determine protease balance, such characteristics are likely not to be simply measurable with determinations of absolute α_1AP level.

Measurements of *functional* activity of α_1AP, as obtained from the bronchoalveolar lavage fluid of smokers and nonsmokers (Abboud et al., 1985), and the measurement of elastin degradation products (Davies et al., 1983) (urinary desmosine levels or serum concentrations of elastin peptides) have been attempted in order to characterize better protease imbalance in smokers and nonsmokers. Whether, in population studies, such determination would identify subjects at risk for augmented elastin degradation with exposure to cigarette smoke cannot be reasonably speculated. To date, such determinations have not shown consistent associations with exposure (smoking) or disease (low FEV_1). In particular, one large epidemiological study of French adults showed no association between *functional* activity of α_1AP and smoking status (Lellouch et al., 1985); however, in this study the relationship of enzyme activity and pulmonary function was not examined. The failure to demonstrate an association of α_1AP, smoking, and pulmonary function may relate to the wide within individual fluctuations of α_1AP activity that also varies according to intensity and interval from exposure to cigarette smoke (Janoff, 1985). Furthermore, previous laboratory studies in which α_1AP activity have been determined have been too small to determine whether the between individual variability in activity could also relate to individual differences in genetic propensity for disease.

Studies of the relationship among urinary desmosine, smoking, and pulmonary function also have failed to reveal consistent associations. These few studies also may have been limited by small numbers and selection biases. For example, one such study population consisted of healthy firemen, a group with generally normal pulmonary function in whom accelerated elastin turnover is unlikely to be prevalent (Davies et al., 1983). Furthermore, determination of urinary desmosine concentrations may not be of sufficient sensitivity to identify abnormalities in lung elastin turnover.

C. Airway Responsiveness

Whether airways hyperresponsiveness predisposes the smoker to chronic airflow obstruction is a question under active investigation. Augmented airway responsiveness is found in subjects with chronic bronchitis (Bahous et al., 1984; Ramsdell et al., 1982). Furthermore, airway responsiveness may be elevated in subjects with COPD who demonstrate accelerated rates of decline in FEV_1 (Kanner, 1984; Taylor et al., 1985). The details that implicate airway hyperresponsiveness as a risk factor for COPD are provided in Chapter 9.

Familial Aggregation of Airway Responsiveness

A genetic basis for airway responsiveness was suggested in two twin studies. Konig and Godfrey (1974) demonstrated a greater concordance rate for airway responsiveness with exercise among 8 MZ(62.5%) than with 7(14.3%) DZ twinships. Responsiveness to methacholine challenge tests among a larger population (61 MZ, 46 DZ pairs), selected in part because of the presence of asthma or allergy, similarly demonstrated greater pairwise correlations in responsiveness among MZ than DZ twins (0.67 and 0.34, for MZ and DZ, respectively) (Hopp et al., 1984). In a smaller study of methacholine reactivity among healthy nonsmoking twins, however, no differences in the magnitude of intrapair differences were demonstrated for MZ and DZ twins, which the authors interpreted as evidence for an environmental rather than genetic basis for airway responsiveness (Zamel et al., 1984). However, the degree of responsiveness, as well as size of this sample, was not sufficient to allow computation of concordance rates for hyperresponsiveness, an analysis that may have demonstrated greater similarities in MZ than in DZ twins.

A familial aggregation of airway hyperresponsiveness has been demonstrated most convincingly in families of asthmatics. An increased prevalence of exercise-induced bronchial lability, consisting of abnormal bronchodilation in the early stages of exercise, has been described in the relatives of patients with asthma who were otherwise normal (32% prevalence) or who had hayfever (40% prevalence) (Konig and Godfrey, 1973a). Similar abnormalities in airway responsiveness were described by these investigators in the relatives of infants with wheezy bronchitis, which were not present among relatives of infants without this history (Konig and Godfrey, 1973b). Townley and associates (1976) demonstrated in approximately 500 subjects that the distribution of airway responsiveness to methacholine inhalation differed in relatives of asthmatic patients compared with relatives of nonatopic nonasthmatics (Townley et al., 1986). Among the relatives of "normals," a unimodal distribution of responsiveness was observed; in contrast, among the relatives of asthmatic patients, a bimodal distribution was present that identified a subsample of relatives with augmented airway responsiveness. Pedigree analysis of these data did not demonstrate a strict Mendelian mode of inheritance nor the sole effects of environmental influences. Airway responsiveness, similar to the data for wheeze and asthma, was suggested as following a multifactorial mode of inheritance.

There are few data available regarding the aggregation of AR in family members of subjects with COPD. Britt and associates (1980) reported the prevalence of airway hyperresponsiveness to methacholine to be 45% among 20 adult male offspring of patients with COPD (Britt et al., 1980). However, such findings could relate to effects of active or passive smoking, or to the selection of families with asthma rather than with COPD. Additionally, studies in a control population were not performed.

The Genetic Basis for Airway Responsiveness

The studies cited above suggest that there is not a single gene or haplotype responsible for airway hyperresponsiveness. The major histocompatability complexes HLA- A1 and B8 have been found to occur at increased frequency in some asthmatic persons (Proust et al., 1987; Morris et al., 1977; Thornsby et al., 1971); however, there may be limited ability to generalize this finding to the general population.

The associations of airway hyperresponsiveness with various manifestations of allergy, which include allergic asthma and rhinitis, eczema, skin tests reactivity, eosinophilia, IgE elevations, and the familial aggregation of asthma/allergy, suggests the possibility that multiple genetic factors that influence immediate-type hypersensitivity may be important in determining airways responsiveness.

The airway hyperresponsiveness that has been observed in smokers with chronic bronchitis and/or airflow obstruction may represent a manifestation of allergy. In smokers, immunological abnormalities consisting of elevations in systemic and lung leukocyte counts (Bridges et al., Wyatt, and Rehm, 1985; Reynolds and Newball, 1974), peripheral IgE levels (Burrows et al., 1981), specific IgE responses to occupational aeroallergens (Venables et al., 1985), and skin test reactivity (Welty et al., 1984) have been observed. Whether these findings are due to systemic and pulmonary reactions to cigarette smoke and pulmonary infection that occur independently of an allergic predisposition, or whether they preferentially occur in subjects with a genetic propensity for allergy, is not known. Population studies have not yet clarified the relationships of allergy, airway responsiveness, and COPD.

The genetic basis for immunological mechanisms that influence lymphocyte and mast cell function and target organ sensitivity has not been extensively studied in population research. An Italian study of 291 cases of children with wheeze, bronchiolitis, or asthma, and 1417 unmatched normal controls, suggested that a genetic basis for wheeze in atopic children may relate to adenosine deaminase 2-1 phenotype, an enzyme that influences utilization of a protein (adenosine) that may modulate histamine release from basophils (Ronchetti et al., 1984). However, the association of a specific phenotype with clinical states was relatively weak, and the differences in the age, sex, and selection processes for the identification of cases and controls weaken these findings. Further studies of the distribution of biochemical markers in the population are needed.

The genetics of the IgE response have been more extensively investigated. Based on the twin studies of Basarel, 59% of the variability of basal IgE level in adults and 79% of the variability in children is determined by genetic factors (Basarel et al., 1974). The genetic control of the allergic response appears to be complex and multifactorial (Marsh et al., 1980; Marsh et al., 1981), and may involve three different genetic controls that are either antigen nonspecific or specific. The antigen-nonspecific effect of the postulated IgE regulator gene may be strongly influenced by environmental antigens. However, the genetic control of IgE secretion has not been systematically evaluated in any epidemiological investigation.

Environmental Modifications of Airway
Responsiveness and Allergy

The degree to which a familial aggregation of airway responsiveness and/or allergy is determined by a common genetic substrate rather than common pre- and postnatal exposures (e.g., smoking and respiratory infection) is unclear. The specific clinical manifestations of allergy in given individuals or given families appear to be determined by as yet poorly understood interactions between genetic factors and the environment. This is consistent with the finding that specific clinical manifestations of allergy (e.g., asthma, allergic rhinitis, eczema) often differ among first-degree relatives (Sibbald et al., 1980). Furthermore, in MZ twins, although there is almost a 100% concordance for the presence of *any* allergic disease, there is only a 20–60% concordance specifically for asthma (Falliers et al., 1971; Criep, 1942; Konig and Godfrey, 1974).

The potential importance of environmental factors in influencing the expression of airway responsiveness in given individuals is also supported by recent evidence that suggests that airway hyperresponsiveness may be regularly found in normal newborns. At least three reports have noted very marked increases in airway responsiveness in small numbers of normal newborn infants during the first year of life when tested with methacholine (Tepper, 1987), histamine (Landau, 1987), and eucapneic hyperpnea to sub-freezing air (Geller et al., 1985). Whether this finding relates to artifacts of test performance, mechanical factors of the developing lung and chest wall, auto-nomic nervous system development, or other unknown factors is unclear. If these preliminary observations are confirmed it may suggest that the genetics of airway responsiveness is less important and environmental events may play a more permissive role in maintaining this physiological trait. Much further work will be necessary to understand the significance of these preliminary observations.

D. Autonomic Function

Inherited abnormalities to autonomic nervous system function could poten-tially explain familial occurrences of chronic bronchitis and asthma, and perhaps COPD. Baseline airway smooth muscle tone and bronchial mucus secretion are modulated by input from the autonomic nervous system (Cabezas et al., 1971; Boat and Kleinman, 1975). Beta-adrenergic hyporesponsiveness, and α-adrenergic and cholinergic hyperresponsiveness are variably found in asthmatics (Henderson et al., 1979; Apold and Aksnes, 1977; Lang et al., 1978; Davis, 1986), allergic nonasthmatics (Kaliner, 1976; Bruce et al., 1975), and subjects with cystic fibrosis (Davis et al., 1980, 1983). Airway responsiveness to methacholine characteristically is abnormal in these groups of subjects. In subjects with cystic fibrosis and their asymptomatic relatives there are abnormalities in pupillary responses to cholinergic stimula-tion that suggest that, in at least these subjects, a generalized abnormality in autonomic function that may be inherited (Davis, 1984).

Autonomic nervous system dysfunction also has been implicated in COPD based on the observation of airway hyperresponsiveness to cholinergic agents (Bahous et al., 1984). However, unlike in asthmatics, airway respon-siveness does not appear to increase following α-adrenoreceptor stimulation or diminish with pretreatment with ipratropium bromide (Yan et al., Woolcock, 1985). These findings may suggest that the mechanisms responsi-ble for airway hyperresponsiveness differ in asthma and COPD and that the autonomic system may not play a similar role in these conditions. Further-more, in COPD the finding of airway hyperresponsiveness to cholinergic agents could occur as a consequence of disease rather than be an endogenous host characteristic that acts as a risk factor for disease.

E.   ABO Blood Groups and ABH Secretor Status

Blood group phenotype and secretor status may influence antibacterial defense mechanisms. Bacteria have antigens that cross-react with blood groups A and B, and the presence of anti-A and anti-B antibodies in type O individuals has been hypothesized to protect against respiratory tract infection and to decrease the risk of developing COPD (Viskum, 1973). ABH secretor status also may influence respiratory tract defense mechanisms; this action may be mediated by mucosal secretions of certain glycoproteins and alterations in the activity of the secretory immunoglobulin IgA (Kinane et al., 1982).

The results of studies relating ABO and ABH secretor phenotypes with COPD have been reviewed in detail by Kauffmann (1984). In several studies, an increased frequency of respiratory illness in infancy has been found in children with blood group A compared to those with O, the relative risk ranging from 1.3 to 2.2 (Bubnov et al., 1973; Struthers, 1951; Carter and Heslop, 1957). The relationship of blood group and reduced FEV_1 in adults has not been consistently demonstrated, however. Kauffmann compared a number of blood group polymorphisms in 99 subjects selected to represent individuals genetically predisposed to (nonsmokers with low FEV_1 levels) or genetically protected from (smokers with high levels of FEV_1) COPD (Kauffmann et al., 1983). A modest increase in the frequency of A antigen carriers compared to non-A carriers was demonstrated (odds ratio 1.6) in those subjects considered to be genetically predisposed to develop COPD. Among a subset of subjects in whom secretor status was determined, an odds ratio of 2.5 for low FEV_1 was found for nonsecretors. These associations were based on small numbers of subjects and did not reach statistical significance.

The relationship of blood antigens and secretor status to pulmonary function has been studied in a larger Baltimore population (n = 192). Pulmonary function was determined on two occasions approximately 5 years apart. Level of FEV_1/FVC was modestly reduced and decreased more rapidly among women, but not men, with blood group A antigen. ABH nonsecretor status was related to reduced FEV_1 in an initial cross-sectional survey, (Cohen, 1980) but was not found in a somewhat smaller follow-up study (Khoury et al., 1986). Thus, if a relationship of ABO antigens and ABH secretor status and pulmonary function exists, it appears to be relatively weak and may explain only a small proportion of the variability in the distribution of pulmonary function. Although the differences in the findings of studies of women versus men, or of cross-sectional versus longitudinal samples, may relate to random error or differences in sample size, such differences also may indicate the operation of yet poorly defined interactions between these markers and other host characteristics.

F. Male Sex

Males have an increased incidence of asthma and allergic diseases (Croner et al., 1982; Naeye et al., 1971), more respiratory infections (Weiss, 1985), a higher incidence of infant respiratory distress syndrome (Khoury, 1985), and have lower size compensated flows (Tepper et al., 1986) than females. Increased male susceptibility to respiratory disease in early life suggests the possibility that male sex confers a greater risk of lung disease in adulthood for a given level of cigarette smoke exposure. The nature of this increased male susceptibility is unknown, but may relate to in utero or genetic differences. This hypothesis deserves further investigation.

G. Smoking Behavior

Smoking behavior is clearly a complex trait that is influenced by multiple social and economic factors (McKennell, 1970). However, the significantly higher correlations for smoking behavior in MZ than DZ twins found in several large studies suggest the possibility that genetic factors, in addition to environmental factors, may influence both the initiation and perpetuation of smoking habits (Hannah et al., Mathews, 1985; Friberg et al., 1970; Raaschau-Nielson, 1960; Crumpacker et al., 1979). Such genetic factors may relate to inherited personality traits; for example, the genetic basis of extraversion and neuroticism have been addressed in the psychiatric literature (Vandenberg, 1967). Genetic factors that relate to specific reactions to nicotine and propensity for addiction possibly may be important in the perpetuation of smoking; thus, exposure per se to cigarette smoking may have a genetic basis.

IV. Prenatal and Early Postnatal Environmental Influences That May Aggregate Within Families

A number of environmental exposures that are common to family members may cause phenotypic similarities in pulmonary function in families (Table 2). Certainly, viral respiratory infection, often commonly transmitted within families, may cause transient airway hyperresponsiveness (Aquilina et al., 1980). Such infections, especially when occurring in early childhood, may predispose to airway hyperresponsiveness and atopy in adulthood, and the subsequent development of respiratory disease (Leeder, 1975; Burrows and Taussig, 1980). However, these suggestions are based predominantly on retrospective data that demonstrate associations between lower respiratory tract infection before age 2 years and respiratory symptoms and asthma in later life (Colley et al., 1973; Kiernan et al., 1976; Leeder et al., 1976b), and that demonstrate a relationship between childhood respiratory infection and subsequent atopy (Frick et al., 1979). The potential problems in these data have been discussed extensively (Burrows and Taussig, 1980; Samet et al., 1983) and include preferential recollection of disease in symptomatic subjects; the possible misdiagnosis

Table 2 Environmental Factors
Operating in Utero or During
the First Year of Life

Passive cigarette smoke exposure
Breast feeding
Respiratory illness

of the first episode of asthma as a respiratory infection (i.e., bronchitis and bronchiolitis; and the lack of physiological data collected prior to the putative "infection."

A. Postnatal Passive Smoke Exposure

The effects of passive smoke exposure may cause similarities in respiratory symptoms, an increase in respiratory infections, and a modest reduction in lung function among family members (Tager et al., 1983; Schenker et al., 1983; Ware et al., 1984). Airway responsiveness assessed with methacholine and eucapnic hyperventilation with cold air also has been demonstrated to be greater among children, especially asthmatics, exposed to parental cigarette smoking (Martinez et al., 1985; O'Connor et al., 1987). This could be related to a greater prevalence of respiratory infections in families exposed to passive cigarette smoke, to other socioeconomic factors, or to a common genetic propensity for disease.

B. Prenatal Smoke Exposure

The health effects of passive smoking may be mediated through in utero exposure. The prenatal effects of maternal smoking on fetal lung development are an area of active research. Animal studies suggest that fetal lung development is adversely affected by maternal smoking (Bassi et al., 1984; Collins et al., 1985). It has been speculated that lung hypoplasia may result from in utero exposure to carbon monoxide, nicotine, and cadmium (Daston, 1981). Longitudinal assessment of the relationship of maternal smoke exposure with lung growth in children also suggest that these effects may extend to the prenatal period (Tager I.B., personal communication).

One interesting hypothesis is that maternal smoking influences the expression of atopy and leads to an elevation of cord blood IgE level (Magnusson, 1986). Kjellman and co-workers have studied a large cohort of Swedish mothers and found that mothers who smoked during pregnancy had children with elevated levels of cord blood IgE (Hattevig et al., 1984) that was not secondary to maternal IgE transfer (Zeiger, 1985). Instead, IgE may be produced in response to placental transfer of antigens and in utero sensitization (Kauffmann, 1971) that may occur as early as 11 weeks of gestation (Miller et al., 1973). The importance of this finding is related to the ability of cord blood IgE to predict allergic diseases of childhood (asthma, hayfever, and eczema). In fact, cord blood IgE is a better predictor of early childhood atopy than is family history (Croner et al., 1982).

C. Breast Feeding

Breast feeding could potentially influence the lung function of neonates by altering the propensity for or the severity of respiratory infections, or by influencing atopy and airway responsiveness.

Breast Feeding and Respiratory Infections

Breast milk supplies the infant with maternal antibodies, particularly, secretory IgA, that may prevent or reduce the severity of infection (Chandra, 1979; Watkins et al., 1974). However, despite these observations there is little epidemiological evidence to support a significant protective effect of breast feeding.

In the Houston Family Study, the incidence and severity of viral respiratory infections were determined in 81 infants evaluated for 6 months (Frank et al., 1982). Although the results did not reach statistical significance, in this study as in others, (Taylor et al., 1982; Pullan et al., 1980) the breast-fed infants had lower exposure to passive smoking and came from families with higher socioeconomic class than did the bottle-fed infants. No differences in the number of viral infections in the first 3 months or 6 months of life were found in infants fed with cow's or breast milk. However, diminished morbidity, consisting of fewer cases of pneumonia and bronchitis, was observed in breast-fed infants. The lack of more significant findings may relate to the relatively small sample studied.

A larger British study also examined the relationship of breast feeding and respiratory illness (Taylor et al., 1982). The prevalence of respiratory disease in the first year and in the first 5 years of life was examined in 13,135 children in this retrospective cohort study. Data regarding both breast feeding and respiratory illness were collected when the child reached age 5 years. No relationship between respiratory illness in the first year of life and breast feeding was found after adjustments for maternal age, sex of the child, and socioeconomic class. More admissions due to respiratory illness were observed in association with lower socioeconomic class, parental smoking, and low birth weight. Whether the discrepancies between these studies relate to incomplete adjustments for variables associated with socioeconomic class in the former study, or for misclassification of respiratory illness and breast feeding patterns in the latter study, is not clear.

Breast Feeding and Atopy

Immune tolerance in the neonate may be particularly susceptible to modification, and the minimization of antigenic exposure that is potentially achieved with breast feeding may reduce atopy in high-risk infants.

Studies from Australia, (Van Asperen et al., 1984) Sweden, (Hattevig, et al., 1984; Kjellman et al., 1984; Juto and Bjorksten, 1980) and Great Britain (Taylor et al., 1983) of infants drawn from the general population or selected on the basis of family history for atopy have shown no protective effect of breast feeding on the development of atopic disease, including asthma, or elevated IgE levels in infancy when mothers followed unrestricted diets. One large British study showed a significant increase in the incidence of eczema in children who had been breast fed (Taylor et al., 1983). Other studies have shown specific IgE levels to food proteins to be present in atopic infants fed exclusively breast milk (Kaplan and Solli, 1979; Bjorksten and Saarinen, 1978); furthermore, occasionally breast-fed infants develop severe allergic reactions with their first cow's milk feeding. This suggests that small amounts of food antigens ingested by the mother can be transmitted in breast milk to infants and can cause sensitization. One Italian study of 101 newborns with a family history of atopy found a significant reduction in the occurrence of atopic disease in the first 2 years of life in breast-fed infants of mothers who avoided dietary exposure to eggs and milk (Businco et al., 1983).

V. Summary

Epidemiological studies clearly demonstrate an aggregation of pulmonary function and disease within families, which, not completely explained by common household exposures, suggests the operation of genetic factors. However, the probable heterogeneity in mechanisms capable of producing significant reductions in FEV_1 and FEV_1/FVC levels limits the ability of population studies to identify precisely specific modes of inheritance and the specific biochemical or physiological properties responsible for aggregation. Despite such limitations, a number of factors have been identified that may modify levels of lung function in adulthood and increase susceptibility to cigarette smoke. In particular, those genetic factors that determine lung size in childhood and early adulthood may influence whether a clinically significant degree of pulmonary impairment will be produced in response to any given reduction in lung function caused by exposure to cigarette smoke. The extent to which lung dimensions in childhood are influenced by prenatal and early postnatal exposures (e.g., nutritional factors and smoking exposures), in addition to genetic factors, is unknown. Furthermore, the degree to which such influences are mediated through alterations in immune responsiveness is not clear. A better understanding of the significance of such factors on fetal and postnatal lung development may allow the development of strategies to modify the risk associated with inheriting "small" lungs or lungs that grow less rapidly.

Some epidemiological evidence suggests individual variability in specific physiological reactions (manifest as protease imbalance and/or atopic diatheses) to oxidants and other irritants in cigarette smoke, aeroallergens, and infections, has a genetic basis. The degree to which such variability in biological responses to environmental exposures significantly predispose to COPD is less certain. A disturbance in elastin homeostasis occurring with cigarette smoke exposure only has been demonstrated unequivocally in a small minority of subjects with severe α_1AP deficiency. More refined assessments of subtler abnormalities in elastin homeostasis may demonstrate populations at risk for disease, but also may be considerably more difficult to determine in general populations. The possibility that there are additional genetic markers for emphysema linked to the α_1AP gene presents an exciting challenge to both the epidemiologist and molecular geneticist.

Airway hyperresponsiveness seems to have a familial basis in subjects with allergic backgrounds, and also has been observed in subjects with COPD. However, there are not sufficient data to determine if the airway hyperresponsiveness observed in COPD represents an inherited risk factor for this disease, or whether it occurs secondary to other derangements in lung function. Family studies of airway responsiveness, atopy, and autonomic function in the healthy family members of patients with COPD may help to elucidate this problem and shed further light on the interactions and relationships between these three factors and COPD.

To date, examination of blood markers and their associations with pulmonary infections and pulmonary disease have shown no or rather weak relationships. These factors, if occurring in the absence of other risk factors, probably do not significantly influence the distribution of disease in the population.

A more comprehensive understanding of potentially inherited factors that influence behavioral responses to cigarette smoke is certainly important and also may facilitate the design of smoking intervention programs suited for the needs of the particular subject or population.

There is some understanding of the distribution of gross phenotypes within and between families. In the future, however, the genetic epidemiologist may need to identify patterns of distribution of distinct physiological and/or biochemical properties of the lung and relate such specific traits to potential familial and environmental risk factors and exposures.

Acknowledgment

We gratefully thank Peter V. Tishler and Frank E. Speizer for their critical comments, and Christine Harrington for excellent secretarial assistance.

References

Abboud, R. T., Fera, T., Richter, A., Tabona, M. Z., and Johal, S. (1985). Acute effect of smoking on the functional activity of alpha$_1$-proteinase inhibitor in bronchoalveolar lavage fluid. *Am. Rev. Respir. Dis.* **131**:79–85.

Apold, J., and Aksnes, L. (1977). Correlation between increased bronchial responsiveness to histamine and diminished plasma cyclic AMP response after epinephrine in asthmatic children. *J. Allergy Clin. Immunol.* **59**:343–347.

Aquilina, A. T., Hall, W. J., Douglas, R. G., and Utell, M. J. (1980). Airway reactivity in subjects with viral upper respiratory tract infections: the effects of exercise and cold air. *Am. Rev. Respir. Dis.* **122**:3–10.

Astemborski, J. A., Beaty, T. H., and Cohen, B. H. (1985). Variance components analysis of forced expiration in families. *Am. J. Genet.* **21**:747–753.

Bahous, J., Cartier, A., Ouimet, G., Pineau, L., and Malo, J. L. (1984). Nonallergic bronchial hyperexcitability in chronic bronchitis. *Am. Rev. Respir. Dis.* **129**:216–220.

Bassi, J. A., Rosso, P., Moessinger, A. C., Blanc, W. A., and James, L. S. (1984). Fetal growth retardation due to maternal tobacco smoke exposure in the rat. *Pediatr. Res.* **18**:127–130.

Bazarel, M., Orgel, V. A., and Hamburger, R. N. (1974). Genetics of IgE and allergy: serum IgE levels in twins. *J. Allergy Clin. Immunol.* **54**:288–304.

Beaty, T. H., Menkes, H. A., Cohen, B. H., and Newill, C. A. (1984). Risk factors associated with longitudinal change in pulmonary function. *Am. Rev. Respir. Dis.* **129**:660–667.

Boat, T. F., and Kleinman, J. I. (1975). Human respiratory tract secretions: effect of cholinergic and adrenergic agents on in vitro release of protein and mucous glycoprotein. *Chest* **67**:325–335.

Bjorksten, F., and Saarinen, U. M. (1978). IgE antibodies to cow's milk in infants fed breast milk and formulae. *Lancet* **2**(8090):624–625.

Bridges, R. B., Wyatt, R. J., and Rehm, S. R. (1985). Effects of smoking on peripheral blood leukocytes. *Eur. J. Respir. Dis.* **66**(S) 139:24–33.

Britt, E. J., Cohen, B., Menkes, H., Bleeker, E., Permutt, S., Rosenthal, R., and Norman, P. (1980). Airways reactivity and functional deterioration in relatives of COPD patients. *Chest* **77**(S):260–261.

Bruce, C. A., Rosenthal, R. R., Lichtenstein, L. M., and Norman, P. S. (1975). Quantitative inhalational bronchial challenge in ragweed hayfever patients. A comparison with ragweed allergic asthmatics. *J. Allergy Clin. Immunol.* **56**:331–337.

Bruce, R. M., Cohen, B. H., Diamond, E. L., Fallat, R. J., Knudson, R. J., Lebowitz, M. D., Mittman, C., Patterson, C. D., and Tockman, M. S. (1984). Collaborative study to assess risk of lung disease in Pi MZ phenotype subjects. *Am. Rev. Respir. Dis.* **130**:386–390.

Bubnov, Y. I., Turkova, T. I., and Ereinyan, A. V. (1974). Influence of infectious diseases on hereditary polymorphism with respect to the blood groups of the ABO system. *Sov. Genet.* **9**:105–108.

Burrows, B., and Taussig, L. M. (1980). "As the twig is bent, the tree inclines (perhaps)." *Am. Rev. Respir. Dis.* **122**:813–816.

Burrows, B., Habnen, M., Barbee, R. A., and Lebowitz, M. D. (1981). The relationship of serum immunoglobulin E to cigarette smoking. *Am. Rev. Respir. Dis.* **124**:523–525.

Businco, L., Marchetti, F., Pellegrini, G., Cantani, A., and Perlini, R. (1983). Prevention of atopic disease in "at-risk newborns" by prolonged breast-feeding. *Ann. Allergy* **51**:296–299.

Cabezas, G. A., Graf, P. D., and Nadel, J. A. (1971). Sympathetic versus parasympathetic nervous regulation of airways in dogs. *J. Appl. Physiol.* **31**:651–655.

Carter, C., and Heslop, B. (1957). ABO blood groups and bronchopneumonia in children. *Br. J. Soc. Med.* **11**:214–216.

Cederlof, R., Edfors, M. L., Friberg, L., and Jonsson, E. (1967). Hereditary factors, "spontaneous cough" and "smoker's cough." *Arch. Environ. Health* **14**:401–406.

Chandra, R. K. (1979). Prospective studies of the effect of breast feeding on incidence of infection and allergy. *Acta Paediatr. Scand.* **68**:691–694.

Cohen, B. H. (1980). Chronic obstructive pulmonary disease: a challenge in genetic epidemiology. *Am. J. Epidemiol.* **112**:274–288.

Colley, J. R. T., Douglas, J. W. B., Reid, D. D. (1973). Respiratory disease in young adults: influence of early childhood lower respiratory tract illness, social class, air pollution, and smoking. *Br. Med. J.* **3**:195–198.

Collins, M. H., Moessinger, A. C., Kleinerman, J., Bassi, J., Rosso, P., Collins, A. M., James, L. S., and Blanc, W. (1985). Fetal lung hypoplasia associated with maternal smoking: a morphometric analysis. *Pediatr. Res.* **19**:408–412.

Criep, L. H. (1942). Allergy in identical twins. *J. Allergy* **13**:591–598.

Croner, S., Kjellman, N.-I.M., Ericksson, B., and Roth, A. (1982). IgE screening in 1701 newborn infants and the development of atopic disease during infancy. *Arch. Dis. Child.* **57**:364–368.

Crumpacker, D. W., Cederlof, R., Friberg, L., Kimberling, W. J., Sorenson, S., Vandenberg, S. G., Williams, J. S., McClearn, G. E., Grever, B., Iyer, H., Krier, M. J., Pedersen, N. L., Price, R. A., and Roulette, I. (1979). A twin methodology for the study of genetic and environmental control of variation in human smoking behavior. *Acta Genet. Med. Gemellol.* **28**:173–195.

Daston, G. P. (1981). Effects of cadmium on the prenatal ultrastructural maturation of rat alveolar epithelium. *Teratology* **23**:75–84.

Davies, S. F., Offord, K. P., Brown, M. G., Campe, H., and Niewoehner, D. (1983). Urine desmosine is unrelated to cigarette smoking or to spirometric function. *Am. Rev. Respir. Dis.* **128**:473–475.

Davis, P. B., Shelhamer, J., and Kaliner, M. (1980). Abnormal adrenergic and cholinergic sensitivity in cystic fibrosis. *N. Engl. J. Med.* **302**:1453–1456.

Davis, P. B., Dieckman, L., Boat, T. F., Stern, R. C., and Doershuk, C. F. (1983). Beta-adrenergic receptors on lymphocytes and granulocytes from patients with cystic fibrosis. *J. Clin. Invest.* **71**:1787–1795.

Davis, P. B. (1984). Autonomic and airway reactivity in obligate heterozygotes for cystic fibrosis. *Am. Rev. Respir. Dis.* **129**:911–914.

Davis, P. B. (1986). Pupillary responses and airway reactivity in asthma. *J. Allergy Clin. Immunol.* **77**:667–672.

Devor, E. J., and Crawford, M. H. (1984). Family resemblance for normal pulmonary function. *Ann. Hum. Biol.* **11**:439–448.

Dockery, D. W., Berkey, C. S., Ware, J. H., Speizer, F. E., and Ferris, B. G. (1983). Distribution of forced vital capacity and forced expiratory volume in one second in children 6 to 11 years of age. *Am. Rev. Respir. Dis.* **128**:405–412.

Dockery, D. W., Ware, J. H., Ferris, B. G., Glicksberg, D. S., Fay, M. E., Spiro, A., and Speizer, F. E. (1985). Distribution of forced expiratory volume in one second and forced vital capacity in healthy, white, adult never-smokers in six U.S. cities. *Am. Rev. Respir. Dis.* **131**:511–520.

Eriksson, S. (1964). Pulmonary emphysema and alpha-1-antitrypsin deficiency. *Acta Med. Scand.* **175**:197–205.

Fabsitz, R., Feinleib, M., and Hubert, H. (1985). Regression analysis of data with correlatd errors: an example from the NHLBI twin study. *J. Chron. Dis.* **38**:165–170.

Fagerhol, M. K., and Cox, D. W. (1981). The Pi polymorphism. Genetic, biochemical and clinical aspects of human alpha$_1$-antitrypsin. *Adv. Hum. Genet.* **11**:1–62.

Falliers, C. J., de A Cardoso, R. R., Bane, H. N., Coffey, R., and Middleton, E. (1971). Discordant allergic manifestations in monozygotic twins: genetic identity versus clinical, physiologic, and biochemical differences. *J. Allergy* **47**:207–219.

Fanta, C. H., and Ingram, R. H., Jr. (1981). Airway responsiveness and chronic airway obstruction. *Med. Clin. North Am.* **65**:473–487.

Fletcher, C., Peto, R., Tinker, C., and Speizer, F. E. (1976). *The Natural History of Chronic Bronchitis: An Eight Year Follow-Up Study of Working Men in London.* Oxford, Oxford University Press.

Frank, A. L., Taber, L. H., Glezen, W. P., Kasel, G. L., Wells, C. R., and Paredes, A. (1982). Breast-feeding and respiratory virus infection. *Pediatrics* **70**:239–245.

Friberg, L., Cederlof, R., Lundman, T., and Olsson, H. (1970). Mortality in smoking discordant monozygotic and dizygotic twins. *Arch. Environ. Health* **21**:508–513.

Frick, O. L., German, D. F., and Mills, J. (1979). Development of allergy in children. I. Association with virus infections. *J. Allergy Clin. Immunol.* **63**:228–241.

Geller, D. E., Morgan, K. J., Cota, K. A., and Taussig, L. M. (1985). Response of maximal expiratory flow (VmaxFRC) to breathing cold dry air (CDA) in normal infants. *Am. Rev. Respir. Dis.* **131**:A256.

Hannah, M. C., Hopper, J. L., and Mathews, J. D. (1985). Twin concordance for a binary trait. Nested analysis of ever-smoking and ex-smoking traits and unnested analyses of a "committed smoking" trait. *Am. Hum. Genet.* **37**:153–165.

Hattevig, G., Kjellman, B., Johansson, S. G. O., and Bjorksten, B. (1984). Clinical symptoms and IgE responses to common food proteins in atopic and healthy children. *Clin. Allergy* **14**:551–559.

Henderson, W. R., Shelhamer, J. H., Reingold, D. B., Smith, L. J., Evans, R., Kaliner, M. (1979). Alpha-adrenergic hyperresponsiveness in asthma. Analysis of vascular and pupillary responses. *N. Engl. J. Med.* **300**:642–647.

Higgins, M., and Keller, J. (1975). Familial occurrence of chronic respiratory disease and familial resemblance in ventilatory capacity. *J. Chron. Dis.* **28**:239–251.

Hinman, L. J., Stevens, C. A., Matthay, R. A., and Gee, B. L. (1980). Elastase and lysozyme activities in human alveolar macrophages. *Am. Rev. Respir. Dis.* **121**:263–271.

Hopp, R. J., Bewtra, A. K., Watt, G. D., Nair, N. M., and Townley, R. G. (1984). Genetic analysis of allergic disease in twins. *J. Allergy Clin. Immunol.* **73**:265–270.

Janoff, A. (1985). Elastases and emphysema. *Am. Rev. Respir. Dis.* **132**:417–433.

Johnson, D., and Travis, J. (1979). The oxidative inactivation of human alpha 1-proteinase inhibitor: further evidence for methionine at the reactive center. *J. Biol. Chem.* **254**:4022–4026.

Juto, P., and Bjorksten, B. (1980). Serum IgE and influence of type of feeding. *Clin. Allergy* **10**:593–600.

Kaliner, M. (1976). The cholinergic nervous system and immediate hypersensitivity. Eccrine sweat responses in allergic patients. *J. Allergy Clin. Immunol.* **58**:308–315.

Kalsheker, N., Hodgson, I., White, J., Morrison, H., Burnett, D., and Stockley, R. (1987). Alpha₁-antitrypsin polymorphism: a new marker for genetic predisposition to bronchiectases and pulmonary emphysema. *Am. Rev. Respir. Dis.* **133**:A219.

Kanner, R. E. (1984). The relationship between airways responsiveness and chronic airflow limitation. *Chest* **86**:54–57.

Kaplan, M. S., and Solli, N. J. (1979). Immunologlobulin E to cow's milk protein in breast-fed atopic children. *J. Allergy Clin. Immunol.* **64**:122–126.

Kaufman, H. S. (1971). Allergy in the newborn: skin test reactions confirmed by the Prausnitz-Kustner test at birth. *Clin. Allergy* **1**:363–367.

Kauffmann, F. (1984). Genetics of chronic obstructive pulmonary diseases. Searching for their heterogeneity. *Bull. Eur. Physiopathol. Respir.* **20**:163–210.

Kauffmann, F., Kleisbauer, J. P., Cambon-de-Mouzon, A., Mercier, P., Constans, J., Blanc, M., Rouch, Y., and Feingold, N. (1983). Genetic markers in chronic airflow limitation. *Am. Rev. Respir. Dis.* **127**:263–269.

Kawakami, Y., Kosaka, H., Nishimura, M., and Abe, S. (1986). Trachea and lung dimensions in nonsmoking twins: morphologic and functional studies. *J. Appl. Physiol.* **61**:495–499.

Khoury, M. J., Marks, J. S., McCarthy, B. A., and Zaro, S. M. (1985). Factors effecting the sex differential in neonatal mortality: The role of respiratory distress syndrome. *Ann. Obstet. Gynecol.* **151**:777–782.

Khoury, M. J., Beaty, T. H., Newill, C. A., Bryant, S., and Cohen, B. H. (1986). Genetic-environmental interactions in chronic airways obstruction. *Int. J. Epidemiol.* **15**:65–73.

Kiernan, K. E., Colley, J. R. T., Douglas, J. W. B., and Reid, D. D. (1976). Chronic cough in adults in relation to smoking habits, childhood environment, and chest illness. *Respiration* **33**:236–244.

Kinane, D. F., Blackwell, C. C., Brettle, R. P., Weir, D. M., Winstanley, F. P., and Elton, R. A. (1982). ABO blood group, secretor status, and susceptibility to recurrent urinary tract infection in women. *Br. Med. J.* **285**:7–9.

Kjellman, N.-I.M., Croner, S. (1984). Cord blood IgE determination for allergy prediction—a follow-up to seven years of age in 1651 children. *Ann. Allergy* **53**:167–171.

Konig, P., and Godfrey, S. (1973a). Prevalence of exercise-induced bronchial lability in families of children with asthma. *Arch. Dis. Child.* **48**:513–518.

Konig, P., and Godfrey, S. (1973b). Exercise-induced bronchial lability and atopic status in families of infants with wheezy bronchitis. *Arch. Dis. Child.* **48**:942–946.

Konig, P., and Godfrey, S. (1974). Exercise-induced bronchial lability in monozygotic (identical) and dizygotic (nonidentical) twins. *J. Allergy Clin. Immunol.* **54**:280–287.

Kueppers, F., Fallat, R., and Larson, R. K. (1969). Obstructive lung disease and alpha$_1$-antitrypsin deficiency gene heterozygosity. *Science* **165**:899–901.

Kueppers, F., Miller, R. D., Gordon, H., Hepper, N. G., and Offord, K. (1977). Familial prevalence of chronic obstructive pulmonary disease in a matched pair study. *Am. J. Med.* **63**:336–342.

Landau, L. I., Morgan, S. E. G., Turner, D. J., and LeSouef, P. N. (1987). Bronchial hyper-reactivity but lack of bronchodilator response in infants with chronic airway pathology. *Am. Rev. Respir. Dis.* **135**:A381.

Lang, P., Goel, Z., and Grieco, M. H. (1978). Sensitivity of T-lymphocytes to sympathomimetic and cholinergic stimulation in bronchial asthma. *J. Allergy Clin. Immunol.* **61**:248–254.

Larson, R. K., Barman, M. L., Kueppers, F., and Fudenberg, H. H. (1970). Genetic and environmental determinants of chronic obstructive pulmonary disease. *Ann. Intern. Med.* **72**:627–632.

Laurent, P., Janoff, A., and Kagan, H. M. (1983). Cigarette smoke blocks cross-linking of elastin in vitro. *Am. Rev. Respir. Dis.* **127**:189–192.

Leeder, S. R. (1975). Role of infection in the cause and course of chronic bronchitis and emphysema. *J. Infect. Dis.* **131**:731–742.

Leeder, S. R., Corkhill, R. T., Irwig, L. M., Holland, W. W., and Colley, J. R. T. (1976a). Influence of family factors on asthma and wheezing during the first five years of life. *Br. J. Prev. Soc. Med.* **30**:213–218.

Leeder, S. R., Corkhill, R., Irwig, L. M., Holland, W. W., and Colley, J. R. T. (1976b). Influence of family factors on the incidence of lower respiratory illness during the first year of life. *Br. J. Prev. Soc. Med.* **30**:203–212.

Lellouch, J., Claude, J.-R., Martin, J.-P., Orssaud, G., Zaoui, D., and Bieth, J. G. (1985). Smoking does not reduce the functional activity of serum alpha-1-proteinase inhibitor. *Am. Rev. Respir. Dis.* **132**:818–820.

Lewitter, F. I., Tager, I. B., McGue, M., Tishler, P. V., and Speizer, F. E. (1984). Genetic and environmental determinants of level of pulmonary function. *Am. J. Epidemiol.* **120**:518–529.

Lieberman, J. (1971). Heterozygous and homozygous alpha₁-antitrypsin in patients with pulmonary emphysema. *N. Engl. J. Med.* **281**:279–284.

Lubs, M. L. E. (1971). Allergy in 7000 twin pairs. *Acta Allergol.* **26**:249–285.

Magnusson, C. G. M. (1986). Maternal smoking influences cord serum IgE and IgD levels and increases the risk for subsequent infant allergy. *J. Allergy Clin. Immunol.* **78**:898–904.

Marsh, D. G., Hou, S. H., Hunan, R., Meyers, D. A., Freidhoff, L. R., and Bias, W. B. (1980). Genetics of human immune response to antigens. *J. Allergy Clin. Immunol.* **65**:322–332.

Marsh, D. G., Meyers, D. A., and Bias, W. B. (1981). The epidemiology and genetics of atopic allergy. *N. Engl. J. Med.* **305**:1551–1559.

Martinez, F., Antognoni, G., Macri, F., Lebowitz, M., and Ronchetti, R. (1985). Distribution of bronchial responsiveness to a constrictive drug in a random pediatric population sample. *Am. Rev. Respir. Dis.* **131** (4,part 2):A242.

McKennell, A. C. (1970). Smoking motivation factors. *Br. J. Soc. Clin. Psychol.* **9**:8–22.

Miller, D. L., Hirvanen, T., and Gitten, D. (1973). Synthesis of IgE by the human conceptus. *J. Allergy Clin. Immunol.* **52**:182–188.

Mittman, C., Lieberman, J., and Rumsfeld, J. (1974). Prevalence of abnormal protease inhibitor phenotypes in patients with chronic obstructive lung disease. *Am. Rev. Respir. Dis.* **109**:295–296.

Morris, M. Y., Vaughnan, H., Lane, D. J., and Harris, P. J. (1977). HLA in asthma. *Monogr. Allergy* **11**:30–34.

Morse, J. O., Lebowitz, M. D., Knudson, R. J., and Burrows, B. (1977). Relation of protease inhibitor phenotypes to obstructive lung disease in a community. *N. Engl. J. Med.* **296**:1190–1194.

Morse, J. O. (1978). Alpha₁-antitrypsin deficiency. *N. Engl. J. Med.* **299**: 1045.

Naeye, R. L., Burt, L. S., Wright, D. L., Blanc, W. A., and Tatter, D. (1971). Neonatal mortality, the male disadvantage. *Pediatrics* **48**:902–906.

O'Connor, G. T., Weiss, S. T., Tager, I. B., and Speizer, F. E. (1987). The effect of passive smoking on pulmonary function and nonspecific bronchial responsiveness in a population-based sample of children and young adults. *Am. Rev. Respir. Dis.* **135**:800–804.

Proust, A., Dewitte, J. D., Ferece, C., Clavier, J., and Saleun, J. P. (1987). A genetic marker for a severe form of asthma. *Med. Sci. Res.* **15**:131.

Pullan, C. R., Toms, G. L., Martin, A. J., Webb, J. K. G., and Appleton, D. R. (1980). Breast feeding and respiratory syncytial virus infection. *Br. Med. J.* **2**:1034–1036.

Raaschau-Nielson, E. (1960). Smoking habits in twins. *Dan. Med. Bull.* **7**:82.

Ramsdell, J. W., Nachtwey, F. J., and Moser, K. M. (1982). Bronchial hyperreactivity in chronic obstructive bronchitis. *Am. Rev. Respir. Dis.* **126**:829–832.

Redline, S., Tishler, P. V., Lewitter, F. I., Tager, I. B., Munoz, A., and Speizer, F. E. (1987). Assessment of genetic and nongenetic influences on pulmonary function. A twin study. *Am. Rev. Respir. Dis.* **135**:217–222.

Redline, S., Tishler, P. V., Lewitter, F. I., Weiss, S. T., Vandenberg, M., and Speizer, F. E. (1989). Genotypic and phenotypic similarities in pulmonary function. *Am. J. Epidemiol.* (in press).

Reynolds, H. Y., and Newboll, H. H. (1974). Analysis of proteins and respiratory cells obtained from human lung by bronchial lavage. *J. Lab. Clin. Med.* **84**:559–573.

Ronchetti, R., Lucarini, N., Lucarelli, P., Martinez, F., Macri, F., Carapella, E., and Bottini, E. (1984). A genetic basis for heterogeneity of asthma syndrome in pediatric ages: adenosine deaminase phenotypes. *J. Allergy Clin. Immunol.* **74**:81–84.

Samet, J. M., Tager, I. B., and Speizer, F. E. (1983). The relationship between respiratory illness in childhood and chronic airflow obstruction in adulthood. *Am. Rev. Respir. Dis.* **127**:508–523.

Schenker, M. B., Samet, J. M., and Speizer, F. E. (1983). Risk factors for childhood respiratory disease. The effect of host factors and home environmental exposures. *Am. Rev. Respir. Dis.* **128**:1038–1043.

Shigeoka, J. W., Hall, W. J., Hyde, R. W., Schwartz, R. H., Mudholkar, G. S., Spears, D. M., and Lin, C.-C. (1976). The prevalence of alpha$_1$-antitrypsin heterozygotes (PiMZ) in patients with obstructive pulmonary disease. *Am. Rev. Respir. Dis.* **114**:1077–1085.

Sibbald, B., Horn, M. E., and Gregg, I. (1980). A family study of the genetic basis of asthma and wheezy bronchitis. *Arch. Dis. Child.* **55**:354–357.

Speizer, F. E., Rosner, B., and Tager, I. (1976). Familial aggregation of chronic respiratory disease: use of a national health interview survey data for specific hypothesis testing. *Int. J. Epidemiol.* **5**:167–172.

Struthers, D. (1951). ABO groups of infants and children dying in the west of Scotland (1949–1951). *Br. J. Soc. Med.* **5**:223–228.

Tager, I. B., Rosner, B., Tishler, P. V., Speizer, F. E., and Kass, E. H. (1976). Household aggregation of pulmonary function and chronic bronchitis. *Am. Rev. Respir. Dis.* **114**:485–492.

Tager, I., Tishler, P. V., Rosner, B., Speizer, F. E., and Litt, M. (1978). Studies of the familial aggregation of chronic bronchitis and obstructive airways disease. *Int. J. Epidemiol.* **7**:55–62.

Tager, I. B., Weiss, S. T., Munoz, A., Rosner, B., and Speizer, F. E. (1983). Longitudinal study of the effects of maternal smoking on pulmonary function in children. *N. Engl. J. Med.* **309**:699–703.

Taylor, B., Golding, J., Wadsworth, J., and Butler, N. (1982). Breast-feeding, bronchitis, and admissions for lower respiratory illness and gastroenteritis during the first five years. *Lancet* 1:1227–1229.

Taylor, B., Wadsworth, J., Golding, J., and Butler, N. (1983). Breast-feeding, eczema, asthma, and hayfever. *J. Epidemiol. Commun. Health* 37:95–99.

Taylor, R. G., Joyce, H., Gross, E., Holland, F., and Pride, N. B. (1985). Bronchial reactivity to inhaled histamine and annual rate of decline in FEV_1 in male smokers and ex-smokers. *Thorax* 40:9–16.

Tepper, R. S., Morgan, W. Y., Coke, K., Wright, A., Taussig, L. M., and GHMA Pediatricians (1986). Physiologic growth and development of the lung during the first year of life. *Am. Rev. Respir. Dis.* 134:513–519.

Tepper, R. S. (1987). Airway reactivity in infants: a positive response to methacholine and metaproteranol. *J. Appl. Physiol.* 62:1155–1159.

Thornsby, E., Engeset, A., and Lie, S. O. (1971). HLA polymorphism of Norwegian Lapps. *Tissue Antigens* 1:147–152.

Townley, R. G., Bewtra, A., Wilson, A. F., Hopp, R. J., Elston, R. C., Nair, N., and Watt, G. D. (1986). Segregation analysis of bronchial response to methacholine inhalation challenge in families with and without asthma. *J. Allergy Clin. Immunol.* 77:101–107.

Van Asperen, P. P., Kemp, A. S., and Mellis, C. M. (1984). Relationship of diet in the development of atopy in infancy. *Clin. Allergy* 14:525–532.

Vandenberg, S. G. (1967). Hereditary factors in normal personality traits (as measured by inventories). In *Recent Advances in Biological Psychiatry*. Edited by J. Wort. New York, Plenum, pp. 5–104.

Venables, K. M., Topping, M. D., Howe, W., Luczynska, C. M., Hawkins, R., and Newman-Taylor, A. J. (1985). Interactions of smoking and atopy in producing specific IgE antibody against a hapten protein conjugate. *Br. Med. J.* 290:201–206.

Viskum, K. (1973). Respiratory disease and ABO and rhesus blood groups. *Scand. J. Respir. Dis.* 54:97–102.

Ware, J. H., Dockery, D. W., Spiro, A., Speizer, F. E., and Ferris, B. G. (1984). Passive smoking, gas cooking and respiratory health of children living in six cities. *Am. Rev. Respir. Dis.* 129:366–374.

Watkins, C. J., Leeder, S. R., and Cockhill, R. T. (1979). The relationship between breast and bottle feeding and respiratory illness in the first year of life. *J. Epidemiol. Commun. Health* 33:180–182.

Weiss, S. T., Tager, I. B., Munoz, A., and Speizer, F. E. (1985). The relationship of respiratory infections in early childhood to the occurrence of increased levels of bronchial responsiveness and atopy. *Am. Rev. Respir. Dis.* 131:573–578.

Welty, C., Weiss, S. T., Tager, I. B., Munoz, A., Becker, C., Speizer, F. E., and Ingram, R. H. (1984). The relationship of airways responsiveness to cold air, cigarette smoking, and atopy to respiratory symptoms and pulmonary function in adults. *Am. Rev. Respir. Dis.* **130**:198–203.

Yan, K., Salome, C. M., and Woolcock, A. J. (1985). Prevalence and nature of bronchial hyperresponsiveness in subjects with chronic obstructive pulmonary disease. *Am. Rev. Respir. Dis.* **132**:25–29.

Zamel, N., Leroux, M., and Vanderdoelen, J. L. (1984). Airway response to inhaled methacholine in healthy nonsmoking twins. *J. Appl. Physiol.* **56**:936–993.

Zeiger, R. S. (1985). Atopy in infancy and early childhood: natural history and role of skin testing. *J. Allergy Clin. Immunol.* **75**:633–639.

9

The Relationship of Airway Reactivity to the Occurrence of Chronic Obstructive Pulmonary Disease: An Epidemiological Assessment

SUSAN REDLINE

Roger Williams General Hospital
Brown University Medical School
Providence, Rhode Island

IRA B. TAGER

University of California, San Francisco
VA Medical Center
San Francisco, California

I. Basic Concepts

Epidemiological studies of respiratory disease have sought to identify host characteristics and environmental exposures that increase the risk of the development of chronic obstructive pulmonary disease (COPD). Exposure to tobacco smoke, the risk factor most clearly associated with the development of COPD, causes severe pulmonary dysfunction in only a minority of apparently susceptible smokers (Fletcher et al., 1976; U.S. Dept. HEW, 1979). The susceptible smoker has been hypothesized to suffer airway inflammation manifest as mucus hypersecretion and recurrent pulmonary infections (Fletcher et al., 1976; Petty et al., 1976; Annesi and Kauffman, 1986). An alternative theory of susceptibility has emphasized the risk related to an allergic predisposition manifest as airway hyperresponsiveness (AH) (Orie et al., 1961; van der Lende, 1970). However, airway hyperresponsiveness may be caused by airway inflammation, and it may be difficult to determine whether AH is an inherent host characteristic that precedes the development of disease or is acquired concurrently with or subsequent to the development of disease. Understanding the role of AH, considered either as an inherent host characteristic or as a secondary manifestation of other exposures, has been the objective of many studies of chronic respiratory disease pathogenesis and susceptibility. This chapter examines the relationship of AH and COPD as defined in epidemiological studies.

A. Interest in Assessment of Airway Responsiveness: A Clinical Tool

Approximately 40 years ago, investigators observed that the systemic or inhalational administration of cholinergic agents resulted in airway constriction among predominantly asthmatic subjects (Starr et al., 1933; Curry, 1947; Dubois and Dautrebrebande, 1958). In addition to suggesting disease mechanisms, the results of these studies led to the development of bronchoprovocation tests for the clinical identification of asthmatic persons with atypical symptoms. It was observed that the degree of bronchoconstriction induced by chemical mediators correlated with severity of wheeze symptoms and requirements for bronchodilator medication (Ryan et al., 1982; Juniper et al., 1981), and varied among asthmatic persons with different allergic backgrounds and clinical presentations (Bhagat and Grunstein, 1984). Thus, bronchoprovocation testing with nonspecific agents also was proposed as a means to diagnose asthma, assess the severity of asthma, and to gauge response to therapy in a manner analogous to the use of the measurement of blood pressure in the detection and management of hypertension (Murray et al., 1981; Juniper et al., 1981). For these purposes, it was assumed that an "abnormal" response to bronchoprovocation testing could be defined, that such a response correctly identified the majority of asthmatic persons (i.e., high test sensitivity), and that it was not found in "normal" subjects (i.e., high test specificity).

The distributional characteristics of airway responsiveness in general population samples, however, suggest that AH is not uniquely and necessarily found in subjects diagnosed with asthma (Hopp et al., 1984; Weiss et al., 1984). A schematic of the population distribution of airway responsiveness is shown in Figure 1. It demonstrates that there is a 40-fold range in airway responsiveness in the population, which is skewed with a long tail that consists of small numbers of highly responsive subjects (Fanta and Ingram, 1981; Simonsson, 1984). Population and laboratory studies suggest that this distribution actually is composed of several distinct distributions of responsiveness for groups of symptomatic and asymptomatic asthmatic persons, atopic nonasthmatic persons, chronic bronchitic subjects, and nonatopic nonsmokers—groups that may differ quantitatively, but perhaps not qualitatively, from each other (Stevens and Vermeire, 1980; Bahous et al., 1984; Yan et al., 1985). An overlap of responsiveness among clinically distinct groups has been found to exist in

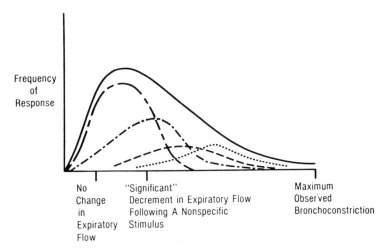

Figure 1 Schematized frequency distribution of airway responsiveness for the general population (solid line); nonatopic nonasthmatics (———); bronchitics (---), asymptomatic asthmatics (····); and symptomatic asthmatics (dotted line). The area represented between the origin and the point "no change in FEV_1" consists of individuals in whom FEV_1 appears to increase following the challenge test. The area to the right of the "no change" point represents increasing decrements in measured flow rate following the airway challenge. The exact magnitude of relative change in flow rate at these various points varies according to the inhalational challenge and choice of flow measurement. For FEV_1, the origin identifies an increase in flow of between 5 and 12%; the point considered to indicate a "significant decrement" varies from 9 to 20%; and the maximum observed bronchoconstriction varies from approximately 25 to 70%.

varying degrees regardless of the method (histamine, carbachol, or methacholine administration; exercise testing; or hyperventilation with subfreezing air) used to induce bronchoconstriction (Chatham et al., 1982; Muranaka et al., 1974; Garcia-Herreios et al., 1980).

Measurement of nonspecific airway responsiveness, rather than identifying the presence or absence of a unique pathophysiological state, may gauge the intensity of interactions among a number of pathways that influence airway function. Airway responsiveness may be augmented as a result of varying degrees of alteration in the function of the autonomic nervous system, including b-adrenergic hyporesponsiveness and a-adrenergic hyperresponsiveness (Szentivanyi, 1986; Simonsson et al., 1967; Henderson et al., 1979); smooth muscle, leading to a propensity for sensitization and greater contractile responses (Stephens, 1987); the epithelium, allowing greater mucosal penetrance of particles and greater exposure of irritant receptors (Simonsson, 1984; Hogg, 1983); and immunological responsiveness, allowing for specific sensitization to environmental agents (Bryant et al., 1976; Cockcroft et al., 1979). Whether AH is expressed at a given time may depend on the attainment of a critical level of susceptibility as determined by the interactions among multiple factors. Such interactions may vary over time in given individuals. For example, occasionally "normal" degrees of responsiveness are found among subjects with a history of asthma (Weiss et al., 1984). It has been hypothesized that, in these circumstances, AH may not be a cause, but a *consequence* of specific allergic reactions that alter the local availability of chemical mediators in the airway and transiently increase responsiveness in susceptible (atopic) individuals (Simonnson, 1984; Boulet et al., 1983; Hargreave et al., 1986). This might explain why AH only can be measured in the pollen season (Stanescu and Frans, 1982), or at harvest time (Hensley et al., 1988) in certain asthmatics. Conversely, AH may be present in nonasthmatic persons after viral respiratory infections (Aquilina et al., 1980; Empey et al., 1976) or after exposure to ozone (Holtzman et al., 1979), influences that transiently injure the respiratory epithelium in normal, nonatopic subjects. If airway responsiveness is an expression of multifactorial influences that vary over time, it may not be possible to identify precisely a degree of AH that consistently differentiates asthmatic from nonasthmatic persons. This may put limitations on the clinical and epidemiological usefulness of tests of nonspecific airway responsiveness, especially in regard to the evaluation of less symptomatic asthmatics who may have variable degrees of AH over time and subjects with nonasthmatic obstructive lung disease who also may wheeze.

B. Tests of Airway Responsiveness: Epidemiological Applications

The continuum of responsiveness observed in population-based studies (perhaps composed of several overlapping distributions for groups with different risk factors) could be explored by epidemiologists to understand better the natural history of lung disease. For these purposes, the identification of a discrete value of responsiveness that directly correlates with a known disease state may be less important than the description of the distributional characteristics of airway responsiveness among groups of individuals who differ in regard to symptom constellations, environmental exposures, and longitudinal behavior of pulmonary function change. For maximum utility, assessment of airway responsiveness ideally would provide unique information about airway function that could not be derived by questionnaire alone and would express some property of airway function that is related directly or indirectly to pulmonary disease. Whether the assessment of airway responsiveness provides information about pathogenetic mechanisms and risk will be evaluated in the subsequent review of epidemiologic data. A review of animal data and in vitro work is beyond the scope of this chapter.

C. Uniqueness: Relationship of AH and Wheeze/Asthma Symptoms

Variable degrees of correlation have been demonstrated between level of AH and asthma and wheeze symptoms. Most subjects with histories compatible with persistent wheeze symptoms and asthma that require medication demonstrate AH (Townley et al., 1975); fewer subjects with wheezing that occurs with and occasionally apart from colds, or with a more remote history of asthma, have AH (Weiss et al., 1984; Sears et al., 1986). With the use of eucapnic hyperventilation with subfreezing air in a population-based study, Weiss and associates (1984), found that only 43% of 28 subjects with a history of asthma demonstrated significant airway constriction and that 51% of all responders to the cold air challenge had no history of asthma or wheeze symptoms. Lee and colleagues (1983) and Sears and co-workers (1986) demonstrated similar findings with the use of methacholine challenge testing. In an attempt to quantify the relationship between symptoms and level of airway responsiveness, Cookson and associates (1986) estimated that the level of responsiveness explained 31% of the variability in the distribution of asthma and 32% of the variability in the distribution of wheeze symptoms in a sample of 105 subjects aged 15–30 years. Mark and associates (1986), in a study of a younger population (8–12 years), found that the relative risk of having wheeze symptoms or of having a doctor's diagnosis of asthma given a positive response to cold air challenge testing was 8.7. In contrast, a study by Redline et al. (1989) found the odds of any wheeze or persistent wheeze, given a positive cold air response, were somewhat lower (2.3 and 2.5, respectively) in a larger population that included children and young adults as old as 24 years. Furthermore, these later investigators demonstrated that although the presence of asthma/wheeze and AH overlapped in a considerable number of subjects, wheeze symptoms and the physiological measurement of airway responsiveness were not each predicted by the same risk factors. Thus, these population studies suggest that asthma/wheeze symptoms and AH may be described as a Venn diagram (Fig. 2), and there may be unique epidemiological information contained in the identification of AH in asymptomatic subjects.

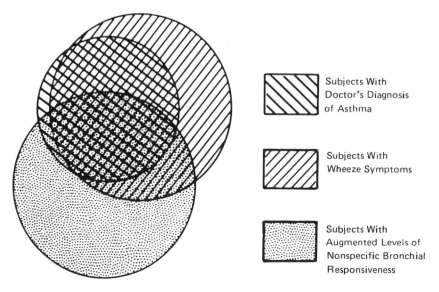

Figure 2   Relationship between asthma, wheeze, and bronchial responsiveness in the population. Although there is a considerable overlap between asthma/wheeze and airway hyperresponsiveness, approximately 1/2 of subjects with airway hyperresponsiveness may be asymptomatic, and between 1/6 and 1/3 of those with asthma/wheeze may not be observed to have airway hyperresponsiveness.

An interesting example of the epidemiological assessment of airway responsiveness for the identification of unique subsets of individuals is found in a British study that related bronchial responsiveness to respiratory symptoms (Mortagy et al., 1986). These investigations identified a cluster of symptoms—bronchial irritability (shortness of breath or wheezing to inhaled irritants), nocturnal dyspnea, and prolonged morning chest tightness—that uniquely identified subjects with the greatest levels of responsiveness (PC$_{20}$ histamine -0.5g/L). Approximately 70% of subjects with the syndrome of "bronchial irritability" had not been diagnosed as asthmatic. The description of bronchial hyperresponsiveness occurring in predominantly nonasthmatic subjects with recognizable symptoms may help clinically to identify patients who require specific therapy, and, in epidemiological research, may provide insights into disease mechanisms.

The ability of tests of nonspecific airway responsiveness to identify *nonasthmatic* subjects at risk for the development of chronic airflow obstruction also has been investigated. Among 184 children and young adults evaluated for up to 12 years as part of a longitudinal epidemiological study of risk factors for COPD, Redline and colleagues (1989) identified 35 nonasthmatic subjects with augmented airway responsiveness measured on at least one survey who had significantly lower levels of FEF_{25-75} and higher levels of FVC when measured longitudinally than subjects with less responsiveness. The clinical and epidemiological implications of these findings are as yet uncertain, but they do support the notion that physiological measurements of airway responsiveness provide complimentary information to that provided by data derived from standard respiratory symptom questionnaires.

II. Interpretation of Data: Relationships Among Challenge Characteristic, Definition of Response, and Outcome

A. Choice of Agonist

A variety of bronchoprovocation tests have been utilized in clinical, laboratory, and population-based epidemiological studies that may have different degrees of sensitivity, specificity, and reproducibility. The choice of agonists that have been used in various studies historically has been determined by feasibility issues (cost, time involved, acceptability to subjects, and safety), systemic side effects (e.g., histamine-induced flushing, headaches, and laryngospasm), and the experience of the investigator. In an attempt to standardize bronchial challenge testing, the European Society for Clinical Respiratory Physiology in 1983 published a review of the potential sources of variability in the collection of airway responsiveness data related to laboratory differences in methods of challenge and measurement of response (Eiser et al., 1983). Consideration of such differences may be particularly important when relating the findings of laboratory-based to population-based studies and in the comparisons of different epidemiological surveys.

Bronchoconstriction can be induced nonspecifically with synthetic choline esters (carbachol, methacholine chloride), or with histamine chloride, agonists that excite postganglionic parasympathetic nerve endings and/or directly alter smooth muscle membrane calcium permeability (Koelle, 1975; Douglas, 1975). Bronchoprovocation testing also can utilize physical stimuli, such as exercise hyperventilation with dry cooled air (Deal et al., 1980), or inhalation of nonisotonic aerosols (Anderson et al., 1983). Osmotic changes in the airways may increase alpha-adrenoreceptor activity and cause smooth muscle contraction (Walden et al., 1984) or may lead to bronchoconstriction via other mechanisms such as mediator release.

The extent to which the pharmacodynamic properties of different agonists differentially affect airways of different size or in different subsets of the population is not clearly understood. Nonetheless, comparisons of small groups of subjects have demonstrated that, in general, the dose of aerosol (histamine vs. methacholine) and degree of respiratory heat loss (cold air hyperventilation) required to induce a given fall in pulmonary function are correlated. For example, correlation coefficients that relate the log dose of agonist causing a 20% drop in FEV_1 for methacholine to that for histamine vary from 0.70 to 0.95 (Aquilina, 1983; Juniper et al., 1978; Chatham et al., 1982), and the maximal degree of airway narrowing (as measured with the plateau of the dose–response curve) induced by methacholine and histamine have not been found to differ in asthmatics (Sterk et al., 1986). Similarly, there is a correlation of 0.86 between the dose of methacholine and the degree of respiratory heat loss induced by cold air hyperventilation that is required to cause a significant reduction in pulmonary function in asthmatics (O'Byrne et al., 1982). Comparisons of responses to chemical challenges with response to exercise, however, show lesser degrees of correlation (0.44–0.55) (Chatham et al., 1982), a finding that may relate to a more complex pattern of physiological responses that is induced by exercise.

The comparability of different physiological tests, however, can be overestimated with the use of correlation coefficients and may be assessed better with the use of statistics that estimate the predictive abilities of different tests. For example, studies of small numbers of subjects suggest that response to methacholine challenge may be more useful to differentiate asthmatics from nonasthmatics than is a histamine response (Chatham et al., 1982), and, among asthmatics, may better identify subjects with different clinical features. The responses to exercise testing or hyperventilation with room air do not predict asthma to the extent predicted by pharmological challenges (Chatham et al., 1982). However, the predictive ability of cold air challenge testing appears to be comparable to methacholine challenge; both tests are able to differentiate current asthmatics from nonatopic normals, and each is less useful to differentiate atopic nonasthmatic subjects from subjects with asthma (Deal et al., 1980; Aquilina, 1983; Garcia-Herreios et al., 1980; Townley et al., 1975; Stevens and Vermeire, 1980). Therefore, generally comparable data appear to be collected with the use of methacholine, histamine, or cold air hyperventilation challenge tests. There may be some differences in the ability of these tests to identify specific clinical syndromes or to demonstrate differences in the distribution of bronchial responsiveness in symptomatic subsets of the general population, perhaps limiting the comparability of various studies. Such differences may be greatest in nonasthmatic subjects with chronic airflow limitation who may require greater molar doses of methacholine than of histamine for given degrees of bronchoconstriction. However, the data that suggest such differences are based on studies of small numbers of highly selected subjects and may well be explained by chance alone or by technical factors involved in the construction of the dose–response relationships.

An alternative method for the assessment of nonspecific bronchial responsiveness is to measure the change in pulmonary function that occurs following a bronchodilator. In several population-based studies, the distributional characteristics of airways responsiveness (AR) to isoproterenol have been found to be similar to the distributional characteristics of AR to pharmacological and cold air challenges; the majority of subjects demonstrate small postchallenge changes in FEV_1 that appear to relate to the "noise" in repetitive determinations, and a small number of subjects show larger changes that cause the distribution to appear to be skewed toward increasing responsiveness (Lorber et al., 1978; Vollmer et al., 1985). Furthermore, the degree of change in airway function that occurs following challenge with either a bronchoconstrictor or bronchodilator is associated with similar sets of risk factors: the subject's baseline FEV_1, asthma (wheeze) history, and smoking exposure. In some studies, responsiveness to either a bronchodilator or bronchoconstrictor also predicted more rapid rates of decline in FEV_1 (Kanner, 1984; Vollmer et al., 1985).

The relationship between response to nonspecific bronchoconstrictors and response to bronchodilators, however, may be more complex than the previously described relationships among different bronchoconstrictors. In a large study of nonasthmatic adults in which both responses were assessed, there was no relationship demonstrated between response to histamine and response to salbutamol (Taylor et al., 1985a). Unfortunately, in this study, the response to different challenges was measured in different surveys performed 1 year apart. The degree to which the poor correlation between these measures was due to temporally related changes in responsiveness is not clear. In contrast, a laboratory study of 28 subjects with chronic bronchitis demonstrated a significant relationship among responsiveness to histamine, methacholine, and ipratroprium bromide when each was assessed within several days of the other (Bahous et al., 1984). Barter and Campbell (1976) also showed that methacholine and isoproterenol responses were correlated ($r = 0.59$), although to a lesser degree than was found in studies that compared various bronchoconstrictors with each other. Furthermore, the ability to bronchodilate with isoproterenol measured immediately following methacholine-induced bronchoconstriction appears to relate directly to the degree of acute bronchoconstriction induced by the methacholine challenge. Among nonasthmatic subjects, functional changes induced by either challenge (bronchodilation or bronchoconstriction) have been found to be of almost equivalent magnitude (Townley et al., 1975). In asthmatics, however, the bronchodilatory response has been observed to be somewhat less than the bronchoconstrictor response, which suggests the possibility of different mechanisms that induce and reverse bronchial constriction among different populations. Thus, while the relationship between bronchodilator and bronchoconstrictor challenges may relate to the characteristics of the study population (i.e., the prevalence of asthma), the information derived from the use of these different challenges, at least on theoretical grounds, provides different information regarding airway function: bronchodilator responses provide information about the presence of potentially reversible smooth muscle constriction, whereas the previously described tests utilizing bronchoconstrictors broadly assess the vasomotor, inflammatory, and smooth muscle airway responses to nonspecific stimulation.

B. Protocol Variability

Technical differences in the methods used for methacholine, histamine, or cold air hyperventilation challenge (dosing pattern, i.e., cumulative vs. noncumulative, total dose delivered, and pulmonary distribution of dose) also can contribute to apparent discrepancies among the results of bronchoprovocation studies performed in different laboratories (Eiser et al., 1983). Aerosol distribution within the lungs is influenced by particle size such that the smaller the particle, the greater the likelihood of pulmonary rather than nasopharyngeal or tracheobronchial deposition (Hounam and Morgan, 1977). Breathing patterns (including variations in inspiratory flow rate) and duration of breath holding also can influence the dose of agonist delivered to the lungs (Brain and Valberg, 1979; Palmes et al., 1973; Ryan et al., 1981a,b). Variations of up to twofold in the particle size produced by different commercial nebulizers (Eiser et al., 1983; Massey et al., 1982) and variability in the methods of delivery (e.g., tidal breathing of aerosol from a continuous nebulizer vs. vital capacity maneuvers with mechanical dosimeters or hand-activated systems) also affect particle deposition. Tidal breathing methods may result in more peripheral deposition of aerosol than methods using a dosimeter (Ryan et al., 1981a). Investigators also have varied the dosing schedule for histamine and methacholine challenges, often choosing different initial concentrations and variably altering the initial concentrations presented to asthmatic and nonasthmatic subjects, actions that may have an impact on the interpretation of response to cumulative dose or of threshold for response (discussed below).

The degree to which such technical sources of variability contribute to the overall variability in outcome among studies that use different methods of bronchoprovocation testing is not clear. Technical variations in test administration appear to be minimized if, regardless of protocol and equipment used, there is careful assessment of total aerosol output (assessed by determination of the quantity of solution used), maintenance of particle size to within a range of 1–4 μm and use of an inspiratory duration between 1 and 5 sec (Eiser et al., 1983; Ryan et al., 1981a,b). Laboratory studies have suggested that, within these guidelines, the doses required to cause a fixed reduction in pulmonary function are highly correlated among protocols that use different nebulizer systems and patterns of breathing. Despite adherence to these guidelines, the slopes of the dose–response curves may be steeper and, among asthmatics, the dose of agonist required to cause broncho-constriction may be lower, for protocols that utilize a dosimeter and vital capacity maneuvers (O'Connor et al., 1988).

Similar considerations may apply to bronchoprovocation tests with cold dry air. This challenge may be administered as an exposure to a fixed dose of cold air attained by a constant level of hyperventilation, or by pro-gressive increments in ventilation attained by varying tidal volume and respiratory frequency. The latter is an attempt to establish a dose–response relationship, which, in epidemiological studies, may be technically difficult to accomplish. The effect of cold air hyperventilation appears to be cumulative, and significant variability in response does not appear to be related to variations in pattern of breathing (Malo et al., 1986). However, among protocols that use a single dose challenge, there may be variability in measured response because of differences in levels of ventilation achieved (Weiss et al., 1984; Welty et al., 1984). These levels usually have been deter-mined either by having the subject freely breathe at his or her maximal capacity or by predetermining this level to be a fixed percentage of his or her baseline FEV_1. Although these two rates should be comparable in most sub-jects, both rates may vary considerably between subjects of different size and baseline function. Dose–response curves to cold, dry air suggest that there may be a threshold level of hyperventilation required to cause broncho-constriction in asthmatics. This level may vary from 29 to 68 L/min (O'Byrne et al., 1982; Malo et al., 1986). Thus, there is the possibility of misclassification of response in instances in which higher levels of hyperven-tilation are not achieved (e.g., in subjects with lower baseline FEV_1 levels or who are not able to be fully cooperative).

C. Definitions of Response

The choice of which pulmonary function parameter is used as an index of responsiveness also may influence the characteristics of the data. Changes in smooth muscle contractility only can be indirectly inferred from changes in maximal expiratory flow rates or airways resistance. However, these measurements reflect a composite picture of changes in large and small airways induced by changes both in the smooth muscle and airway secretions. There may be differences in the degree to which maximal expiratory flow rates and measurements of resistance are sensitive to these effects and, to this extent, may identify subjects who differ in the sensitivities of their large vs. small airways, or who preferentially show either smooth muscle, vasomotor, or inflammatory responses to the challenge.

The effects of a deep inspiration may be to increase bronchoconstriction in asthmatic persons and to attenuate induced bronchoconstriction in nonasthmatic persons. These effects of volume history would accentuate differences between asthmatic and nonasthmatic subjects when forced vital capacity maneuvers are used, in contrast to protocols that use partial expiratory or panting maneuvers (Nadel and Tierney, 1961; Liu et al., 1985).

There also are differences in the intrinsic variability of various pulmonary function measures; the within-subject coefficient of variation for FEV_1 and for partial expiratory flow rates are approximately one-half that for airway conductance; differences in the ability to detect significant functional changes would be expected to vary accordingly. Greater variability in AR as assessed with measures of airway resistance rather than with FEV_1 or partial expiratory maneuvers has been shown in laboratory studies of highly selected subjects as well as in a population-based study. Various protocols require the performance of different numbers of measurements of pulmonary function after any given dose of agonist for the calculation of a mean level of response or the determination of a "best" effort. This factor also potentially introduces variability in AH data (Orehek et al., 1981; Scott and Kong, 1985).

In summary, response to a bronchoprovocation challenge as evaluated by change in airway resistance minimizes the effects of volume history (Habib et al., 1979; Orehek 1982) and is highly sensitive to changes in large airways (as may occur in asthma); however, this measurement is highly variable and poorly reproducible because of its technical complexity (Madsen et al., 1985). Measurement of response with FEV_1 has the advantage of low intrinsic variability (Dehaut et al., 1983) and ease in measurement, although this measurment is not sensitive to localized airway effects and requires a deep inspiration (Orehek, 1982). Utilization of partial expiratory flow maneuvers may be the best outcome variable to measure, since it avoids volume history effects and has acceptable variability (Bouhuys et al., 1969). However, it is somewhat more difficult to measure outside the laboratory setting.

D. Statistical Treatment of Data

There is not yet a universally acceptable method for the characterization of dose–response relationships between pulmonary function and bronchoconstrictor stimulae (Eiser et al., 1983; Eiser, 1983). There appears to be considerable interindividual variability in the shape of dose–response curves: straight, convex, or sigmoid (O'Connor et al., 1988; Woolcock et al., 1984; Bellia et al., 1983). Statistically, such data are limited by the small number of data points used in the construction of these curves and by the collection of a different number of measurements in different people. Furthermore, in regard to subjects in whom levels of baseline function differ, there is not a consensus as to whether pulmonary function should be expressed in absolute terms or as a percentage of baseline function (Eiser, 1983; Antonisen et al., 1986). Statistically, these data may be limited by the phenomenon of "regression to the mean," that is, those subjects whose pre-challenge level are most different from the population average would be predicted to have postchallenge levels that more closely approach the mean level and, therefore, to show a large absolute or relative change that is not necessarily physiologically meaningful. There also may be significant differences in the biological interpretation of absolute vs. relative changes in pulmonary function; these data may not be interpretable in subjects with compromised lung function in whom small absolute changes would produce large relative changes. Anthonisen and colleagues (1986), based on data from the IPPB trial, discussed this problem and recommended that AR be expressed both in absolute and relative terms. This issue is also relevant to assessment of outcome of treatment in patients with COPD (see Chapter 14).

Most commonly, bronchial responsiveness has been expressed as the dose of agonist required to induce a fixed reduction in function (PD_x). The magnitude of the reduction usually is related empirically to the inherent variability of the measure of function selected (Orehek, 1982; Eiser et al., 1983). The use of PD_x as an expression of AH appears to be more reproducible than the use of other techniques (Dehaut et al., 1983). PD_x is determined by interpolation of dose–response curves expressed semilogarithmically or as double reciprocals. However, responsiveness in subjects who do not attain a fixed reduction (10 or 20%) in flow rates cannot be completely characterized and may result in a censorship of data. Exclusion of data for "hyporesponders" necessarily alters the distribution of AR and may bias results. New attempts to characterize responsiveness more completely have led to determination of values for threshold (Habib et al., 1979), slope (Orehek et al., 1977), plateau (Sterk et al., 1986), and area under the curves (Townley et al., 1979), and to the fitting of polygonal functions to the data (Neijens et al., 1982; Woolcock et al., 1984). However, often there is not a flat baseline to determine threshold level, models may be overparameterized for given numbers of data points, and curve shapes differ unpredictably among people (Eiser, 1983). A summary dose–response slope simply constructed by drawing a line from the point of origin of the dose–response curve to the point at which the curve crosses the dose or response limits of the protocol recently has been proposed as a means of quantitating AH without censoring data on hyporesponders (O'Connor et al., 1988). This approach was found to differentiate asthmatics from nonasthmatics accurately. More work is needed to identify the extent to which different individuals are identified as "abnormal" based on the use of different statistical treatments of such data.

In protocols that involve bronchoconstrictors, an additional statistical concern relates to the necessity for exclusion from the study of subjects with severely low levels of FEV_1 ($< 60-70\%$) or subjects who demonstrate bronchoconstriction to saline or distilled water. The result is a "truncated" population sample in whom "deceased" subjects are likely to be excluded. A relationship between reduced baseline FEV_1 and AH would be diminished. Further studies of the effects of such exclusions on apparent epidemiological associations are needed.

E. Stability of Response

Laboratory studies suggest that there is a high level of short-term reproducibility and somewhat less long-term reproducibility in tests of airway responsiveness (Madsen et al., 1985). Short-term reproducibility (< 2 weeks) of the provocative dose of histamine or of ventilation (cold air challenge) among small numbers of asthmatics when expressed as within-individual correlation coefficients, has been found to range from 0.63 to 0.91 (Juniper et al., 1978; Dehaut et al., 1983; O'Byrne et al., 1982). Intraclass correlations, which are an expression of the proportion of total variability in a measure attributable to differences between individuals rather than within individuals (i.e., the higher the correlation coefficient, the more the variation is due to that between subjects) have been measured to be 0.88 for PD_{20} histamine (Dehaut et al., 1983) and > 0.90 for cold air challenge (Tessier et al., 1986). The subjects in these studies have been restricted to volunteer asthmatics whose baseline FEV_1 values varied by no more than 10% between studies, a criterion that may have selected individuals with inherently less variable performance. Indeed, when bronchial provocation testing is performed on less selected samples of the general population and on asymptomatic and variably symptomatic subjects, lesser degrees of correlation have been found. Redline and associates (1989a) found the week-to-week correlation in $\Delta FEV_1/FEV_1$ following cold air challenge testing to be 0.49 in a sample ($n = 23$) drawn from their larger cohort of children and young adults. The year-to-year correlation (measured over a maximal interval of 6 years) in 184 subjects was only 0.31

and was not improved with adjustments for age, atopic status, baseline lung function, and smoking exposure. Similarly, Sears and associates (1986) in a population-based sample of children, found significant variability in responsiveness to methacholine; this was especially notable among subjects with intermittent wheeze symptoms.

These findings may reflect a real temporal variability in airway responsiveness that may be biologically significant. In subjects with severe COPD, large intraindividual variability in AR has been related to large initial brochodilator responses and variability of FEV_1 with time (Anthonisen et al., 1986). In a generally healthy population of children and young adults, high intraindividual variability in AR was related to asthma history and a subsequent slower growth rates of FEV_1 (Redline et al., 1989a). However, variability in data may also relate to technical variability in the collection of such data. Additional work is needed to determine if, on a population level, the choice of bronchial challenge test, method of administration, and expression of data can reduce the long-term variability of these data. At the present time, however, an appreciation of the factors that contribute to the variability in airway responsiveness data, as well as the magnitude of variability that has been measured longitudinally, may improve interpretation of population-based studies. Characterization of airway responsiveness with a single cross-sectional assessment may be of limited value since it does not allow for the identification of individuals with more labile responses.

III. Cross-sectional and Longitudinal Uses of Tests of Bronchial Responsiveness for the Characterization of Airway Responsiveness in Population Samples

A number of studies have attempted to determine the prevalence of nonspecific airway responsiveness in general population samples and to describe the relationship of AH to age, sex, respiratory symptoms, level of lung function, smoking exposure, atopy, and occupational exposures. An understanding of these relationships is important for the interpretation of studies of airway responsiveness in relationship to COPD. This section briefly reviews several of the larger cross-sectional and longitudinal studies that provide data that may be generalizable to larger populations. However, even in these selected studies, there are considerable differences in methods of subject recruitment, the characteristics of the study population (e.g., ethnicity, age distribution, and disease prevalence), definitions of symptoms and disease, and methods of ascertaining a "positive" challenge test. As alluded to in previous sections, these differences among studies may limit their comparability and generalizability.

A. Prevalence of Hyperresponsiveness and Relations to Age and Gender

Assessment of the prevalence of nonspecific airway hyperresponsiveness in the population may provide information on the distribution of a unique physiological trait and the relationship of this trait to symptoms, disease status, and other physiological parameters. Alternatively, assessment of AH has been proposed as an objective means for determining the prevalence of asthma, a condition that is difficult to define and is inconsistently identified by questionnaire information.

Burney and associates (1987) examined the prevalence of AH in a large population of adults (n = 511) drawn from two villages and one town in Southampton. These investigators used an abbreviated histamine challenge test that provided a maximal dose of histamine of 4 μmol delivered via a hand-held nebulizer. Those individuals in whom FEV_1 dropped by at least 20% to a concentration of 8 mol of histamine (determined in some by back extrapolation) were defined as "responders." According to this definition, 14% of their population demonstrated AH. Significant predictors of AH were age, smoking status, atopic status, area of residence, and gender. Specifically, they described a U-shaped age-dependent distribution of AH, with the greatest prevalence of AH occurring in subjects 18–24 and 55–64 years of age, and the lowest (10%) occurring in those subjects 35–44 years of age. An increased prevalence of AH among the younger subjects was positively associated with a history of atopy and, among the oldest subjects, with smoking exposure. Males were more likely to demonstrate AH than were females. These findings are consistent with those of Hopp and associates (1985) who demonstrated similar relationships with gender and age in a more selected population of patients and hospital volunteers challenged with methacholine.

A higher prevalence of AH (24.5%) to histamine challenge was demonstrated in a large (n = 1905) randomly selected population sample from The Netherlands (Rijcken et al., 1987). Although the differences in the prevalence rate of AH between this study and the previously cited British study could be due to inherent differences (genetic and environmental) in the two populations, a more likely explanation relates to the different definitions of "positive response" utilized: a 10% decrease in FEV_1 was defined as "positive" in the Dutch study, which increased the likelihood of classifying any given subject as a responder. Similarly to the previous two studies, the Dutch study also demonstrated a greater prevalence of AH among males (26.1%) than females (22.5%) and a greater prevalence of AH among older than middle-aged subjects. However, greater AH was not demonstrated in the younger subjects (14–24 years) of this cohort, a finding that may be dependent partly on the criterion utilized for defining responder status.

A high prevalence (29.9%) of AH to methacholine (defined as a 20% decrease in FEV_1) has been demonstrated among 458 male veterans with a mean age of 60 years who participated in a longitudinal study (Sparrow et al., 1987). The prevalence of AH in this cohort would support a significant association of AH with male gender and older age.

Turner and colleagues (1986) used histamine challenge tests to determine the prevalence of asthma among children and adults of Papua New Guinea. These investigators defined a PD_{20} (FEV_1) < 5 μmol as indicating a positive response and the presence of asthma. They demonstrated 7% of adults and 0.5% of children as "positive." This relationship with age, different from that observed in the previously described studies, most certainly relates to the environmental or genetic factors peculiar to this population, and underscores the importance of detailing the characteristics of the study population.

The prevalence of AH to cold air challenge was assessed by Weiss and associates (1984) in a representative population of 213 children and 134 adults from East Boston, MA. Responders were defined as subjects who, following one level of hyperventilation, demonstrated a 9% decline in postchallenge FEV_1 expressed as a fraction of prechallenge FVC. In this population, 19% of nonasthmatics and 43% of asthmatics were identified as responders. The distributional characteristics of AH indicated a greater degree of responsiveness for children than adults; these findings, however, were based on a relatively small amount of data for older subjects. No relationship of AH with gender was demonstrated; wheeze symptoms, however, were more common among males. It is possible that the asthmatics in this study (who were predominantly male) received a less intense ventilatory challenge because of lower baseline levels of FEV_1 or suboptimal effort.

Response to a bronchodilator may provide somewhat different information about the prevalence of airway responsiveness than the previously described challenges. Lorber and associates (1978) assessed response to isoproterenol in a population of 1063 healthy subjects from Tucson, AZ, with no known cardiac disease or history of regular bronchodilator use. These investigators demonstrated a significant airway response among 20% of nonasthmatics with normal levels of FEV_1 and 51% of nonasthmatics with reduced levels of FEV_1; these prevalence rates of response may be higher than rates of AH to nonspecific bronchoconstrictors. In contrast, Vollmer and colleagues (1985) found a lower prevalence of responsiveness to isoproterenol in a general population from Portland, OR (3.4%), however, they observed a higher prevalence (9.5%) of responsiveness in a volunteer population attending an emphysema screening clinic. These investigators used an identical definition of responsiveness (a 7.7% increase in FEV_1) as the Tucson group. These disparate findings as well as data from the IPPB trial that demonstrated that the majority of subjects with severe COLD increase significantly their FEV_1 with isoproterenol inhalation, suggest that population composition (particularly the prevalence of respiratory impairment) substantially influences prevalence rates of bronchodilator responsiveness.

B. Relationship of the Prevalence of Airway Hyperresponsiveness and the Prevalence of Asthma

Prevalence rates of AH as determined in the general population do not appear to be equivalent to prevalence rates of asthma. In laboratory studies of subjects with current asthma, virtually all subjects are found to have AH (Deal et al., 1980). In contrast, studies based on general population samples show a less clear association between AH and the presence of wheeze/asthma. For example, Sears and associates (1986) have demonstrated that AH to methacholine was present in 8% of asymptomatic children and was absent in 35% of children with wheeze/asthma. Similar findings with cold air challenge testing in children were demonstrated by Redline and associates (1989a). In a Dutch cohort of adolescents and adults, only 56% of subjects with a history of asthma had a positive histamine challenge test, and 59% of the subjects with a positive response were asymptomatic (Rijcken et al., 1987).

The degree to which the prevalence of AH and relationship of AH to wheeze symptoms are influenced by the selected criterion for response and disease is seen in a study by Cookson and associates (1986). Among 105 adolescents and young adults from western Australia, an 11% prevalence of asthma and a 24% prevalence of wheeze was found. Ten percent of subjects had a "significant" bronchoconstrictor response, defined as a 20% reduction in FEV_1 to < 4 μmol of methacholine, and 30% were considered to be positive based on a $PD_{20} \leq 15$ μmol of methacholine. Clearly, the overall prevalence rate of AH and the relationship of AH with symptoms will vary according to the levels of responsiveness considered to be "significant."

C. Relationship of Smoking, Chronic Bronchitis, and Airway Responsiveness

Recurrent episodes of bronchoconstriction associated with increased AR have been hypothesized to contribute to the development of irreversible airflow obstruction (Weiss and Speizer, 1984). Assessment of the influence of AR on the natural history of lung disease, however, requires an understanding of the association of AR with smoking, chronic bronchitis, and baseline lung function.

A number of theoretical mechanisms exist that might increase AR in cigarette smokers. AR might be truly elevated in smokers by such mechanisms as an increase in airway mucosal permeability that allows greater access of chemical mediators to smooth muscle effector sites (Simani et al., 1974); airway inflammation and an alteration in the local milieu of chemical mediators (Muller et al., 1986); a systemic alteration in immunological reactions, for example, manifest by elevated peripheral blood eosinophilia and IgE levels (Taylor et al., 1985b) and alteration of antibody response to aeroallergens with increased production of IgE compared to nonsmokers (Venables et al., 1985); and increasing airway smooth muscle mass and causing a greater contractile response to a given stimulus (Macklem, 1979). Smoking might *factitiously* elevate AR by decreasing peripheral airway size and causing greater central deposition of aerosol to sites with greater concentrations of irritant receptors and where the effect of reduced airway caliber would cause a proportionately greater reduction in maximal expiratory flow rates than would occur had more peripheral airways been narrowed (Brown et al., 1977); causing a diffuse reduction in baseline airway caliber and a disproportionate absolute reduction in flow rates (inversely proportionate to a power function of airway radius) (Boushey et al., 1980). Alternatively, excess mucus production induced by cigarette smoke might dilute the concentration of aerosol challenge and thus might diminish the measured level of AR. The effects of a general disruption of the normal length–tension and force–velocity relationships caused by the chronic effects of cigarette smoke on lung structure are less clear.

Accordingly, studies of AR among smokers with and without chronic bronchitis have suggested that smoking, chronic bronchitis, and AR are related. In particular, smokers with chronic bronchitis often have levels of AR greater than are found among nonsmokers but less than those found among asthmatics (Ramsdell et al., 1982, 1985; Bahous et al., 1984; Yan et al., 1985). However, convincing evidence that these relationships are not solely due to the relationship of AR with lower baseline level of FEV_1 has not been provided consistently.

There is a significant correlation between increasing airway responsiveness and increasing degree of airway obstruction. Ramsdale and associates (1985) have shown a significant relationship between PC_{20} methacholine and baseline FEV_1 among 22 adults with chronic cough, all of whom had an FEV_1 less than 70% of the predicted level. Such a relationship was not seen for subjects classified as asthmatic. Bahous and associates (1984) studied 28 subjects with chronic bronchitis and similarly demonstrated a correlation of + 0.54 between PC_{20} (histamine and methacholine) and FEV_1/FVC level. This relationship was found in subjects with only moderate pulmonary impairment; only one subject had an FEV_1/FVC less than 75%. Greater degrees of airway responsiveness, expressed as the relative increase in FEV_1 following inhalation of a β-agonist, in subjects with greater airflow obstruction also have been demonstrated in longitudinal studies of smokers. In subjects with COPD drawn from a randomly selected Australian population (Yan et al., 1985) and subjects with severe airways obstruction participating in the IPPB trial (Anthonisen et al., 1986), significant relationships between baseline lung function and AH were demonstrated among nonasthmatic subjects. Although augmented airway responsiveness may be postulated to be causally related to obstructive disease, it is possible, as previously discussed, that AR was factitiously elevated as a result of altered aerosol deposition and airway mechanics that occur with airflow obstruction. Alternatively, statistical associations between baseline function and change in function following a bronchodilator in part may be a consequence of "regression to the mean." An understanding of the relationship between smoking and AR therefore requires consideration of the difference in baseline function that may be anticipated to occur among smokers and nonsmokers.

A comparison of airway responsiveness to histamine challenge of 17 smokers and 17 nonsmokers matched for age and initial level of airway conductance demonstrated greater responsiveness among the smokers (Gerard et al., 1980). A study of 227 nonasthmatic adults demonstrated greater airway responsiveness among smokers than nonsmokers (Taylor et al., 1985a). The baseline function in these groups was significantly different and may, at least in part, explain these observations. However, exclusion of subjects with FEV_1 levels less than 80% of the predicted value did not substantially alter the relationship of smoking and AH. Furthermore, among two healthy occupational cohorts, a greater prevalence of AH to methacholine (Tabona et al., 1984) and to acetylcholine (Pham et al., 1984) was demonstrated in smokers than in nonsmokers.

A dose–response relationship between the number of cigarettes smoked per day and the prevalence of AH was suggested among smokers in The Netherlands general population cohort (Rijcken et al., 1987). However, in this study there were no differences in AH according to smoking status, and it is not clear to what degree such a dose–response relationship was influenced by differences in the baseline lung function between the lighter and heavier smokers. Furthermore, in subjects with severely reduced lung function ($FEV_1 < 60\%$), a negative association between smoking exposure and degree of AH observed with β-agonist-induced bronchodilation was demonstrated (Anthonisen et al., 1986), which suggests that heavy smoking diminishes bronchial responsiveness. The severe degree of impairment in these subjects, however, limits the generalizability of this finding.

In COPD, it is important to assess the degree to which a relationship between smoking and AH is restricted to subjects with symptoms of mucus hypersecretion. Chronic bronchitis was found to be present in 47% of smokers found to have AH in two Portland, OR, cohorts (Vollmer et al., 1985). Furthermore, the previously cited studies of AR in subjects with COPD were concerned predominantly with subjects who also had evidence of mucus hypersecretion. It is possible that in smokers AH may accompany the airway inflammation characteristic of chronic bronchitis but that AH may not be manifest in smokers with predominant emphysema. Further studies of the relationship of smoking with AH need to address the influence of baseline FEV_1 as well as differences in clinical disease states on the observed associations.

Studies of small numbers of younger subjects have shown smokers to have the same or lesser degree of airway responsiveness as nonatopic nonsmokers (Brown et al., 1977). Furthermore, a study of a volunteer group of asthmatics and subjects with allergic rhinitis (a group who may be more susceptible to the effects of tobacco smoke) demonstrated no difference in responsiveness between smokers and nonsmokers (Garcia-Herreios et al., 1980). However, a selection bias may also be operative in this study. Asthmatics with the greatest degree of responsiveness may refrain from smoking; those who are able to smoke may have inherently less airway reactivity. In support of an effect of smoking on increasing responsiveness in asthmatics is the observation that passive smoking, an exposure that a susceptible individual is less able to avoid actively, has been associated with augmented airway responsiveness among asthmatic subjects (O'Connor et al., 1987).

Other studies have examined the relationship of AR and longitudinal decline in pulmonary function with attempts to control for differences in baseline lung function or smoking exposure. Barter and Campbell (1976) first demonstrated that annual rate of decline in FEV_1 in 34 subjects with chronic bronchitis was significantly related to AH to methacholine and isoproterenol, but baseline level of function was not controlled for. Kanner (1984) evaluated a large number of (n = 84) of subjects with obstructive airways disease for a mean of 4.4 years. More rapid rates of decline of FEV_1 were demonstrated in individuals with greater bronchodilator responses to aerosolized isoetharine, a relationship that persisted after adjustment for initial level of FEV_1. However, the influence of smoking on these relationships was not detailed. In a British study, a greater decline in FEV_1 was demonstrated in smokers with AR to histamine challenge, but such a relationship between AR and longitudinal change in lung function was not found among exsmokers or nonsmokers (Taylor et al., 1985a). This suggests that there may be an interaction between AR and current smoke exposure that accelerates loss of lung function; that is, smokers with augmented AR may be at the greatest risk for developing COPD.

Of considerable interest are the somewhat disparate findings from the IPPB trial concerning AH and longitudinal rate of decline in FEV_1 (Anthonisen et al., 1986). In this study, subjects with large responses to isoproterenol had slower rates of decline in lung function than subjects with less responsiveness: 7 ml vs. 49 ml decreases in FEV_1 per year for subjects with the greatest and least AH, respectively. Differences in longitudinal decline in FEV_1 in these groups may relate to differences in smoking exposures in subjects with different degrees of AH. However, it is interesting to speculate that the more favorable outcome observed in subjects with greater AH occurred as a result of effective intervention with bronchodilator medication.

D. Occupational Exposures

Airway responsiveness has been tested in several populations of workers thought to be at risk for occupational asthma (TDI, red cedar, colophony) or COPD (grain dust, cotton dust) (Chan-Yueng et al., 1984; Enarson et al., 1985; Hendrick et al., 1986). Tests of AH may be useful to predict which subjects are likely to develop symptoms; to define the physiological impairment associated with exposure; and to study the long-term sequelae of such exposures. It should be noted, however, that AR may vary dramatically with changes in exposure to offending substances, such as occurs seasonally in grain handlers (Hensly et al., 1988). The relationship of occupational exposures is detailed further in Chapter 11.

IV. Summary and Conclusions

Despite a substantial body of epidemiological data that associates the presence of nonspecific airway responsiveness with the occurrence of COPD, a causal link between AR and COPD has yet to be established conclusively. The cross-sectional nature of many of the studies and the frequently observed correlation of AR and lowered levels of lung function in subjects with COPD complicate the interpretation of these data. Existing longitudinal studies have not resolved this problem completely, since all of these studies have made their initial observations in midlife, a time that may be relatively late in the natural history of COPD. The extent to which AR contributes to the risk of COPD independently of its association with cigarette smoking also requires additional investigation.

Continued epidemiological investigation of the relationship of AR to the occurrence of COLD seems appropriate not only to provide a more complete understanding of the natural history of COLD but also to determine whether AR is a useful marker to identify smokers at high risk for the occurrence of COLD. To facilitate the resolution of these questions, future epidemiological studies will need to address a number of remaining issues:

1. Definition of a "positive" response that accounts for the statistical problem of "regression to the mean" and permits interpretation of data derived from patients with different levels of baseline lung function

2. Determination of the degree to which intraindividual variability in AR represents a biologically important trait and/or represents technical limitations inherent in the protocols to evaluate AR

3. Determination of the minimum number of measurements of AR and the optimal timing of these measurements required to characterize the AR status of study subjects

4. Interrelationships between AR, smoking exposure and atopy

5. More complete characterization of the distribution of AR in various populations that accounts for lack of data for subjects with greatly reduced baseline lung function and/or for subjects who fail to demonstrate significant bronchoconstriction to the challenge protocol used and for the considerable interindividual variability in the shapes of the dose–response curves to nonspecific bronchoconstrictors.

References

Anderson, S. D., Schoeffel, R. E., and Finney, M. (1983). Evaluation of ultrasonically nebulized solutions for provocation testing in patients with asthma. *Thorax* **38**:284–291.

Annesi, I., and Kauffman, F. (1986). Is respiratory mucus hypersecretion really an innocent disorder? *Am. Rev. Respir. Dis.* **134**:688–693.

Anthonisen, N. R., Wright, E. C., and the IPPB Trial Group. (1986). Bronchodilator response in chronic obstructive pulmonary disease. *Am. Rev. Respir. Dis.* **133**:814–819.

Aquilina, A. T., Hall, W. J., Douglas, R. G., and Utell, M. J. (1980). Airway reactivity in subjects with viral upper respiratory tract infections: the effects of exercise and cold air. *Am. Rev. Respir. Dis.* **122**:3–10.

Aquilina, A. T. (1983). Comparison of airway reactivity induced by histamine, methacholine and isocapnic hyperventilation in normal and asthmatic subjects. *Thorax* **38**:766–770.

Bahous, J., Cartier, A., Ouimet, G., Pineau, L., and Malo, J. L. (1984). Nonallergic bronchial hyperexcitability in chronic bronchitis. *Am. Rev. Respir. Dis.* **129**:216–220.

Barter, C. E., and Campbell, A. H. (1976). Relationship of constitutional factors and cigarette smoking to decrease in 1-second forced expiratory volume. *Am. Rev. Respir. Dis.* **113**:305–314.

Bellia, V., Rizzo, A., Amoroso, S., Mirabella, A., and Bonsignore, G. (1983). Analysis of dose–response curves in the detection of bronchial hyperreactivity. *Respiration* **44**:10–18.

Bhagat, R. G., and Grunstein, M. M. (1984). Comparison of the responsiveness to methacholine, histamine, and exercise in subgroups of asthmatic children. *Am. Rev. Respir. Dis.* **129**:221–224.

Boushey, H. A., Holtzman, M. J., Sheller, J. R., and Nadel, J. A. (1980). Bronchial hyperreactivity. *Am. Rev. Respir. Dis.* **121**:389–413.

Bouhuys, A., Hurt, V. R., Kion, B. M., and Zapletal, A. (1969). Maximum expiratory flow rates in induced bronchoconstriction in man. *J. Clin. Invest.* **48**:1159–1168.

Boulet, L. P., Cartier, A., Thomson, N. C., Roberts, R. S., Dolovich, J., and Hargreave, F. E. (1983). Asthma and increases in nonallergic bronchial responsiveness from seasonal pollen exposure. *J. Allergy Clin. Immunol.* **71**:399–406.

Brain, J. D., and Valberg, P. A. (1979). Deposition of aerosol in the respiratory tract. *Am. Rev. Respir. Dis.* **120**:1325–1373.

Brown, N. E., McFadden, E. R., and Ingram, R. H. (1977). Airway responses to inhaled histamine in asymptomatic smokers and nonsmokers. *J. Appl. Physiol.* **42**:508–513.

Bryant, D. H., and Burns, M. W. (1976). Bronchial histamine reactivity: its relationship to the reactivity of the bronchi to allergens. *Clin. Allergy* **6**:523–532.

Burney, P. G. J., Britton, J. R., Chinn, S., Tattersfield, A. E., Papacosta, A. O., Kelson, M. C., Anderson, F., and Corfield, D. R. (1987). Descriptive epidemiology of bronchial reactivity in an adult population: results from a community study. *Thorax* **42**:38–44.

Chan-Yeung, M., Vedal, S., Kus, J., Maclean, L., Enarson, D., and Tse, K. S. (1984). Symptoms, pulmonary function and bronchial hyperreactivity in western red cedar workers compared with those in office workers. *Am. Rev. Respir. Dis.* **130**:1038–1041.

Chatham, M., Bleecker, E. R., Smith, P. L., Rosenthal, R. R., Mason, P., and Norman, P. S. (1982). A comparison of histamine, methacholine, and exercise airway reactivity in normal and asthmatic subjects. *Am. Rev. Respir. Dis.* **126**:235–240.

Chung, K. F., Morgan, B., Keyes, S. J., and Snashall, P. D. (1982). Histamine dose-response relationships in normal and asthmatic subjects. *Am. Rev. Respir. Dis.* **126**:849–854.

Cockcroft, D. W., Reyfin, R. D. E., Frith, P. A., Cartier, A., Juniper, E. F., Dolovich, J., and Hargreave, F. E. (1979). Determinants of allergen-induced asthma: dose of allergen, circulating IgE antibody concentration and bronchial responsiveness to inhaled histamine. *Am. Rev. Respir. Dis.* **120**:1053–1058.

Cookson, W. O. C. M., Ryan, G., MacDonald, S., and Musk, A. W. (1986). Atopy, non-allergic bronchial reactivity, and past history as determinants of work related symptoms in seasonal grain handlers. *Br. J. Indust. Med.* **43**:396–400.

Curry, J. J. (1947). Comparative action of acetyl-beta-methacholine and histamine on the respiratory tract in normals, patients with hay fever, and subjects with bronchial asthma. *J. Clin. Invest.* **26**:430.

Deal, E. C., McFadden, E. R., Ingram, R. H., Breslin, F. J., and Jaeger, J. J. (1980). Airway responsiveness to cold air and hyperpnea in normal subjects and in those with hay fever and asthma. *Am. Rev. Respir. Dis.* **121**:621–628.

Dehaut, P., Rachiele, A., Martin, R. R., and Malo, J. L. (1983). Histamine dose-response curves in asthma: reproducibility and sensitivity of different indices to assess response. *Thorax* **38**:516–522.

Douglas, W. W. (1975). Histamine. In *The Pharmacologic Basis of Therapeutics*. Edited by L. S. Goodman, A. Gilman. New York, Macmillan.

Dubois, A. B., and Dautrebrebande, L. (1958). Acute effects of breathing inert dust particles and of carbachol aerosol on the mechanical characteristics of the lungs in man, changes in response after inhaling sympathomimetic aerosols. *J. Clin. Invest.* **37**:1746.

Eiser, N. M., Kerrebijn, K. F., and Quanjer, P. H. (1983). Guidelines for standardization of bronchial challenges with (nonspecific) bronchoconstricting agents. *Eur. J. Physiopathol. Respir.* **19**:495–514.

Eiser, N. M. (1983). Airway hyperreactivity. Calculation of data. *Eur. J. Respir. Dis.* (Suppl.) **131**:241–265.

Empey, D. W., Laitinen, L. A., Jacobs, L., Gold, W. M., and Nadel, J. A. (1976). Mechanisms of bronchial hyperreactivity in normal subjects after upper respiratory tract infection. *Am. Rev. Respir. Dis.* **113**:131–139.

Enarson, D. A., Chan-Yeung, M., Tabon, M., Kus, J., Vedal, S., and Lum, S. (1985). Predictors of bronchial hyperexcitability in grain handlers. *Chest* **87**:452–455.

Fanta, C. H., and Ingram, R. H. J. (1981). Airway responsiveness and chronic airway obstruction. *Med. Clin. North Am.* **68**:473–487.

Fletcher, C., Peto, R., Tinker, C., and Speizer, F. E. (1976). *The Natural History of Chronic Bronchitis and Emphysema.* London, Oxford University Press.

Garcia-Herreros, P. G., Azama, M., Van Steenberghe, J. V., Bracomonte, M., Sergysels, R., DeCoster, A., and Yernault, J. C. (1980). Bronchial hyperreactivity to histamine in allergic and non-allergic asthma, allergic rhinitis and chronic bronchitis. *Prog. Respir. Res.* **14**:78–86.

Gerard, J. W., Cockcroft, D. W., Mink, J. T., Cotton, D. J., Poonawala, R., and Dosman, J. A. (1980). Increased nonspecific bronchial reactivity in cigarette smokers with normal lung function. *Am. Rev. Respir. Dis.* **122**:577–581.

Habib, M. P., Pare, P. D., and Engel, L. A. (1979). Variability in airway responses to inhaled histamine in normal subjects. *J. Appl. Physiol.* **47**:51–58.

Hargreave, F. E., Dolovich, J., O'Byrne, P. M., Ramsdale, E. H., and Daniel, E. E. (1986). The origin of airway hyperresponsiveness. *J. Allergy Clin. Immunol.* **78**:825–832.

Henderson, W. R., Shelhamer, J. H., Reingold, D. B., Smith, L. F., Evans, R., and Kaliner, M. (1979). Alpha-adrenergic hyperresponsiveness in asthma. *N. Engl. J. Med.* **300**:642–647.

Hendrick, D. J., Fabbri, L. M., Hughes, J. M., Banks, D. E., Burkman, H. W., Connolly, M. J., Jones, R. N., and Weill, H. (1986). Modification of the methacholine inhalation test and its epidemiologic use in polyurethane workers. *Am. Rev. Respir. Dis.* **133**:600–604.

Hensley, M. J., Schittitano, R, Saunders, N. A., Cripps, A. W., Ruhno, J., Sutherland, D. and Clancy, R. L. (1988). Seasonal variation in nonspecific bronchial reactivity: a study of wheat workers with a history of wheat associated asthma. *Thorax* **43**:103–107.

Hogg, J. C. (1983). Bronchial mucosal permeability in airways hyperreactivity. In *Airway Hyperreactivity. A symposium organized by the Swedish Association for Allergology, Stolkholm, 1982.* Edited by B. G. Simonsson. *Eur. J. Respir. Dis.* **64**:131.

Holtzman, M. J., Cunningham, J. H., Sheller, J. R., Irsigler, G. B., Nadel, J. A., and Boushey, H. A. (1979). Effect of ozone on bronchial reactivity in atopic and nonatopic subjects. *Am. Rev. Respir. Dis.* **120**:1059–1067.

Hopp, R. J., Bewtra, A. K., Nair, N. M., and Townley, R. G. (1984). Specificity and sensitivity of methacholine inhalation challenge in normal and asthmatic children. *J. Allergy Clin. Immunol.* **74**:154–158.

Hopp, R. J., Bewtra, A., Nair, N. M., and Townley, R. G. (1985). The effect of age on methacholine response. *J. Allergy Clin. Immunol.* **76**:609–613.

Hounam, R. F., and Morgan, A. (1977). Particle deposition. In *Respiratory Defence Mechanisms*. Edited by J. O. Brain. New York, Marcel Dekker, pp. 125–156.

Juniper, E. F., Frith, P. A., Dunnet, C., Cockcroft, D. W., and Hargreave, F. E. (1978). Reproducibility and comparison of responses to inhaled histamine and methacholine. *Thorax* 33:705–710.

Juniper, E. F., Frith, P. A., and Hargreave, F. E. (1981). Airway responsiveness to histamine and methacholine: relationship to minimum treatment to control symptoms of asthma. *Thorax* 36:575–579.

Kanner, R. E. (1984). The relationship between airways responsiveness and chronic airflow limitation. *Chest* 86:54–57.

Koelle, G. B. (1975). Parasympathomimetic agents. In *The Pharmacologic Bases of Therapeutics*. Edited by L. S. Goodman and A. Gilman. New York, Macmillan.

Lee, D. A., Winslow, N. R., Speight, A. W. P., and Hey, E. N. (1983). Prevalence and spectrum of asthma in childhood. *Br. Med. J.* 286:1256–1258.

Liu, Y-N., Sosaki, H., Sekizawa, K., Hida, W., Ichinose, M., and Takishima, T. (1985). Effect of circadian rhythm on bronchomotor tone after deep inspiration in normal and asthmatic subjects. *Am. Rev. Respir. Dis.* 132:278–282.

Lorber, D. B., Kaltenborn, W., and Burrows, B. (1978). Responses to iso-proterenol in a general population sample. *Am. Rev. Respir. Dis.* 118:855–861.

Macklem, P. T. (1979). Discussion-session I. In *Mechanisms of Airways Obstruction in Human Respiratory Disease: Proceedings of the International Symposium, Tyerberg, South Africa, 1978*. Edited by M. A. de Kock, J. A. Nadel, and C. M. Lewis. Capetown, A. A. Balkema, p. 146.

Madsen, F., Rathlow, H. H., Frolund, L., Svendsen, U. G., and Weeke, B. (1985). Short and long term reproducibility of responsiveness to inhaled histamine: R_+ compared to FEV_1 as measurement of response to challenge. *Eur. J. Respir. Dis.* 67:193–203.

Malo, J. L., Cartier, A., L'Archeveque, J., Ghezzo, H., and Martin, R. R. (1986). Cold air inhalation has a cumulative bronchospastic effect when inhaled in consecutive doses for progressively increasing degrees of ventilation. *Am. Rev. Respir. Dis.* 134:990–993.

Mark, J. D., McBride, J. T., Brooks, J. G., McConnochie, K. M., and Hall, W. J. (1986). Airway hyperreactivity and a history of clinical manifestations of asthma in childhood. *Pediatr. Pulmonol.* 2:170–174.

Massey, D. G., Miyauchi, D., and Fournier-Massey, G. (1982). Nebulizer function. *Bull. Europ. Physiopathol. Respir.* 18:665–671.

Mortagy, A. K., Howell, J. B. L., and Waters, W. E. (1986). Respiratory symptoms and bronchial reactivity: identification of a syndrome and its relation to asthma. *Br. Med. J.* **293**:525–529.

Muller, J. B. M., Wigg, B. R., Wright, J. L., Hogg, J. C., and Pare, P. D. (1986). Nonspecific airway reactivity in cigarette smokers. *Am. Rev. Respir. Dis.* **133**:120–125.

Muranaka, M., Suzuki, S., Miyamoto, T., Takeda, K., Okumura, H., and Makino, S. (1974). Bronchial reactivities to acetylcholine and IgE levels in asthmatic subjects after long-term remissions. *J. Allergy Clin. Immunol.* **54**:32–40.

Murray, A. B., Ferguson, A. C., and Morrison, B. (1981). Airway responsiveness to histamine as a test for overall severity of asthma in children. *J. Allergy Clin. Immunol.* **68**:119–124.

Nadel, J. A., and Tierney, D. F. (1961). Effect of a previous deep inspiration on airway resistance in man. *J. Appl. Physiol.* **16**:717–719.

Neijens, H. F., Hofkamp, M., Degenhart, H. J., and Kerrebijn, K. F. (1982). Bronchial responsiveness as a function of inhaled histamine and the method of measurement. *Bull. Europ. Physiopathol. Respir.* **18**:427–438.

O'Byrne, P. M., Ryan, G., Morris, M., McCormick, D., Jones, N. L., Morse, J. L. C., and Hargreave, F. E. (1982). Asthma induced by cold air and its relation to nonspecific bronchial responsiveness to methacholine. *Am. Rev. Respir. Dis.* **125**:281–285.

O'Connor, G. T., Weiss, S. T., Tager, I. B., and Speizer, F. E. (1987). The effect of passive smoking on pulmonary function and nonspecific bronchial responsiveness in a population-based sample of children and young adults. *Am. Rev. Respir. Dis.* **135**:800–804.

O'Connor, G., Sparrow, D., Taylor, D., Segal, M., and Weiss, S. T. (1987). Analyses of dose-response curves to methacholine: an approach suitable for population studies. *Am. Rev. Respir. Dis.* **136**:1412–1417.

Orehek, J., Gayrard, P., Smith, A. P., and Charpin, J. (1977). Airway response to carbochol in normal and asthmatic subjects. *Am. Rev. Respir. Dis.* **115**:937–943.

Orehek, J., Nicoli, M. M., Delpierre, S., and Beauprett, A. (1981). Influence of the previous deep inspiration on the spirometric measurement of provoked bronchoconstriction in asthma. *Am. Rev. Respir. Dis.* **123**:269–272.

Orehek, J. (1982). Measurement of airway hyperresponsiveness in man. *Eur. J. Respir. Dis.* **63**:42–60.

Orie, N. G. M., Sluiter, H. J., de Vries, K., Tammeling, G. J., and Witkop, J. (1961). The host factor in bronchitis. In *Bronchitis.* Edited by W. G. M. Orie and H. J. Sluiter. Assen, Royal Van Gorcum, pp. 43–59.

Palmes, E. D., Wang, C., Golding, R. M., and Alishuler, B. (1973). Effect of depth of inhalation on aerosol persistance during breath holding. *J. Appl. Physiol.* **34**:351–360.

Petty, T. L., Pierson, D. J., Dick, N. P., Hudson, L. D., and Walker, S. H. (1976). Follow-up evaluation of a prevalence study for chronic bronchitis and chronic airway obstruction. *Am. Rev. Respir. Dis.* **114**:881–890.

Pham, Q. T., Mur, J. M., Chau, N., Gabiano, M., Henquel, J. C., and Teculescu, D. (1984). Prognostic value of acetylcholine challenge test: a prospective study. *Br. J. Indust. Med.* **41**:267–271.

Ramsdell, J. W., Nachtwey, F. J., and Moser, K. M. (1982). Bronchial hyperreactivity in chronic obstructive bronchitis. *Am. Rev. Respir. Dis.* **126**:829–832.

Ramsdale, E. H., Roberts, R. S., Morris, M. M., and Hargreave, F. E. (1985). Differences in responsiveness to hyperventilation and metacholine in asthma and chronic bronchitis. *Thorax* **40**:422–426.

Redline, S., Tager, I. B., Speizer, F. E., Rosner B., and Weiss, S. T. (1989a) Longitudinal variability in airway responsiveness in a population-based sample of children and young adults: intrinsic and extrinsic factors. *Am. Rev. Respir. Dis.* (In press).

Redline, S., Tager, I. B., Segal, M. R., Gold, D. R., Speizer, F. E., and (1989b). The relationship between longitudinal change in pulmonary function and nonspecific airway responsiveness in children and young adults *Am. Rev. Respir. Dis.* (In press).

Rijcken, B., Schouten, J. P., Weiss, S. T., Speizer, F. E., and van der Lende, R. (1987). The relationship of nonspecific bronchial responsiveness to respiratory symptoms in a random population sample. *Am. Rev. Respir. Dis.* **136**:62–68.

Ryan, G., Dolovich, M. B., Roberts, R. S., Frith, P. A., Juniper, E. F., Hargreave, F. E., and Newhouse, M. T. (1981a). Standardization of inhalation provocation tests: two techniques of aerosol generation and inhalation compared. *Am. Rev. Respir. Dis.* **123**:195–199.

Ryan, G., Dolovich, M. B., Juniper, E. F., Hargreave, F. E., and Newhouse, M. T. (1981b). Standardization of inhalation provocation tests: influence of nebulizer output, particle size and method of inhalation. *J. Allergy Clin. Immunol.* **67**:156–161.

Ryan, G., Latimer, K. M., Dolovich, J., and Hargreave, F. E. (1982). Bronchial responsiveness to histamine: relationship to diurnal variation of peak flow rate, improvement after bronchodilator and airway caliber. *Thorax* **37**:423–429.

Scott, G. C., and Kong, M. (1985). How many spirograms for a histamine challenge? *Am. Rev. Respir. Dis.* **132**:268–271.

Sears, M. R., Jones, D. T., Holdaway, M. D., Hewitt, C. J., Flannery, E. M., Herbison, G. P., and Silva, P. A. (1986). Prevalence of bronchial reactivity to inhaled methacholine in New Zealand children. *Thorax* **41**:283–289.

Simani, A. S., Inuue, S., and Hogg, J. C. (1974). Penetration of the respiratory epithelium of guinea pig following exposure to cigarette smoke. *Lab. Invest.* **31**:75–81.

Simonsson, B. G., Jacobs, F. M., and Nadel, J. A. (1967). Role of autonomic nervous system and cough reflex in the increased responsiveness of airways in patients with obstructive airways disease. *J. Clin. Invest.* **46**:1812–1818.

Simonsson, B. G. (1984). Nonspecific bronchial hyperreactivity: correlation to asthma and modifying factors. *Europ. J. Respir. Dis.* **65**:17–24.

Sparrow, D., O'Connor, G., Colton, T., Barry, C. L., and Weiss, S. T. (1987). The relationship of nonspecific bronchial responsiveness to the occurrence of respiratory symptoms and decreased levels of pulmonary function. *Am. Rev. Respir. Dis.* **135**:1255–1260.

Stanescu, D. C., and Frans, A. (1982). Bronchial asthma without increased airway reactivity. *Eur. J. Respir. Dis.* **63**:5–12.

Starr, I., Elsom, K. A., Reisinger, J. A., and Richards, H. N. (1933). Acetyl-beta-methacholine. I. The action on normal persons with a note on the action of ethyester of beta-methacholine. *Am. J. Med. Sci.* **186**:313.

Stephens, N. L. (1987). Airway smooth muscle. *Am. Rev. Respir. Dis.* **135**:960–975.

Sterk, P. J., Timmers, M. C., and Dijkman, J. H. (1986). Maximal airway narrowing in humans *in vivo*. *Am. Rev. Respir. Dis.* **134**:714–718.

Stevens, W. J., and Vermeire, P. A. (1980). Bronchial responsiveness to histamine and allergen in patients with asthma, rhinitis, cough. *Eur. J. Respir. Dis.* **61**:203–212.

Szentivanyi, A. (1968). The beta-adrenergic theory of the atopic abnormality in bronchial asthma. *J. Allergy* **42**:203–223.

Tabona, M., Chan-Yeung, M., Enarson, D., MacLean, L., Dorken, E., and Schulzer, M. (1984). Host factors affecting longitudinal decline in lung spirometry among grain elevator workers. *Chest* **85**:782–786.

Taylor, R. G., Joyce, H., Gross, E., Holland, F., and Pride, N. B. (1985a). Bronchial reactivity to inhaled histamine and annual rate of decline in FEV_1 in male smokers and ex-smokers. *Thorax* **40**:9–16.

Taylor, R. G., Gross, E., Joyce, H., Holland, F., and Pride, N. B. (1985b). Smoking, allergy and the differential white blood cell count. *Thorax* **40**:17–22.

Tessier, P., Cartier, A., L'Archeveque, J., Ghezzo, H., Martin, R. R., and Malo, J. L. (1986). Within- and between-day reproducibility of isocapnic cold air challenges in subjects with asthma. *J. Allergy Clin. Immunol.* **78**:379–387.

Townley, R. G., Ryo, U. Y., Kolotkin, B. M., and Kang, B. (1975). Bronchial sensitivity to methacholine in current and former asthmatic and allergic rhinitis patients and control subjects. *J. Allergy Clin. Immunol.* **56**:429–442.

Townley, R. G., Bewtra, A. K., Nair, N. M., Brodkey, F. D., Watt, G. D., and Burke, K. M. (1979). Methacholine inhalation challenge studies. *J. Allergy Clin. Immunol.* **64**:569–574.

Turner, K. J., Dowse, G. K., Stewart, G. A., and Alpers, M. P. (1986). Studies on bronchial hyperreactivity, allergic responsiveness, and asthma in rural and urban children of the highlands of Papua, New Guinea. *J. Allergy Clin. Immunol.* **77**:558–566.

U.S. Dept. of HEW (1979). *The Health Consequences of Smoking.* OSGPG, Washington, D.C.

van der Lende, R., de Kroon, J. P. M., van der Meulen, G. G., Tammeling, G. J., Visser, B. F., de Vries, K., and Orie, N. G. M. (1970). Possible indicators of endogenous factors in the development of WSLD. In *Bronchitis III.* Edited by N. G. M. Orie and R. van der Lende. Assen, Royal Van Gorcum, pp. 52–70.

Venables, K. M., Toppling, M. D., Howe, W., Luczynska, C. M., Hawkins, R., and Taylor, J. N. (1985). Interaction of smoking and atopy in producing specific IgE antibody against a hapten protein conjugate. *Br. Med. J.* **290**:201–204.

Vollmer, W. M., Johnson, L. R., and Buist, A. S. (1985). Relationship of response to a bronchodilator and decline on forced expiratory volume in one second in population studies. *Am. Rev. Respir. Dis.* **132**:1186–1193.

Walden, S. M., Bleecker, E. R., Chahol, K., Britt, E. J., and Permutt, S. (1984). Effect of alpha-adrenergic blockade on exercise-induced asthma and conditioned air. *Am. Rev. Respir. Dis.* **130**:357–362.

Weiss, S. T., Tager, I. B., Weiss, J. W., Munoz, A., Speizer, F. E., and Ingram, R. H. (1984). Airways responsiveness in a population sample of adults and children. *Am. Rev. Respir. Dis.* **129**:898–902.

Weiss, S. T., and Speizer, F. E. (1984). Increased levels of airways responsiveness as a risk factor for development of chronic obstructive lung disease. *Chest* **86**:3–4.

Welty, C., Weiss, S. T., Tager, I. B., Munoz, A., Becker, C., Speizer, F. E., and Ingram, R. H. (1984). The relationship of airways responsiveness to cold air, cigarette smoking, and atopy to respiratory symptoms and pulmonary function in adults. *Am. Rev. Respir. Dis.* **130**:198–203.

Woolcock, A. J., Salome, C. M., and Yan, K. (1984). The shape of the dose–response curve to histamine in asthma and normal subjects. *Am. Rev. Respir. Dis.* **130**:71–75.

Yan, K., Salome, C. M., and Woolcock, A. J. (1985). Prevalence and nature of bronchial hyperresponsiveness in subjects with chronic obstructive pulmonary disease. *Am. Rev. Respir. Dis.* **132**:25–29.

10

Epidemiological Evidence for Aggravation and Promotion of COPD by Acid Air Pollution

DOUGLAS W. DOCKERY and FRANK E. SPEIZER

Harvard School of Public Health
Harvard Medical School
Brigham and Women's Hospital
Boston, Massachusetts

I. Introduction

The public and scientific debate over acid rain and its precursors has focused on the ecological effects of the removal of acid from the atmosphere. A substantial body of evidence indicates that deposition of acids through precipitation processes is responsible for the acidification of poorly buffered lakes in portions of Scandinavia and North America, and for forest decline in many industrialized countries. There is also evidence that the deposition of acids has increased over the last 20 years despite progress in the control of air pollution. Oxidation of primary pollutants (sulfur and nitrogen oxides) to acidic gases and particles is clearly identified as the main source of these agents.

Far less concern has been shown for direct human health effects, either acute or chronic, due to acid aerosols (Maugh, 1984). There are remarkably few data on the health impact of either current or past exposures to acidic air pollution. The large-scale pollution disasters in the middle of this century in the Meuse Valley in 1930, in London in 1952, and in Donora, Pennsylvania, in 1948, likely involved acid aerosols as well as primary pollutants such as SO_2 and smoke. From what has been learned subsequently about the acute effects of these pollutants, it is likely that the offending agent in those episodes was the acidity of particles in the stagnating air masses.

Fortunately, levels of acid aerosol exposure that occurred in the episodes identified in the 1930s–1950s are not likely to occur again in the United States or Great Britain. However, it is unknown whether less severe daily or cumulative exposures to acid aerosols and gases can affect respiratory symptoms either by themselves or in conjunction with other pollutants. Animal and clinical studies suggest the possibility of such adverse effects at sulfuric acid concentrations of 100 $\mu g/m^3$, which are comparable to concentrations being measured in North America. Whether entire populations or only sensitive groups are affected is not known.

Although epidemiological studies suggest that groups of free-living individuals may be affected by air pollution in general, remarkably few population-based studies have directly measured acid aerosol exposure and response. Part of the problem has been the lack of an operational monitoring system for the measurement of gaseous and aerosol acidity in ambient air.

Because of this our knowledge of the temporal and spatial distribution of aerosol acidity concentrations is extremely limited. In a recent review, Lippmann (1985) found less than 20 reports of acid aerosol measurements, all of which were for brief periods (a few days or less) except for an extended record of 6–12 months in three communities (Ferris and Spengler, 1985). Only in recent years have epidemiological studies including acid aerosol measurements been attempted (e.g., Bock et al., 1985; Lioy et al., 1985; Spektor et al., 1988).

In this chapter, we describe the atmospheric processes that produce acid aerosols, describe several population based studies to test the hypothesis that acid aerosols were the causative agent in the air pollution mix, and describe recent controlled studies of acid aerosol exposure among animals and humans.

II. Acid Aerosol Chemistry

Although natural sources of acid aerosols exist, their primary origin in North America is sulfur and nitrogen oxides released into the atmosphere from anthropogenic sources and oxidized during airborne transport to sulfuric and nitric acids. Sulfur oxides (SO_x) are produced by industrial processes and coal- and oil-fixed power plants. Nitrogen oxides (NO_x) come primarily from transportation and electric utilities.

Three sets of conditions are associated with acid aerosol exposures (Fig. 1). The first is the direct emission of acids. Acids are important

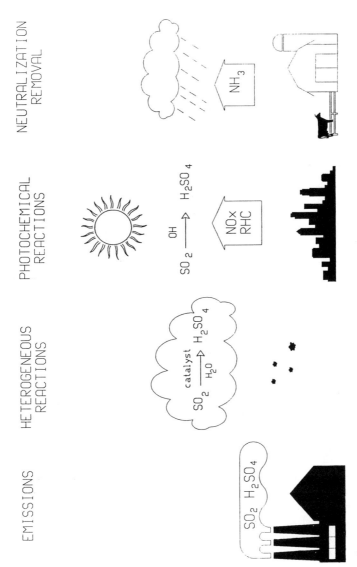

Figure 1 Schematic representation of atmospheric chemistry for sulfur oxides.

byproducts of many industrial processes and are minor byproducts of fossil fuel combustion. Sulfur is a natural contaminant of all fossil fuels. During combustion, the sulfur is oxidized primarily to sulfur dioxide, SO_2. A low percentage of the sulfur is oxidized and reacts with water vapor, a primary combustion product, to form sulfuric acid, H_2SO_4. Population exposures in these conditions will depend on local industry and local dispersion characteristics.

In areas with multiple industrial or fossil fuel combustion sources (including residential heating), the second mechanism, heterogeneous reactions (Fig. 1) can be important. A stagnating, foggy air mass in which sulfur oxides and particulate pollution build up is conducive to the rapid production of acid aerosols. The transformation of SO_2 into H_2SO_4 is catalyzed by various metals (e.g., iron, manganese, and zinc) within water droplets and also by carbon on the surface of particles. Reaction rates are relatively fast, 10–30%/hr. These catalyzed reactions require neither sunlight nor warm temperatures, and therefore can produce acid exposures during the foggy conditions associated with the classic air pollution episodes.

The third set of conditions are based on photochemical reactions (Fig. 1). Nitrogen oxides, produced by automobiles and power plants, react in sunlight with reactive hydrocarbons (RHC) from the same sources to produce oxidizing agents such as the hydroxyl radical (OH) and ozone (O_3). SO_2 gas reacts very quickly with the OH radicals to produce H_2SO_4 (see Calvert et al., 1985, for a more complete description of the atmospheric chemistry). Because of the need for solar energy, these reactions are restricted to midday during the summer, and require a rich mix of pollutants, usually from major urban or industrial areas. Maximum reaction rates are slow (1–4%/hr) so that long reaction times, and therefore long travel times, are required before substantial concentrations of acid can accumulate.

Sulfuric as well as nitric acid can be neutralized (Fig. 1) by atmospheric ammonia (NH_3). Ammonia is a common constituent of the atmosphere resulting from biological processes. Fertilizer, animals, humans, and therefore urban areas are major sources of ammonia. Because of its source from biological processes, ammonia is released into the atmosphere from the ground. Thus aerosol acidity tend to increase with elevation above the ground (Ferek et al., 1983; Tanner et al., 1984). As a result, acidic air pollutants can be transported a long distance from their sources, particularly when a temperature inversion protects them from interactions near the ground. Depending on their location, rural or semirural areas can be affected. In rural or semirural areas, where the majority of acidic aerosols and gases are transported from long distances, high acid pollutant concentrations occur during downward mixing of acidic air from higher altitudes. As a result, high concentrations are usually observed in the late morning when stratified air near the ground is dissipated by thermal instability in the convective boundary layer.

Measurement of the acidity of aerosols in the ambient environment is very difficult (Lippmann, 1985). The species of interest are highly reactive so that they will readily react with all but the most inert sampling medium. Special care must be taken so that air passing over the collected acid does not neutralize the sample. Because humans produce ammonia in their breath and from their skin, great care must be taken that the technicians do not contaminate the sample in collection or analysis. Finally, acid concentrations tend to be very low, so that sensitive analytic assays are required.

III. Population-Based Studies

Epidemiological studies have in general been based on exposure measurements from available air pollution monitors. Instruments and site locations are often designed to meet regulatory requirements rather than the research needs of an epidemiological study. Because of the difficulty in measuring aerosol acidity, epidemiological studies generally have estimated exposure with these available data. Many of these measures are correlated because of source characteristics. For example, particulates, sulfur oxides, nitrogen oxides, and acid aerosols are all directly produced by the burning of fossil fuels. Other pollutants are correlated because they are released into the same air mass. The air mass over a major metropolitan area will contain emissions from power plants, automobiles, and industry. If dispersion is poor, the concentrations of all of these pollutants will build up together. As the air mass moves over a monitoring station, the pollutant concentrations will rise and fall in unison. Thus epidemiological studies refer to generic measures of pollution such as particulate or sulfur dioxide concentrations, which measure the general level of air pollution and which are presumably correlated with the more toxic agents that may exist in the mix of pollutants. Ambient measures of the total suspended particulate (TSP) mass, the mass of size-fractionated particles (PM_{10} or $PM_{2.5}$), and sulfur dioxide (SO_2) or nitrogen dioxide (NO_2) as well as particulate sulfate (SO_4) have been presumed to represent surrogates for acid aerosols, in the absence of a suitable method for direct measurement of airborne acidity. Lacking direct measurements, we can use the epidemiological studies of the effects of air pollution on COPD if we assume that an association exists with aerosol acidity, and that the reported measurements are surrogates for that acidity.

We will consider some historical and current studies of the acute effects of air pollution (Table 1). Although few direct measures are available, meteorological conditions were consistent with the formation of acid aerosols by one of the three mechanisms outlined in the last section: catalytic reactions in wet air masses; photochemical reactions in air masses transported over long distances; or direct emissions of acid droplets.

A. Meuse Valley, Belgium: 1930

More than 50 years ago, it was suggested that sulfuric acid may have been the component of air pollution responsible for the health effects observed during extreme episodes. Firket (1931, 1936) has described the fog of December 1st–5th, 1930, in a narrow industrial valley of the Meuse in Belgium. More than 60 people died on the 4th and 5th days of the fog after only a few hours' illness. This rate of mortality was more than 10 times normal. Several hundred suddenly developed respiratory disorders that were often accompanied by cardiac insufficiency. Many cattle had to be slaughtered, and others were saved only by being driven up the hillsides.

Examination of patients and questioning of physicians soon after the episode showed that most patients complained of painful irritation and fits of coughing and shortness of breath. Many patients had symptoms of asthma that improved rapidly following treatment with epinephrine or epinephrine-based drugs, although in some the asthma symptoms were followed by cardiac insufficiency and collapse. Patients with a history of asthma or previous signs of heart failure, the elderly, or the debilitated were reported to be especially affected by the fog.

Fifteen autopsies indicated widespread congestion of the tracheal mucous membrane and the main bronchi. Irritation of the mucous membranes of the respiratory tract was superficial, suggesting that irritation did not precede death by many hours. Fine particles of soot were found as deep in the lungs as the alveoli. Firket concluded that the pathophysiological findings were more consistent with sulfuric acid exposure than exposure to any of the other possible pollutants.

Based on a detailed examination of the emissions in the valley, the weather during the episodes, and the atmospheric chemistry required for the production of sulfuric acid, Firket (1936) concluded that as "the SO_2 evolved in the presence of oxidation catalysts, such as ferric acid and zinc oxide, in the fog, the SO_2 must have been partly transformed into sulphuric acid." From our current understanding of the atmospheric chemistry, this conclusion is very plausible.

Although no air pollution measures were available for this episode, the emissions, meteorological findings, chemistry results, and pathophysiological conclusions were consistent with exposure to acid aerosols.

Table 1 Summary of Epidemiological Studies

	Atmospheric Conditions	Response Characteristics	Comments
Acute Epsiodes			
Meuse Valley Belgium December 1930	Cold fog, SO_2, and particles	Irritation, dyspnea, cough	Greatest number of deaths 4 days after start of fog
Donora, PA Octomber 1948	Cold fog, SO_2 particles, and H_2SO_4	Irritation of lower airways, dyspnea, cough	Greatest number of deaths 4 days after start of fog
London, England December 1952	Cold fog, coal burning	Bronchospasms, bronchial irritation, dyspnea	Greatest number of deaths 4 days after start of fog
Time series			
London, England 1963–1972	Winter, direct acid measurements	Daily mortality	Deaths lag acid by at least 1 day
Ontario, Canada 1974–1982	Winter and summer, long-distance transport events	Respiratory admissions	Admissions lag by 1 day
Yokkaichi, Japan 1974–1983	Local source of H_2SO_4 emissions	Annual mortality for bronchial asthma, chronic bronchitis	Bronchial asthma same year, chronic bronchitis lags 5 years

B. Donora, Pennsylvania: 1948

Donora, Pennsylvania, is an industrial town situated in the valley of the Monongahela River. At the time of the episode, the town had a steel and wire plant with blast furnaces and a zinc smelting plant that produced sulfuric acid as a byproduct. The population was about 14,000.

The air pollution episode occurred as a fog settled in the valley on Tuesday, October 26th, 1948. By October 28th, the fog was reported as very irritating to the senses. Many inhabitants reported respiratory illnesses starting on October 29th, but the magnitude of the event was not recognized until the 30th, when there were 17 deaths, followed by 2 more on the 31st. The episode was ended by rain starting on the afternoon of the 31st.

An extensive investigation by the American Public Health Service (Schrenk et al., 1949) found that 43% of the population, 5910 persons, reported some effect of the episode, with 10.5% being characterized as severely affected. The symptoms reported suggested irritation of the respiratory tract and other exposed mucous membranes. Cough was the most common symptom reported. Among the severely affected, shortness of breath was the most common complaint. Two-thirds of affected persons over 55 years of age reported dyspnea as a first symptom. The American Public Health Service report concluded that the larynx, trachea, and large bronchi were not affected, but that the irritating agents acted primarily upon the terminal bronchi, bronchioles, and lung parenchyma.

It was also concluded that sulfur oxides and their oxidation products, plus particulate matter were the major contributors to the observed excess mortality and morbidity. Hemeon (1955) examined the water-soluble fraction of solids on a filter of an electronic air cleaner operating during the episode and concluded that acid salts were an important component.

C. London, England: 1952

On Thursday, December 4, 1952, a slow-moving anticyclone came to a halt over the city of London (Brimblecombe, 1987). Fog developed over the city, and particulate and sulfur pollution began accumulating in the stagnating air mass. Smoke and sulfur dioxide concentrations built up over the following 3 days. On Monday, the pollution fog began to ease, and by Tuesday conditions were back to normal. Mortality records showed that deaths increased in a pattern very similar to that of the pollution measurements (Fig. 2). The maximum number of deaths occurred on the 4th day of the fog. Firket (1936) had estimated that if a pollutant fog were to occur in London similar to that which occurred in the Meuse Valley in 1930, there would be 3200 extra deaths. During the London fog episode of 1952, it was estimated that 4000 extra deaths occurred (Martin, 1964).

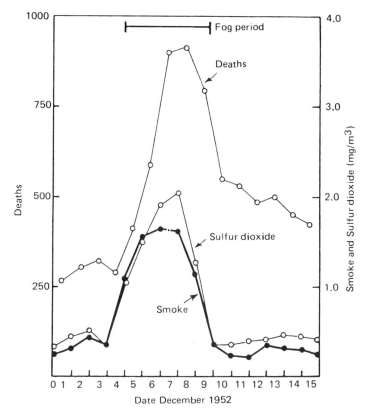

Figure 2 Deaths and pollutant concentrations during the London fog of 1952 (Wilkins, 1954).

The reports from hospital records and general practitioners' reports (Ministry of Health, 1954) indicate bronchial irritation, dyspnea, bronchospasm, and, in some cases, cyanosis among patients seen during the episode. There was a considerable increase in sudden deaths from respiratory and cardiovascular events. Evidence for irritation of the respiratory tract was found frequently.

Waller (1963) reported that sulfuric acid was one of the pollutants considered as a possible cause although no direct measurements were available. Various emergency control measures were attempted, but the only promising technique was placing wicked ammonia bottles in the hospital wards to neutralize the acid aerosols (Waller, 1987; Thurston et al., 1989). Many prize animals at the Smithfield Club's Show in London were affected with acute respiratory symptoms (Ministry of Health, 1954). Sixty cattle required major veterinary treatment, 1 died from suffocation, and 12 had to be destroyed. It has been suggested that the pens of the less affected animals were not frequently cleaned and the ammonia from the decomposing urine and feces neutralized the effects of the acid fog droplets (Meetham, 1964).

D. London, England: 1963–1972 Mortality Studies

Beginning in 1959, Commins and Waller (1967) began measuring aerosol acidity at a central London site. They reported these measurements as equivalent concentrations of sulfuric acid. Acid aerosol concentrations as high as 199 mg/m^3 for 24 hr in February, 1959, and 1 hr concentrations as high as 388 mg/m^3 in January of that year were reported. The highest reported mean sulfuric acid concentrations were a daily mean of 347 mg/m^3 and a 1 hr maximum of 678 mg/m^3 in December of 1962. During the winter of 1963–1964, they began regular daily measurements, which continued through the winter of 1971–1972.

Thurston and colleagues (1989) have compared daily mortality rates in greater London (MacFarlane, 1976) with daily sulfur dioxide, particulate (BS), and aerosol acidity measurements for the winters from 1963 through 1972. Preliminary analyses indicate that total daily mortality had a higher correlation with the log of aerosol acidity measured at the central sites on the previous day (r = 0.31) than with the log of SO$_2$ (r = 0.17) or with the log of particulate (BS) concentrations (r = 0.14). Significant correlations also were found with temperature, and significant autocorrelation was found, suggesting that a more thorough analysis will be required. Several authors have shown significant associations between mortality and city-averaged daily particulate and SO$_2$ concentrations in these data, even after controlling for confounders (Mazumdar et al., 1982; Ostro, 1984; Schwartz and Marcus, 1989). The analysis with direct aerosol acidity measurements suggests that these other pollutants may only have been surrogates for the more toxic acid concentrations.

E. Ontario, Canada

Bates and Sizto (1983, 1986, 1987) have studied the association of hospital admissions and air pollutant concentrations in southern Ontario between 1974 and 1983. Hospital admissions in all of the 79 acute care hospitals serving the region for 2 winter months, January and February, and 2 summer months, July and August, were classified by International Classification of Disease (ICD) code and age of the patient. Acute respiratory conditions were considered, as well as a group of nonrespiratory conditions for comparison.

In the initial analysis of the period 1974, 1976, 1977, and 1978 (Bates and Sizto, 1983), highly significant associations were found for the summer months between excess respiratory admissions and SO_2, O_3, and temperature, with 24 and 48 hr lags for the environmental variables. For the winter months, only temperature was associated with respiratory admissions. Incidence of nonrespiratory conditions was not associated with the environmental variables.

In subsequent analyses (Bates and Sizto, 1986; 1987), the period of record was extended through 1983, and every 6th day measurements of sulfate (SO_4) particle concentrations included. In these analysis SO_2, O_3, temperature, and SO_4 were correlated with respiratory admissions in the summer months. In a stepwise regression analysis, only SO_4 (lagged by 24 hr) was related to total respiratory admissions. This variable explained 3.5% of the variance in the summer respiratory admissions. Only temperature was associated with respiratory admissions during the winter months. Nonrespiratory conditions were not associated with the environmental variables. Overall asthma admissions were correlated with O_3 and SO_4 lagged by 24 and 48 hrs, but there were no significant correlations of asthma admissions with the environmental variables for children up to 14 years of age.

The average number of respiratory admissions was about 40/day in the summer period and 70/day in the winter. The maximum deviation from the expected number for the same day of the week in the same year in summer was 22 admissions per day.

The SO_4 concentrations were similar in the winter: overall mean 12.4 $\mu g/m^3$, and the summer, 13.3 $\mu g/m^3$. Yet hospital admissions were correlated with SO_4 in the summer but not in the winter. Bates and Sizto (1987) suggest that the health effect may be attributable neither to ozone nor to sulfates, but to some species that "travels" with them over the region in the summer but not in the winter.

Summer sulfates may be more acidic than those of winter. Air masses that have accumulated pollutants from the industrial midwest are often transported across the Great Lakes into Ontario. Secondary pollutants, including ozone, sulfates, and presumably acid aerosols, are produced photochemically. During the summer, the water of the Great Lakes is much cooler than the air moving across it. A surface inversion is formed that prevents the mixing of these secondary pollutants down to the surface, and that also prevents the mixing of neutralizing agents (e.g., ammonia) up from the surface. Thus the air mass may contain a layer of relatively unneutralized acid as it reaches the Canadian shore. Warming of the air mass as it moves over the land will produce fumigation conditions, which will bring this layer of acid aerosols down to the ground. This type of summer acid event was observed by Thurston and Waldman (1987) in Toronto. In contrast, during the winter months the lake water will be relatively warm, promoting vertical mixing, neutralization of the acid aerosol, and surface deposition as it moves over the lakes.

F. Yokkaichi, Japan

Imai and colleagues (1986) studied mortality in the population of Yokkaichi, Japan. They identified an area historically exposed to high sulfur oxide pollution from a nearby industrial complex and a control area in the same prefecture with much lower exposures. Deaths due to bronchial asthma and chronic bronchitis were extracted from ICD coding of death certificates for the 21 years from 1963 through 1983. Age-adjusted mortality rates were calculated for each year, separately for the polluted and non-polluted area. Three-year average mortality from bronchial asthma (Fig. 3) was higher in the polluted area during the period of maximum SO_x exposure and declined back to rates of bronchial asthma mortality characteristic of the nonpolluted area as SO_x levels declined. Mortality from bronchial asthma was highest among those 60 years of age or older: 130 deaths in the polluted area over the study for a rate of 64.7 deaths/10^5 person years, compared to 51.9/10^5 in the nonpolluted area. In the 3 years 1967–1970, mortality in this age group was significantly higher in the polluted area (81.7/10^5) than in the nonpolluted area (46.7/10^5). Between 1963 and 1983 mortality rates also were elevated among those less than 20 years of age in the polluted area (12 deaths, for a rate of 4.4/10^5) compared to the rate in the nonpolluted area (1 death, for a rate of 0.4/10^5). Six of these deaths were reported between 1967 and 1970.

Mortality rates from chronic bronchitis were elevated in the polluted area, but with a lag between SO_x exposure and chronic bronchitis mortality of 4–5 years (Fig. 3). Mortality from chronic bronchitis was primarily among those 60 years or older (116 deaths for a rate of 57.7/10^5 in the polluted area and 30 deaths, 33.8/10^5, in the nonpolluted area). In the 3 years 1971–1974, the difference in rates was 74.9/10^5 in the polluted area versus 17.5/10^5 in the nonpolluted area.

The sulfur oxide concentrations during this period were measured by the lead peroxide method, which is a nonspecific measure of all forms of sulfur pollution, both gaseous and particulate. The Yokkaichi study is of interest because in 1969, when some of the highest sulfur pollution values were observed, Kitagawa (1984) directly measured suspended acid mist in the polluted area described by Imai and colleagues. Kitagawa attributes the acid mists to direct emissions of sulfuric acid mist from specific industries within the industrial complex. Thus the Yokkaichi study shows a temporal correlation of general sulfur oxide level and concurrent bronchial asthma mortality and chronic bronchitis mortality 4–5 years later, and it shows

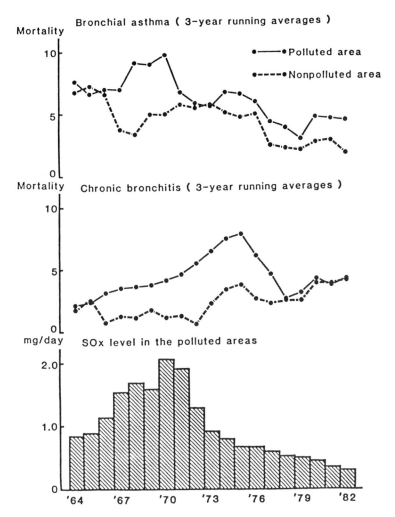

Figure 3 Comparison of SO$_x$ levels and age-adjusted mortality due to bronchial asthma and chronic bronchitis in Yokkaichi, Japan (Imai et al., 1986).

documented acid aerosol exposures during the period of elevated mortality rates.

IV. Controlled Exposure Studies

The epidemiological studies suggest that acid aerosols may aggravate symptoms among subjects with compromised respiratory function. The primary mechanism appears to be irritation of the airways, producing increased symptom reporting and morbidity soon after exposure, and leading to death among apparently sensitive individuals within a few days of initial exposure.

In controlled exposure studies of humans, no changes in pulmonary function have been observed among *normal* subjects after acute exposures to H_2SO_4 of up to 1000 $\mu g/m^3$ (Utell, 1985). However, it appears that "susceptible" subgroups can be identified who are acutely responsive to the effects of H_2SO_4.

Adolescent asthmatics with exercise-induced bronchospasm showed reductions in FEV_1, $Vmax_{50}$, and total resistance after exposure to 100 $\mu g/m^3$ H_2SO_4 during exercise (Fig. 4) (Koenig et al., 1983). Adult asthmatics

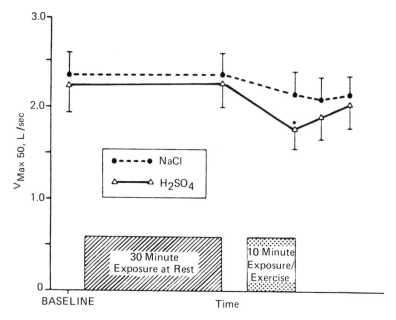

Figure 4   Mean change ($\pm$ SE) in $Vmax_{50}$ in 10 asthmatic adolescent subjects before, during, and following exposure to NaCl and H_2SO_4 aerosols (Koenig et al., 1983).

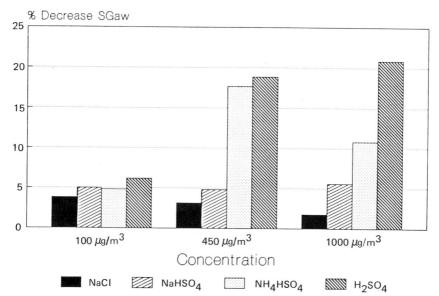

Figure 5 Percentage change in specific airway conductance (SGaw) in 17 asthmatic subjects exposed for 16 min to various sulfate aerosols (after Utell et al., 1983a).

exposed to 450 and 1000 $\mu g/m^3$ H_2SO_4 had reduced specific airway conductance (SG_{aw}) and FEV_1 (Utell et al., 1983a). Exposure to different sulfate aerosols showed that the degree of bronchoconstriction increased with increasing acidity (Fig. 5): H_2SO_4 > NH_4SO_4 > $NaHSO_4$ > $NaCl$. Individual change in SGaw in response to 1000 $\mu g/m^3$ H_2SO_4 was highly correlated with response of 14 ofthese asthmatic subjects to 0.025% carbachol (Fig. 6).

Thus subgroups of the population with demonstrated response to other bronchoconstrictive stimuli have shown significant acute bronchoconstriction following exposure to acid aerosols. These responses are consistent with the observed mortality and morbidity effects observed in epidemiological studies.

Acute exposures of rabbits to sulfuric acid at low concentrations have shown the mean residence time (MRT) in the bronchial region to decrease (i.e., clearance rate increases) following single 1-hr exposures, and MRT to increase (i.e., clearance rate decreases) at higher concentrations (Fig. 7) (Schlesinger et al., 1984). Similar effects were observed among human subjects (Fig. 8) (Leikauf et al., 1981). Studies with other sulfate aerosols (Schlesinger, 1984) indicated that the relative potency was H_2SO_4 > NH_4HSO_4 > $(NH_4)_2SO_4$ or

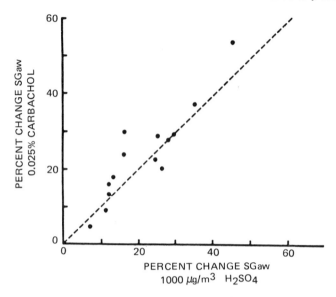

Figure 6   Comparison of change in SGaw after 0.025% carbachol and 1000 μg/m³ sulfuric acid among 14 asthmatic subjects (Utell et al., 1983a).

Na_2SO_4. Since response increased with the strength of these acids, it suggests that the hydrogen ion (H^+) concentration may be the important factor in determining the degree of response.

Proper functioning of the mucociliary transport system requires optimal beating of the cilia and mucus with the appropriate properties. Schlesinger (1985) has suggested that the acceleration of clearance at low concentrations of acid and retardation at higher concentrations may reflect separate effects on the mucus and the cilia. Holma and associates (1977) have shown that acidity "stiffens" the mucus blanket, and therefore may promote the clearance mechanisms. This may occur at low concentrations of acid. At higher concentrations, H_2SO_4 depresses ciliary beat frequency (Holma et al., 1977; Schiff et al., 1979; Grose et al., 1980). Thus, H^+-induced depression of ciliary beating could produce the observed retardation of clearance at higher concentrations.

While the long-term sequelae of these alterations of bronchial clearance are not clear, it is interesting to note that earlier studies have shown that cigarette smoke similarly stimulates mucociliary clearance at low exposures while slowing it at higher concentrations (Albert et al., 1974, 1975).

In the alveolar region, acute exposures of rabbits to sulfuric acid did not increase the number of alveolar macrophages recovered by lavage

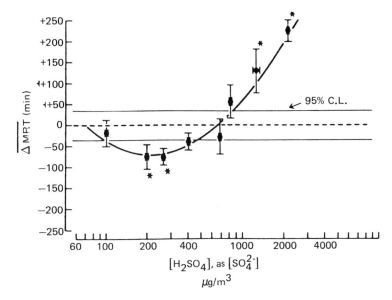

Figure 7 Change in mean residence time (MRT) of tracer particles in rabbits following 1 hr exposures to H_2SO_4 aerosols (Schlesinger et al., 1984).

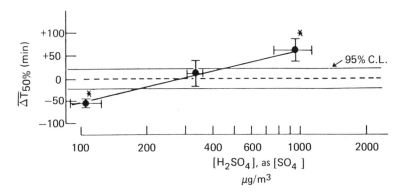

Figure 8 Change in bronchial clearance half-time of tracer particles in humans following 1 hr exposures to H_2SO_4 aerosols (Schlesinger et al., 1984).

(Naumann and Schlesinger, 1985; Shellito and Murphy, 1980), but did significantly increase the number of neutrophils recovered (Shellito and Murphy, 1980) especially between 12 and 24 hr after exposure (Naumann and Schlesinger, 1985). Recruitment of neutrophils is evidence of an inflammatory response. Such a response should not necessarily be considered beneficial, since these cells are involved in the pivotal balance between defense and disease (Schlesinger, 1985). Although the major function of the macrophages is protective, these cells are likely to be involved in the pathogenesis of two classes of chronic disease: interstitial fibrosis and emphysema (Albert et al., 1969; Hunninghake et al., 1979; Brain, 1980; Warheit et al., 1984; Bitterman et al., 1981).

These acute controlled exposures studies give some indication of the mechanisms of, but do not model the exposures of the general population to, ambient exposures. In the classic air pollution episodes, acid concentrations were elevated for several days. It is also clear that the population in these events and in more recent epidemiological studies was repeatedly exposed to low level acid events. The evidence from repeated controlled exposures is therefore especially important.

Repeated low-level exposures of rabbits to sulfuric acid (250 $\mu g/m^3$ for 1 hr, 5 days/week) led to reduced bronchial mucociliary clearance after 4 months of exposure (Gearhart and Schlesinger, 1988). Clearance rates remained depressed even 3 months after the end of the 1 year of repeated exposures. Histological examination of rabbits sacrificed at regular intervals over the course of the experiment showed that the thickness of the epithelia of the small conducting airways was significantly increased, and the number of airways containing epithelial secretory cells was significantly increased after only 1 month of exposure (Schlesinger et al., 1983). Persistent impairment of clearance may increase susceptibility to acute or chronic respiratory disease (Schlesinger, 1985). The appearance of increased secretory cells due to H_2SO_4 exposure is significant since excess mucus production in small airways may be an early feature in the pathogenesis of chronic bronchitis (Hogg et al., 1968).

In addition to producing bronchoconstriction acutely among "susceptible" individuals, there is evidence that H_2SO_4 exposures may promote the development of bronchial hyperreactivity. Normal human subjects exposed to 450 $\mu g/m^3$ H_2SO_4 for 4 hrs during exercise showed no change in pulmonary function immediately following or 24 hrs after inhalation. However, 24 hrs after exposure there was a significant enhancement of carbachol bronchoconstrictive response compared to that following an innocuous exposure (Utell et al., 1983b).

Previously healthy rabbits have been shown to become responsive to acetylcholine challenge following repeated exposures to H_2SO_4 (Gearhart

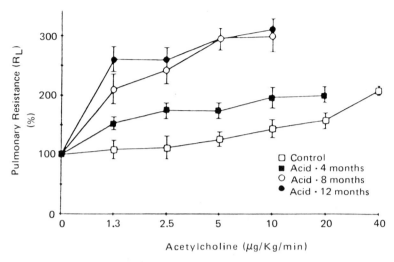

Figure 9 Effect of repeated exposures to H_2SO_4 aerosol on serial bronchoprovocation challenge of pulmonary resistance (R_L) of rabbits. Data are group mean ($\pm$ SE) percentage of baseline R_L for each dose (Gearhart and Schlesinger, 1986).

and Schlesinger, 1986). Group mean pulmonary resistance (R_L) increased in response to bronchoprovocation (Fig. 9) after 4 and 8 months of acid exposure (250 mg/m^3 for 1 hr, 5 days/week). Thus, exposure to acid aerosol not only may produce bronchoconstriction among susceptible individuals, but also repeated exposures may produce hyperreactivity, and therefore sensitivity to H_2SO_4, among previously normal individuals.

The role of airway reactivity in the pathogenesis of COPD is still actively debated (see Chapter 9). Orie et al. (1961) proposed that increased airway reactivity and COPD are manifestations of the same disease. Several epidemiological studies have shown that annual decline of FEV_1 is faster among subjects with asthma (Peat et al., 1987) or with airway hyperreactivity (Barter and Campbell, 1976; Britt et al., 1980). Fish and Menkes (1984) have noted that this association could be based on the observed association of airway reactivity with cigarette smoking or allergy, both of which have been implicated as risk factors for COPD (Burrows et al., 1976). Thus, although the linkage between acid aerosol exposure, promotion of airway hyperreactivity and development of COPD must be considered speculative, it offers an interesting hypothesis for future epidemiological studies.

V. Summary

That acid aerosols present a significant risk of respiratory problems has been hypothesized for many years. Local irritation of the epithelium of the respiratory tract by small droplets of acid may produce a wide range of reversible responses, including aggravation of respiratory symptoms in subjects with COPD, and possibly irreversible responses, such as the promotion of COPD development.

The historic air pollution episodes in the Meuse Valley, Donora, Pennsylvania, and London were all characterized by a stagnating air mass with fog and a buildup of sulfur oxide and particulate pollution. These conditions have been shown to produce catalyzed oxidation of sulfur oxides either on particles or in fog droplets to form acid aerosols. Photochemical processes were apparently not important in these fall and winter events. Commins and Waller (1967) have observed sulfuric acid concentrations greater than 100 $\mu g/m^3$ several years later under similar conditions in London.

While these air pollution episodes occurred several decades ago, it should not be assumed that such events are no longer a problem. Much higher air pollution exposures are routinely observed in developing countries (de Koning et al., 1986), and significant episodes are still observed in developed countries, such as in western Europe in January of 1985 (Wichmann et al., 1989). Moreover, the analysis of the London air pollution episodes by Schwartz and Marcus (1989) indicates that excess mortality can be expected even at much lower levels of particulates and sulfur oxides. These winter episodes are rare because they require a stagnating air mass, with fog, in an area of substantial emissions of sulfur oxides. The region of impact is usually very limited but the effects can be dramatic.

Summer acid events due to photochemical reactions have been observed in Ontario (Thurston and Waldman, 1987), other locations in eastern North America, and in the Los Angeles basin. Excess hospital admissions, in particular excess asthma-related admissions in southern Ontario, have been shown to correlate with summer ozone and sulfate concentrations (Bates and Sizto, 1983, 1986). Based on the atmospheric chemistry, these should be indicators that photochemical oxidation of SO_x and NO_x is taking place. Such acid episodes may have important public health implications because the transported air masses are very large (many hundreds of miles across) and although exposure and effects may be small, the numbers of people exposed will be large. It appears that acid aerosols and ozone occur frequently in otherwise clean air downwind from urban areas and source regions.

In summary, the epidemiological data are only suggestive because measurements of actual acid aerosol exposure are limited. In many respects, the epidemiological research has been led by the technology available for monitoring these pollutants. This is despite the hypothesis first proposed more than 50 years ago that sulfuric acid was the most important component of the mix of pollutants responsible for increased morbidity and mortality in the classic air pollution episodes.

Acknowledgments

Preparation of this manuscript was supported by National Institute of Environmental Health Sciences Grants ES-0002, ES-01108, and ES-04595, Environmental Protection Agency Cooperative Agreement CR 811650, Electric Power Research Institute Contract RP-1001, and the Department of National Health and Welfare, Canada. Dr. Dockery was supported in part by a Mellon Foundation Faculty Development Award. This report has not been subjected to the Environmental Protection Agency's required peer and policy review and therefore does not necessarily reflect the views of the Agency, and no official endorsement should be inferred.

References

Albert, R. E., Lippmann, M., and Briscoe, W. (1969). The characteristics of bronchial clearance in humans and the effects of cigarette smoking. *Arch. Environ. Health* **18**:738–755.

Albert, R. E., Berger, J., Sanborn, K., and Lippmann, M. (1974). Effects of cigarette smoke components on bronchial clearance in the donkey. *Arch. Environ. Health* **29**:96–101.

Albert, R. E., Peterson, H. T., Jr., Bohning, D., and Lippmann, M. (1975). Short-term effects of cigarette smoking on bronchial clearance in humans. *Arch. Environ. Health* **30**:361–367.

Barter, C. E., and Campbell, A. H. (1976). Relationship of constitutional factors and cigarette smoking to decrease in 1-second forced expiratory volume. *Am. Rev. Respir. Dis.* **113**:305–314.

Bates, D. V., and Sizto, R. (1983). Relationship between air pollution levels and hospital admissions in southern Ontario. *Can. J. Publ. Health* **74**:117–122.

Bates, D. V., and Sizto, R. (1986). A study of hospital admissions and air pollutants in southern Ontario. In *Aerosols*. Edited by S. D. Lee, T. Schneider, L. D. Grant, and P. J. Verkerk. Lewis, Chelsea, MI, pp. 767–777.

Bates, D. V., and Sizto, R. (1987). Air pollution and hospital admissions in southern Ontario: the acid summer haze effect. *Environ. Res.* **43**:317–331.

Bitterman, P. B., Rennard, S. I., and Crystal, R. B. (1981). Environmental lung disease and the interstitium. *Chest Med.* **2**:393–412.

Bock, N., Lippmann, M., Lioy, P., Munoz, A., and Speizer, F. E. (1985). The effects of ozone on the pulmonary function of children. In *Evaluation of the Scientific Basis for Ozone/Oxidants Standards: Proceedings of an APCA International Specialty Conference*; November 1984; Houston, TX. Edited by S. D. Lee. Air Pollution Control Association, Pittsburgh, PA; pp. 297–308.

Brain, J. D. (1980). Macrophage damage in relation to the pathogenesis of lung disease. *Environ. Health Perspect.* **35**:21–28.

Britt, J., Cohen, B., Menkes, H. A., Bleeker, E., Permutt, S., Rosenthal, R., and Norman, P. 1980). Airways reactivity and functional deterioration in relatives of COPD patients. *Chest* **77** (Suppl):260–261.

Brimblecombe, P. (1987). *The Big Smoke: A History of Air Pollution in London Since Medieval Times*. Methuen & Co., London, p. 161.

Burrows, B., Lebowitz, M. D., and Barbee, R. A. (1976). Respiratory disorders and allergy skin test reactions. *Ann. Intern. Med.* **84**:134–139.

Calvert, J. G., Lazrus, A., Kok, G. L., Heikes, B. G., Walega, J. G., Lind, J., and Cantrell C. A. (1985). Chemical mechanisms of acid generation in the troposphere. *Nature* **317**:27–35.

Commins, B. T., and Waller, R. E. (1967). Observations from a ten-year study of pollution at a site in the city of London. *Atmos. Environ.* **1**:49–68.

de Koning, H. W., Kretzschmar, J. G., Akland, G. G., and Bennett, B. G. (1986). Air pollution in different cities around the world. *Atmos. Environ.* **20**:101–113.

Ferek, R. J., Lazrus, A. L., Haagenson, P. L., and Winchester, J. W. (1983). Strong and weak acidity of aerosols collected over the northeastern United States. *Environ. Sci. Tech.* **17**:315–323.

Ferris, B. G. Jr. and Spengler J. D. (1985). Problems in the estimation of of human exposure to components of acid precipitation precursors. *Envir. Health Perspect.* **63**:5–9.

Firket, M. (1931). Sur les causes des accients survenus dans la vallée de la Meuse, lors des brouillards de decembre 1930. (The causes of accidents which occurred in the Meuse Valley during the fogs of December 1930). *Bull. Acad. R. Med. Belg.* **11**(Ser 5):683–741.

Firket, J. (1936). Fog along the Meuse Valley. *Trans. Faraday Soc.* **32**: 1192–1197.

Fish, J. E., and Menkes H. A. (1984). Airway reactivity: role in acute and chronic disease. In *Current Pulmonology*, Vol. 5. Edited by D. H. Simmons. New York, pp. 169–199.

Gearhart, J. M., and Schlesinger, R. B. (1986). Sulfuric acid-induced airway hyperresponsiveness. *Fundament. Appl. Toxicol.* **7**:681–689.

Gearhart, J. M., and Schlesinger, R. B. (1988). Response of the tracheobronchial mucociliary clearance system to repeated irritant exposure: effect of sulfuric acid mist on function and structure. *Exp. Lung Res.* **14**:587–605.

Grose, E. C., Gardner, D. E., and Miller, F. J. (1980). Response of ciliated epithelium to ozone and sulfuric acid. *Environ. Res.* **22**:377–385.

Hemeon, W. C. L. (1955). The estimation of health hazards from air pollution. *Arch. Ind. Health* **41**:29–35.

Hogg, J. D., Macklem, P. T., and Thurlbeck, W. W. (1968). Site and nature of airway obstruction in obstructive lung disease. *N. Engl. J. Med.* **278**:1355–1360.

Holma, B., Lindegre, M., and Anderson, J. M. (1977). pH effects on ciliomotility and morphology of respiratory mucosa. *Arch. Environ. Health* **32**:216–226.

Hunninghake, G. W., Gadek, J. E., Kawanami, J. E., et al. (1979). Inflammatory and immune processes in the human lung in health and disease: evaluation by bronchoalveolar lavage. *Am. J. Pathol.* **97**:149–205.

Imai, M., Katsumi, Y., and Kitagawa, M. (1986). Mortality from asthma and chronic bronchitis associated with changes in sulfur oxides air pollution. *Arch. Environ. Health* **41**:29–35.

Kitagawa, T. (1984). Cause analysis of the Yokkaichi asthma episode in Japan. *J. Air Pollution Control Assoc.* **34**:743–746.

Koenig, J. Q., Pierson, W. E., and Horike, M. (1983). The effect of inhaled sulfuric acid on pulmonary function in adolescent asthmatics. *Am. Rev. Respir. Dis.* **128**:221–225, 1983.

Leikauf, G., Yeates, D. B., Wales, K. A., et al. (1981). Effects of sulfuric acid aerosol on respiratory mechanics and mucociliary particle clearance in healthy nonsmoking adults. *Am. Ind. Hyg. Assoc. J.* **43**:273–282.

Lioy, P. J., Vollmuth, T. A., and Lippmann, M. (1985). Persistence of peak flow decrement in children following ozone exposures exceeding the national ambient air quality standard. *J. Air Pollution Control Assoc.* **35**:1068–1071.

Lippmann, M. (1985). Airborne acidity: Estimates of exposure and human health effects. *Environ. Health Perspect.* **63**:63–70.

MacFarlane, A. (1976). Daily deaths in greater London. *Population Trends,* **20**.

Martin, A. E. (1964). Mortality and morbidity statistics and air pollution. *Proc. R. Soc. Med.* **57**:969.

Maugh, T. H., II. (1984). Acid rain's effects on people assessed. *Science* **226**:1408–1410.

Mazumdar, S., Schimmel, H., and Higgins, I. T. T. (1982). Relation of daily mortality to air pollution: an analysis of 14 London winters, 1958/59–1971/72. *Arch. Environ.. Health* **37**:213–220.

Meetham, A. R. (1964). *Atmospheric Pollution.* Pergamon Press, Oxford, p. 231.

Ministry of Health (1954). *Mortality and Morbidity during the London fog of December 1952. Reports on Public Health and Medical Subjects no. 95.* Her Majesty's Stationery Office, London.

Naumann, B. D., and Schlesinger, R. B. (1985). Assessment of early alveolar and macrophage function following acute oral inhalation exposures to sulfuric acid mists. *Toxicologist* **5**:180; 1985.

Orie, N. G. M., Sluter, H. J., DeVries, K., et al., (1961). The host factor in bronchitis. In *Bronchitis.* Edited by N. G. M. Orie and H. J. Sluter. Royal Vangorum, Assen, The Netherlands, pp. 43–59.

Ostro, B. (1984). A search for a threshold in the relationship of air pollution to mortality: a reanalysis of data on London winters. *Environ. Health Perspect.* **58**:397–399.

Peat, J. K., Woolcock, A. J., and Cullen, K. (1987). Rate of decline of lung function in subjects with asthma. *Eur. J. Respir. Dis.* **70**:171–179.

Schiff, L. J., Byrne, M. M., Fenters, J. D., Graham, J. A., and Gardner, D. E. (1980). Cytotoxic effects of sulfuric acid mist, carbon particulates and their mixtures on hamster tracheal epithelium. *Environ. Res.* **22**:377–385.

Schlesinger, R. B., Naumann, B. D., and Chen, L. C. (1983). Physiological and histological alterations in the bronchial mucociliary clearance system of rabbits following intermittent oral and nasal inhalation of sulfuric acid mist. *J. Toxicol. Environ. Health* **12**:441–465.

Schlesinger, R. B., Chen, L. C., and Driscoll, K. E. (1984). Exposure–response relationship of bronchial mucociliary clearance in rabbits following acute inhalations of sulfuric acid mist. *Toxicol. Lett.* **22**:249–254.

Schlesinger, R. B. (1984). Comparative irritant potency of inhaled sulfate aerosols: effects on bronchial mucociliary clearance. *Environ. Res.* **34**:268–279.

Schlesinger, R. B. (1985). Effects of inhaled acids on respiratory tract defense mechanisms. *Environ. Health Perspect.* **63**:25–38.

Schwartz, J., and Marcus, A. H. (1989). Mortality and air pollution in London. A time series analysis. *Am. J. Epidemiol.* (submitted).

Shellito, J., and Murphy, S. (1980). The effect of experimental acid aspiration on alveolar macrophage function in rabbits. *Am. Rev. Respir. Dis.* **122**:551–560.

Shrenk, H. H., Heimann, H., Clayton, G. D., Gafafer, W. M., and Wexler, H. (1949). Air pollution in Donora, PA: epidemiology of the unusual smog episode of October 1948, Preliminary report. Public Health Bulletin No. 306. Public Health Service, Washington, D.C.

Spektor, D. M., Lippmann, M., Lioy, P. J., Thurston, G. D., Citak, K., James, D. J., Bock, N., Speizer, F. E., and Hayes, C. (1988). Effects of ambient ozone on respiratory function in active normal children. *Am. Rev. Respir. Dis.* **137**:313-320.

Tanner, R. L., Kumar, R., and Johnson, S. (1984). Vertical distribution of aerosol strong acidity in the atmosphere. *J. Geophys. Res.* **89**:7149-7157.

Thurston, G. D., and Waldman, J. (1987). Acid aerosol transport episodes in Toronto, Ontario. Paper 87-89.9; Presented at Annual Meeting of Air Pollution Control Association, New York, June 21-26, 1987.

Thurston, G. D., Ito, K., Lippmann, M., and Hayes, C. (1989). Re-examination of London, England mortality in relation to exposure to acidic aerosols during the 1963-1972 winters. Presented at International Symposium on Health Effects of Acid Aerosols, Research Triangle Park, NC Oct 19-21, 1987. *Environ. Health Perspect* **79**:73-82.

Utell, M. J., Morrow, P. E., Speers, D. M., et al. (1983a). Airway responses to sulfate and sulfuric acid aerosols in asthmatics: an exposure–response relationship. *Am. Rev. Respir. Dis.* **128**:444-450.

Utell, M. J., Morrow, P. E., and Hyde, R. W. (1983b). Latent development of airway hyperreactivity in human subjects after sulfuric acid aerosol exposure. *J. Aerosol Sci.* **14**:202-205.

Utell, M. J. (1985). Effects of inhaled acid aerosols on lung mechanics: an analysis of human exposure studies. *Environ. Health Perspect.* **63**:39-44.

Waller, R. E. (1963). Acid droplets in town air. *Int. J. Air Water Pollution* **7**:773.

Waller, R. E. (1987). Urban air pollution and health, the changing scene: a personal reminiscence. Presented at International Conference, Air Pollution Control in European Metropoli. Berlin, 30 Sept-2 Oct 1987.

Warheit, D. V., Chang, L. Y., Hill, L. H., et al. (1984). Pulmonary macrophage accumulation and asbestos-induced lesions at sites of fiber deposition. *Am. Rev. Respir. Dis.* **129**:301-310.

Wichmann, H. E., Mueller, W., and Allhoff, P. (1988). Health effects during a smog episode in West Germany in 1985. Presented at International Symposium on Health Effects of Acid Aerosols, Research Triangle Park, NC Oct 19-21, 1987. *Environ. Health Perspect.* **79**:89-100.

Wilkins, E. T. (1954). Air pollution aspects of the London fog of December 1952. *Q. J. R. Meteorol. Soc.* **80**:267-271.

11

Occupation and Chronic Airflow Limitation

ERIC GARSHICK

Brockton/West Roxbury VA Medical Center
Brigham and Women's Hospital
Harvard Medical School
Boston, Massachusetts

MARC B. SCHENKER

University of California School
of Medicine
Davis, California

I. Introduction

In contrast to the "classic" occupational lung diseases such as asbestosis and silicosis, chronic obstructive pulmonary disease (COPD) continues to be a major source of morbidity and mortality in the United States (Becklake, 1985). Previously, there had not been sufficient evidence to consider occupational exposure to certain dust and fumes to be related to decline in ventilatory function and contributing to clinical COPD occurrence. The current evidence for this relationship will be reviewed in this chapter.

The finding of an accelerated decline in FEV_1, or of an increased prevalence of airflow obstruction in a population, represents a common endpoint attributable to many possible factors, and epidemiological methods are used to identify risk factors. Active cigarette smoking is the environmental exposure most responsible for COPD and must be assessed in epidemiological studies together with the effects of occupational exposures. In blue-collar populations, where occupational exposure to dust and fumes is more prevalent than in white-collar groups, smoking rates generally exceed the rates in white-collar groups (U.S.D.H.H.S., 1985). Concomitant cigarette smoking may modify the effects of occupational exposure (Greaves and Schenker, 1987). In workers who smoke, occupational exposure may result in an effect equal to the effect of the two exposures occurring separately (additive), or an effect greater than expected due to each exposure occurring alone (synergism). A synergism is seen with lung cancer and some occupational lung carcinogens such as asbestos (U.S.D.H.S.S., 1984), but studies reviewed in this chapter indicate that smoking and occupational exposure act most often in an additive fashion to cause a decrement in lung function.

Host factors also may play an important role in determining the effects of occupational exposure, but these factors need to be studied further. For example, workers most susceptible to the effects of cigarette smoking may be similarly more susceptible to an occupational exposure (Hurley and Soutar, 1986). Although decrements in pulmonary function due to occupational exposure are in general less than those due to smoking, in workers with lung function affected by smoking, an additional decrement due to occupation could be clinically important (Marine et al., 1988).

II. Method of Study

A. Study Design

The observed relationship between occupational exposure and ventilatory function is greatly influenced by the method of study. An epidemiological study may fail to detect the true effect of an occupational exposure for a variety of reasons, which may be classified into issues relating to population selection and study design, and relating to the index of exposure measurement used (Tockman, 1982). In the past, mostly cross-sectional or prevalence studies were done to detect occupational pulmonary disease in actively employed workers. A problem with this type of study is that only healthy workers who were physically fit tended to remain at work to be surveyed. Workers ill due to occupational exposure may have already left the work force, as has been observed in workers exposed to cotton dust (Merchant et al., 1973a). Older workers with the opportunity for the most significant exposure may also have other reasons for leaving active employment such as industry layoffs, thus making such a study difficult. In addition, Kauffmann and co-workers (1982) found that younger workers (aged 30–39) in a cohort of Paris workers exposed to dust actually had a higher FEV_1 at the start of a longitudinal study than did unexposed workers of the same age. Thus, exposed workers in some cases might initially be healthier than unexposed workers, which could influence the findings in a cross-sectional survey. Graham and co-workers (1984) in a cross-sectional survey found similarly that currently active potash workers (exposed to potash dust and diesel exhaust fumes) had slightly better pulmonary function than an unexposed comparison group, despite having more bronchitic symptoms. Active steelworkers also had higher values for FEV_1 and FEV_1/FVC compared to an otherwise similar control group at the start of a longitudinal study (Pham et al., 1979).

Cross-sectional surveys may also not detect the effects of an occupational exposure or may minimize the possible effect of an exposure because only the mean level of function in a group of workers is reported. A minority of workers who may be most susceptible to the effects of an exposure might not be detected (Hurley and Soutar, 1986; Becklake et al., 1987). Hurley and Soutar (1986) examined a subgroup of 199 men who had left the coal industry before normal retirement age and found an effect of dust exposure more severe than the average effect previously reported among other miners. In a cross-sectional survey in grain handlers (Chan-Yeung et al., 1980), a small decrement in FEV_1 between grain workers and a comparison group was found. Later follow-up studies (Tabona et al., 1984; Enarson et al., 1985) identified a subgroup of grain handlers with a large annual decline in FEV_1 (> 100 ml/year). Host characteristics identified in these workers and others with a large decrease in FEV_1 were bronchial hyperreactivity (studied at follow-up) and a decline in FEV_1 over a work week. These most severely affected workers were also more likely to have jobs with the highest dust exposure in the grain terminal.

Annual changes in lung function estimated by cross-sectional methods are also susceptible to "cohort" effects that could distort a relationship between pulmonary function and exposure. An effect on lung function unaccounted for by aging or smoking and attributed to occupational exposure, may be observed only because a subject lived in an earlier era and might not be due to the exposure (Glindmeyer et al., 1982).

The longitudinal study has the advantage that pulmonary function measurements (change in pulmonary function) are compared within individuals. This excludes the effects of between-individual variation in pulmonary function unaccounted for by age, height, and smoking that can obscure smaller effects due to occupation (Becklake, 1985). However, a longitudinal study may be insensitive to the effects of an exposure in the past if that exposure no longer influences changes in lung function (Glindmeyer et al., 1982). Complete follow-up of the groups under study, and adequate quality control of the spirometric measurements (Graham et al., 1981) are important in ensuring an ability to detect an effect if one is present. An additional possible pitfall with longitudinal studies is that expected annual declines in FEV_1 (i.e., in the range of 20–40 ml/year in nonsmokers [Fletcher et al., 1976; Glindmeyer et al., 1982; Burrows et al., 1986]) are relatively small in relation to the measurement error of the test (Burrows et al., 1986; Jones, 1984). Therefore follow-up periods of 1–2 years are inadequate to estimate annual change in function. It is also preferable to have more than one follow-up measurement to reduce any source of systematic error (Glindmeyer et al., 1987).

Community-based cross-sectional studies have the advantage of including all individuals without the potential for exclusion based on disability or illness. To assess the health effects of an exposure however, recruitment into the study must be population based and not dependent on health outcome. A case–control design involving community-based cases of respiratory disease has also been used (Kjuus et al., 1981).

B. Exposure Estimation

A weakness of occupational respiratory epidemiology has been the paucity of exposure data in the majority of studies. Methods of estimating exposure should be used that will result in an exposure index representative of the dose actually received by an individual. In workers exposed to dust, measurement of respirable particles (generally less than 5 μm in diameter) is a common component of exposure indices (Dodgson, 1984). Larger particles, but still less than 10–15 μm, are deposited in the tracheobronchial region, whereas the smaller respirable particles are deposited more distally. The measurement of total dust concentration alone might not reflect variations in level of respirable particles. Indeed, measurement of respirable particulate obtained by sampling the general work area may be different from measurements obtained at the breathing zone of workers with personal sampling devices. The composition of the dust may also vary among workers, affecting its biological activity. The dust collected as an index of exposure may also represent a mixture of respirable dusts from a variety of sources, including from cigarette particles or other environmental sources (Woskie et al., 1988), which could confound the measurement of respirable particles attributable to an occupational exposure. It is also not possible to sample every worker in every job, so that representative sampling of workers within a range of job categories must be done, and sufficient measurements made to account for variability in job exposure (Brunekreef et al., 1987).

In some coal and gold mining industry studies, records exist to allow the estimation of a workers' lifetime dust exposure that are suitable for use in epidemiological studies. An index of exposure can be developed that includes the measurement of respirable particles multiplied by a time factor (e.g., years or shifts worked at a particular exposure level). In cross-sectional studies the assumption is usually made that the biological response measured (i.e., level of ventilatory function) is related to the total amount of respirable particles potentially inhaled by a worker. However, the quality of the exposure may vary over a worker's lifetime, such that dust generated during a past period was a more significant health hazard due to its nature. In longitudinal studies, past dust exposure as well as intersurvey dust levels have been used as exposure models (Attfield, 1985; Love and Miller, 1982). The selection of the exposure index used is dependent on the hypothesis under study relating exposure to ventilatory function.

In most industries, however, no past exposure data exist or only inadequate estimates of past exposure are available. Industrial hygiene measurements of current occupational exposure may be the only quantitative measurements available. It also has been a common practice to assume that all workers in an industry (e.g., "coalminers" or "steelworkers") are similarly exposed without recognition of the differences in actual exposure (Wang and Miettinen, 1982). The use of current exposure measurements, current industry/job classification, or years worked in an industry as a surrogate for actual exposure can fail to account for historical trends in exposure intensity and quality. The acceptability of qualitative exposure measurements in an epidemiological study must be assessed based on the group under study. If exposure is homogeneous and jobs are stable in an industry, the use of years "exposed" compared to "unexposed" may be acceptable to determine a relative risk of disease, but may not be suitable to set standards for limiting exposure. It has been suggested that dose–response investigations using years of work should be limited to subgroups of the study population with uniform exposure (Johnson, 1986). Within occupational title job groups, exposure may also vary. In the railroad industry, workers in the diesel engine repair shop exposed to diesel particles had the same job codes (which served as a surrogate of exposure) as workers in other shop areas who were not exposed to diesel particles (Garshick et al., 1987). Uncertainty in the categorization of exposure that results in confusing workers who are exposed with those who are unexposed will make it more difficult to detect an effect of an exposure and will reduce the magnitude of the effect measured.

The source of qualitative exposure data is important. Ideally, exposure information such as job history should be obtained independently of disease outcome, such as from work records in a retrospective study, or be obtained in a prospective fashion. Blinded interview techniques may also minimize recall bias in interviews of exposed and unexposed workers, or healthy and sick workers, if an exposure history must be obtained by interview (Tockman, 1982). The use of objective outcome measurements, such as lung function measurements, or respiratory symptoms elicited after the exposure history, might also minimize this potential for recall bias (Korn et al., 1987).

Similar difficulty exists in the measurement of cigarette smoking but because there are usually stronger pulmonary effects of smoking relative to occupational exposure, the consequences of misclassification of exposure to cigarette smoke on the ability to detect an effect due to smoking are less significant. The usual recording of current and average daily cigarette consumption also does not reflect changes in cigarette brand, differences in smoke inhalation, and temporal changes in tobacco content. FEV_1 level in cross-sectional studies has been found to be dependent on indices of cumulative cigarette consumption, such as pack-years (Burrows et al., 1977; Marine et al., 1988) or duration of smoking and amount smoked daily (Beck et al., 1981). Studies not considering an index of cigarettes smoked may be not adequately assessing the full effect of smoking on lung function.

III. Occupation and Mucus Hypersecretion

In early cross-sectional surveys among dust-exposed workers, large groups of miners and foundry workers were examined and found to have an excess of bronchitic symptoms (i.e., mucus hypersecretion) beyond rates attributable to smoking alone (Gilson, 1970; Higgins, 1973). These findings led to the concept of "occupational" or "industrial" bronchitis. Small decrements in pulmonary function that were also observed have been attributed by some to the "bronchitis" alone (i.e., disease occurring in the larger airways) (Morgan, 1978). For example, investigators (Hankinson, et al., 1977; Morgan, 1978, 1984) argued that in coal miners, coal dust exposure resulted mainly in cough and phlegm but not emphysema and potentially more significant airway obstruction. Hankinson and associates (1977) studied 4 groups of 428 miners matched on age and height selected from 9000 working U.S. miners. Current smokers with and without bronchitis had an elevated residual volume (RV) and total lung capacity (TLC) compared to nonsmokers without bronchitis, whereas nonsmokers with bronchitis presumably due to coal dust exposure alone had a minimally increased RV but no increase in TLC. It was inferred that these changes occurring in smokers but not nonsmokers with only dust exposure were consistent with subclinical emphysema. Mean FEV_1 was slightly decreased in the nonsmoking workers with bronchitis compared to nonsmoking workers without bronchitis.

Other studies also found that active miners had an excess of bronchitis and on average a mild decrement in pulmonary function. For example, Kibelstis and co-workers (1973) found that among nonsmoking U.S. miners, workers at the coal face—the mine location with the highest concentration of respirable particles—had the highest prevalence of chronic bronchitis. The mean FEV_1 was 98.1% of predicted among the nonsmoking face workers (i.e., dust exposed) with an FEV_1/FVC of 101.5% of predicted. Among nonsmoking surface workers (unexposed), the FEV_1 was 102.4% of predicted with an FEV_1/FVC of 102.6%, indicating a mild average decrement in pulmonary function due to dust exposure.

However, completed longitudinal studies and studies that have included retired and exworkers discussed later suggest that the decline in ventilatory function attributable to occupational exposure can be more significant than is suggested by these cross-sectional studies. Pathological evidence of emphysema attributable to dust exposure has subsequently been described in both coal miners (Soutar, 1987) and gold miners (Becklake et al., 1987). Abnormalities have also been described in the small airways of mineral-dust-exposed workers (Churg and Wright, 1984), but without adequate correlation between structure and function. Further work is needed in this area.

The significance of chronic mucus hypersecretion and its relationship to decline in FEV_1 has been subject to intense debate. The "British" hypothesis theorized that mucus hypersecretion with subsequent airway infection was responsible for a decline in lung function (Speizer, 1981). Current evidence suggests that mucus hypersecretion is not related to longitudinal decline in FEV_1 (Fletcher and Peto, 1977; U.S.D.H.S.S., 1984); two separate but parallel processes in the lung may be attributable to a common cause. Cross-sectional studies of coal miners not reporting bronchitis indicate that a decrement in lung function due to dust exposure can be detected exclusive of bronchitis (Rogan et al., 1973; Soutar and Hurley, 1986; Marine et al., 1988).

However, in cross-sectional studies in the general population (Burrows et al., 1977; U.S.D.H.S.S., 1984) the finding of bronchitis indicated on average a lower level of lung function, a finding that is also true in coal miners (Soutar and Hurley, 1986; Marine et al. 1988). Mucus hypersecretion therefore may be a marker of increased susceptibility of some people to excessive decline in FEV_1 but does not imply causality (U.S.D.H.S.S., 1984). Mucus hypersecretion has also been associated with an increased mortality from all causes in some studies, even after adjustment for level of pulmonary function (Annesi and Kauffmann, 1986; Foxman et al., 1986).

IV. Community Surveys of Occupational Exposure and Respiratory Disease

The power of the community survey, as noted above, is that subjects may be studied regardless of their current occupational status. In 1977 Lebowitz reported on a cross-sectional survey of 1195 men in Tucson (Lebowitz,

1977). Fifty-seven percent had one or more occupational exposures. Subjects in the construction industry or with high-intensity exposure to silica, fiberglass, smoke, asbestos, solvents, or sawdust had an increased prevalence of respiratory symptoms compared to subjects without such exposure, after adjustment was made for age and smoking.

In an industrial area of Norway, patients with COPD admitted to a hospital were selected as study cases if they had progressive dyspnea, met clinical criteria suggestive of symptomatic airflow obstruction, and had an FEV_1 less than 2 standard deviations below predicted (Kjuus et al., 1981). Two hospitalized controls free of any lung disease were matched to 36 cases by age and lifetime smoking habits, and occupational exposure was assessed by blinded interview. Most of the occupations selected as exposed to dust or fumes were in the construction, foundry, or mining industries. The odds ratio for work 10 or more years in a workplace where there was regular exposure to dust or vapors was 3.0 (95% CI = 1.2–7.5), but a further exposure–response relationship was not observed, likely due to the crudeness of the exposure data.

Korn and co-workers (1987) have reported changes in FEV_1 and respiratory symptoms in a random sample of 8515 adults residing in six U.S. cities. Lifetime occupational histories were obtained by interviewer-administered questionnaire before the recording of respiratory symptoms, and duration of each job, industry, and specific exposure to dust, gases, or fumes was recorded from the time subjects left school. The prevalence of any occupational dust exposure was 45% among men and 19% among women, and similar prevalences were reported for exposures to gases and fumes. After adjustment for age, gender, current and lifetime smoking, and city of residence, a history of either dust or of gas or fume exposures remained separate and significant predictors of respiratory symptoms. Subjects exposed only to dust had a relative odds of chronic cough, chronic phlegm, persistent wheeze and breathlessness (walking more slowly than others of one's own age on level ground) of 1.33, 1.40, 1.62, and 1.52, respectively. Subjects exposed to fumes or gases only had a similar but slightly smaller increase in relative odds of these symptoms. For subjects reporting both dust and fume exposures the excess risks were roughly additive, suggesting an independent effect of dust and fume exposures on symptom occurrence. There was no evidence of a more than an additive effect of smoking and dust exposure, or of smoking and fume or gas exposures on respiratory symptoms. The odds of chronic phlegm and chronic wheeze significantly increased with increasing years of dust but not fume or gas exposure. The odds of an FEV_1/FVC of less than 60% (an index of chronic airflow obstruction) for workers exposed to dust alone was 1.68, which was similar to the result obtained for combined dust and fume exposures. Gas or fume exposure alone was not a significant predictor of a FEV_1/FVC of less than 60%. Subjects exposed to dust also had similar odds of having an FEV_1/FVC less than 60% regardless of their smoking status.

Krzyzanowski and co-workers (1986) evaluated FEV_1 decline over 13 years among 759 men and 1,065 women in Poland. Occupational exposure was assessed by interview and workers exposed to dust for the 5 years at the start of the study were considered exposed. In men with occupational dust exposure there was a small but statistically significant excess loss of 6.9 ml/year in FEV_1. Men who gave up smoking during the study due to respiratory disease had a 33 ml/year excess decline in FEV_1 relative to nonsmokers, whereas men who continued to smoke had a 9.8 ml/year excess loss in FEV_1 relative to nonsmokers. Interaction between smoking and occupational exposure was not assessed. In women, exposure to dust categorized in this crude fashion was not a significant predictor of FEV_1 loss.

These community-based studies demonstrate an association between decreased pulmonary function and respiratory symptoms, and "categorical" exposure to occupational dust. When assessed, the effect of smoking and occupational exposure on symptom occurrence and reduced pulmonary function was additive.

V. Specific Occupational Exposures

A. Mining

Coal Mining

Coal dust exposure is known to cause coal workers' pneumoconiosis, and pulmonary symptoms and function have been extensively studied among coal miners. Longitudinal studies started in the 1950s have demonstrated a relationship between coal dust exposure and chronic bronchitis as well as airway obstruction. The effect of coal dust on airway function is independent of the radiographic category of simple coal workers' pneumoconiosis. Workers with complicated pneumoconiosis must be excluded when one is studying the effects of coal dust exposure on airway function because airflow obstruction can occur due to the distortion of lung architecture.

In a cross-sectional study of 3581 active British miners with dust exposure at the coal face, lifetime respirable dust exposure was a significant predictor of reduction in FEV_1 (Rogan et al., 1973). Subjects with increasing grades of bronchitis also had more dust exposure. In this large study, exsmokers were excluded and the effects of age, height, weight, cigarettes smoked per day, and dust exposure on FEV_1 were considered in a multiple regression model. Lifetime cumulative exposure to respirable dust was estimated for each worker based on actual measurements. The average lifetime cumulative dust exposure in the group was equivalent to a 100 ml loss in FEV_1, roughly equal to smoking 20 cigarettes/day or aging 2 years. There was no evidence of a greater than additive effect between cigarettes smoked per day and dust exposure on FEV_1. The subgroup of men with bronchitis and history of chest illness and breathlessness while walking on the level ground had an average lifetime decrement in FEV_1 of 430 ml more than predicted based on cigarette use, dust exposure, age, height, and weight. Subjects without symptoms, when analyzed separately, had a decrement in FEV_1 of 87 ml for the average dust exposure.

In the study by Kibelstis and co-workers (1973) of 8555 active U.S. miners, job category was used as a surrogate for exposure. Face workers generally had a higher prevalence of bronchitis than surface workers, if one adjusted for years of mining experience. This finding was more consistent in the nonsmokers than in the ex- or current smokers, probably due to the crude assessment of exposure (job location) and the larger effect of smoking on bronchitis. A mild decrement in FEV_1 and FEV_1/FVC was observed among face workers compared to surface workers who were non- or exsmokers. Face workers in Nigerian coal mines (675 active miners) (Jain and Patrick, 1981) likewise had a slightly lower FEV_1/FVC, and FEF_{25-75} than miners in other job locations with less dust exposure. Smoking was not an adjustment factor, but only 7% of the cohort were smokers and the face workers had the least number of smokers with the shortest duration of smoking, which suggests that the effect was not due to smoking.

In a smaller study of volunteer miners in Utah (136 active and 106 retired miners), years of mining were used as an index of dust exposure and were associated with chronic bronchitis, after adjustment for smoking (Rom et al., 1981). The effects of smoking and chronic bronchitis were additive in their influence on expiratory flow. Pulmonary function was slightly but not significantly lower in nonsmoking miners with bronchitis when compared to those without bronchitis, but the study lacked statistical power (54 nonsmokers).

Recognizing that exminers might have been the workers most affected by dust exposure, Lowe and Khosla (1972) studied 3012 exminers and 9361 nonminers in two South Wales steel companies. When categorized as smokers and nonsmokers, exminers had more chronic bronchitis than nonminers at all ages in both smokers and nonsmokers. Among nonsmokers 55–64 years old, 5.4% of the nonminers had bronchitis compared to 22.4% of the exminers. Among current smokers, 27.3% of the nonminers had chronic bronchitis compared to 35.6% of the exminers. The prevalence of reported chronic bronchitis was roughly additive for the effect of smoking and history of mine work.

Two longitudinal studies have shown a decline in FEV_1 attributable to dust exposure. The 11 year loss in FEV_1 was measured among 1677 active British coal miners based on lifetime cumulative dust exposure obtained from measurements and estimates of past respirable dust. The decline was 42 ml for the average exposure of the group and 223 ml for workers with the maximal observed dust exposure (Love and Miller, 1982). Results were adjusted for mine, height, FEV_1 level, and smoking category (ex-, current, intermittent, and never smokers). Current smokers lost 122 ml of FEV_1 over 11 years compared to nonsmokers. Estimates of cigarette dose were not used in the regression model. In 1072 active U.S. miners, an 11 year decline in FEV_1 ranged from 36 to 84 ml for various indices of dust exposure since total dust exposure was not available (Attfield, 1985). Loss of FEV_1 over 11 years due to current smoking was approximately 100 ml. Cigarette consumption was assessed as never, current, ex-, or intermittent smoking. Pack years smoked between the surveys were used in several regression models without affecting the estimates of dust effect. Both of these studies included only active miners who attended a follow-up survey. If the studies had included miners who had left the industry, the decline in FEV_1 attributed to dust exposure could have been greater. In Attfield's study, the miners who left after the initial survey were older and had more bronchitis and poorer pulmonary function than those remaining.

In a recent study of 4059 subjects (Soutar and Hurley, 1986) including exminers and miners who left the mines before age 65, cross-sectional FEV_1 and FEV_1/FVC were related to increasing level of cumulative dust exposure. For a moderately high lifetime exposure to dust, a 228 ml decline in FEV_1 was predicted after adjustment for smoking, including pack years for current smokers, age, height, and geographic region. Among 199 miners who left the industry (mean age 53) before normal retirement age, had taken other jobs, and who reported symptoms of chronic bronchitis, there was an average lifetime decrement in FEV_1 of 600 ml for the same dust exposure (Hurley and Soutar, 1986). This decrement of FEV_1, given the same exposure as other miners, suggested that these workers were more susceptible to the effects of coal dust.

Marine and co-workers (1988) used logistic regressions in separate analyses of smokers and nonsmokers to adjust for the independent effects of age and lifetime dust exposure. In 543 nonsmoking miners and 2837 smoking miners, lifetime dust exposure was a significant predictor of chronic bronchitis and of FEV_1 levels of 80% and 65% of predicted. Predicted values were internally derived, based on nonsmoking miners without bronchitis. The effect of dust was of similar magnitude in both smokers and nonsmokers. At the average dust exposure of the group, the FEV_1 would have been reduced approximately 200 ml. Based on the logistic models developed, for nonsmokers considered at age 47 at the highest dust exposure, the prevalence of an FEV_1 less than 80% of predicted was 23.9%, and for unexposed nonsmokers the prevalence of an FEV_1 less than 80% of predicted was 9.7%. The prevalence of an FEV_1 of less than 65% of predicted in the same groups was 7.7% and 3.2%, respectively.

Autopsy studies have also demonstrated an excess of emphysema in coal miners, further suggesting a common mechanism for airflow obstruction due to coal dust exposure and smoking. In 39 coal workers and 48 non-coal-workers in South Wales who all died of ischemic heart disease (Cockroft et al., 1982), if one adjusted for age and smoking status, coal workers had a large excess risk of centriacinar emphysema (odds ratio = 10.4, 95% confidence limits 2.7–39.6). If one excluded workers with progressive massive fibrosis, the odds ratio was 5.7. Ruckley and co-workers (1984) found that cumulative lifetime dust exposure was a predictor of postmortem centriacinar emphysema in workers with any palpable dust lesion or with progressive massive fibrosis. Increasing lung dust content was also correlated with the presence of centriacinar emphysema at autopsy. Based on these studies, the presence of (pathological) fibrotic lesions of any type, which are also related to exposure, may be important in determining the presence of centriacinar emphysema in miners.

Other Miners

Miners of other ores are exposed to dust of the particular ore mined, as well as to free silica and other dusts. Workers involved in processing the ore (crushing, milling, smelting) are also exposed to fumes such as sulfur oxides. Underground miners since the 1960s (including coal miners) may also have been exposed to diesel exhaust fumes, which contains respirable particles and oxides of nitrogen.

Hard rock miners in Manitoba are exposed to the fumes and dust related to zinc, copper, and nickel mining and processing (Manfreda et al., 1982). In a cross-sectional survey of 241 mine employees, cough and phlegm were more frequent among smokers and nonsmokers in the mining industry than in a general population sample. The combined effects of occupational exposure and smoking were roughly additive in the prevalence of cough and phlegm. A 7-year follow-up of 972 industry workers presented in an abstract indicated a significant excess decline in FEV_1 among different exposure groups adjusted for age, height, initial FEV_1, and smoking category (Manfreda and Johnston, 1987). The decline in FEV_1 varied from

33 to 69 ml/year, with the highest decline among surface workers in the ore roaster area. Smokers had a 54 ml/year loss of FEV_1, so the effect of occupation in some cases was greater than that of smoking although details of the assessment of smoking were not noted in this preliminary report.

A cross-sectional survey of 116 active Vermont talc miners and millers indicated a trend towards a decreased FEV_1/FVC and FEF_{25-75} when they were stratified by smoking category. No interaction between smoking and exposure was identified (Wegman et al., 1982).

In a community-based survey of 562 South African gold miners and 265 nonminers of similar age, a significant excess of bronchitis was found among smoking dust-exposed miners compared to smokers without a history of dust exposure (50.5% and 28%, respectively), but no effect was observed in nonsmokers. The effect persisted when daily cigarette consumption was considered. (Sluis-Cremer et al., 1967a). No difference in FEV_1 between exposed and unexposed workers was observed in the absence of a history of bronchitis (Sluis-Cremer et al., 1967b). However, FEV_1 was not considered in relation to age and duration of work in a dusty area in a mine. Although this community survey had the potential to include older and former miners, most subjects in this study were active miners, with only 12% older than age 54.

Bronchitis prevalence increased with increasing dust exposure in a cross-sectional survey of 2,209 South African miners aged 45–54 with exposure estimated from measurements of lifetime respirable dust exposure (Wiles and Faure, 1977). FEF_{25-75} fell with increasing dust exposure among non-, ex-, and current smokers, without evidence of an accelerated decline in function in smokers compared to nonsmokers (Table 1). At the highest levels of exposure, the bronchitis prevalence and decline in FEF_{25-75} did not persist, suggestive of a survivor effect in the most heavily exposed subjects.

An autopsy study of South African gold miners has also demonstrated an excess of emphysema due to dust exposure (Becklake et al., 1987). From whole lung sections of miners made at autopsy, 44 cases of emphysema and 42 controls without significant emphysema were selected from miners aged 51–71 who had autopsies in 1980–1981. The decision to have an autopsy was not based on an incentive to establish the presence of disease. Significant predictors of emphysema at autopsy included age, cigarettes smoked/day before 1960, and years worked in high dust-exposed areas of the mine. The odds ratios for emphysema were 12.7 for 20 years of work with high dust exposure, 30.3 for 20 cigarettes smoked/day, and 26.8 for the effects of age (70 relative to age 51). Silicosis grade did not predict the occurrence of emphysema; thus the odds of having emphysema due to dust exposure at postmortem was about half of that attributable to smoking 20 cigarettes/day.

Table 1 Bronchitis Prevalence and Mean Maximal Midexpiratory Flow by Total Respirable Dust Level and Smoking Category in South African Gold Miners

Particle-years ($\times 10^3$)	Nonsmokers		Exsmokers		Smokers	
	N	%	N	%	N	%
10	24	0	57	7.0	88	35.2
17	58	3.4	106	11.3	293	37.8
24	53	17.0	98	23.4	313	44.7
31	50	20.0	96	26.0	297	48.8
38	36	19.4	76	26.3	241	50.2
45	25	16.0	50	20.0	110	53.6
52	14	14.3	31	12.9	93	50.5
Total	260		514		1435	

Mean maximal midexpiratory flow related to dust exposure (L/SEC)

	N	FEF_{25-75}	N	FEF_{25-75}	N	FEF_{25-75}
10	24	4.20	56	3.22	84	2.96
17	57	3.70	101	3.26	274	2.61
24	46	3.66	89	2.91	294	2.61
31	46	3.23	82	2.67	266	2.52
38	28	3.08	72	2.75	213	2.32
45	22	3.60	45	2.92	93	2.30
52	14	3.59	27	2.89	87	2.36
Total	237		472		1311	

Source: Wiles and Faure, 1977.

B. Steelworkers and Cokeworkers

A cross-sectional survey of 10,000 active steelworkers in Wales (Lowe, 1969; Lowe et al., 1970) indicated that when smoking was considered, FEV_1 and bronchitis prevalence were not related to current level of respirable dust, sulfur dioxide level, or years of work in current job. However, lifetime occupational exposure to dust could not be estimated. Job transition from areas of high to low exposure had occurred, making it difficult to use current job only as an index of exposure.

Pham and co-workers (1979) studied a sample of 159 active steel workers and 14 unexposed workers twice over 5 years. The steelworkers had an initial FEV_1 and FEV_1/FVC of 102.2% and 102.8% of predicted, respectively, and 5 years later these values had fallen to an FEV$_1$ of 94.8% and a FEV$_1$/FVC of 94.3% of predicted. The unexposed group had an initial FEV$_1$ of 97.3% and an FEV$_1$/FVC of 96.2% of predicted, which was initially lower than that in the exposed group, and an FEV$_1$ of 96.7% and FEV$_1$/FVC of 94.9% of predicted 5 years later. Thus the steelworkers appeared to lose function faster than the comparison group, but some of this apparent loss could have been due to failure to adjust for level of function (Burrows et al., 1987). Although the smoking habits of the group were similar, the effects of smoking were not taken into consideration directly in the analysis.

Cokeworkers with the most exposure to dust and fumes also have more bronchitis than other cokeworkers (Walker et al., 1971) in both smokers and nonsmokers. The prevalence of bronchitis was also dependent on whether or not the subject had worked in a dusty industry other than the coke industry. Madison and co-workers (1984) more recently studied 3799 active male cokeworkers and used job title as a surrogate of exposure to dust and fumes. They found that among nonsmokers, the mean FEV$_1$ in the supervisors was 4.04 L, and among laborers (who had a higher dust exposure) it was 3.74 L after adjustment for height and age. Similar differences were seen among smokers. Sputum histological findings were examined, and workers with an excess of polymorphonuclear leukocytes (suggestive of bronchitis) tended to have a lower FEV$_1$.

C. Other Silica- and Mineral-Dust-Exposed Workers

Karava and co-workers (1976) studied 861 foundry workers. Smokers with current jobs in high dust areas had almost twice the bronchitis prevalence of smokers with the least exposure (30% vs. 16%). Nonsmokers with high dust exposure had a 9% prevalence of bronchitis compared to a 2% prevalence in nonsmoking workers with less exposure. These results suggest a slightly more than additive effect of smoking and foundry dust in causing bronchitis.

Kauffmann and co-workers (1979, 1982) have reported on the follow-up of respiratory symptoms and pulmonary function among Paris area workers exposed primarily to mineral dust (such as silica), gas, and heat. In 1960-1961 a survey of respiratory symptoms and lung function among men in 11 factories involved with metallurgy, chemicals, printing, and flour milling was performed. Qualitative assessments of exposure in the workplace were recorded after worker interviews and observation of the workplaces. In 1972-1973, follow-up spirometry was done that included 575 men who were aged 30-54 in 1960. Ninety percent were still working, half at the same job. Men with any exposure, broadly defined as exposure to dust, gases, or heat, had a significantly steeper decline in FEV_1 compared to unexposed workers, which was independent of smoking habits. Exposed and nonexposed nonsmokers lost FEV_1 at 40 ml and 31 ml/year, respectively. Among heavy smokers, the decline in FEV_1 among workers with any exposure was 55 ml/year compared to 41 ml/year among nonexposed smokers. Similar results were obtained for decline in FEV_1/FVC but not for FVC. Respiratory symptoms such as cough, phlegm, and dyspnea were not related to decline in FEV_1 after adjustment for level of function, exposure, and smoking habits. In a more detailed analysis of the exposures, workers with mineral dust exposure such as to silica, abrasives, coal, and iron had the greatest FEV_1 decline. FEV_1 slope was also steeper for workers exposed to grain dust (Table 2). No interaction of cigarette smoking and dust exposure was observed.

Airways have also been examined histologically in other, smaller groups of workers exposed to mineral dusts. Small airway lesions have been found histologically in the lungs of workers with exposure to nonasbestos mineral dusts such as iron oxide, aluminum oxide, mica, and silica (Churg and Wright, 1983, 1984). In these patients, the terminal bronchioles, respiratory bronchioles, and alveolar ducts show pigment deposition and fibrous tissue deposition, which are usually not observed in unexposed persons (Churg et al., 1985). These lesions are similar to the lesions seen in the airway of asbestos-exposed workers. However, the functional significance of these small airway lesions need to be determined further (Churg et al., 1985; Kennedy et al., 1985).

D. Asbestos Exposure

The earliest changes of asbestosis observed in animals include peribronchiolar inflammation with compression of the peripheral airways (Begin et al., 1982). Long-term chrysotile asbestos miners without histological evidence of interstitial fibrosis at autopsy had significantly more fibrosis of the terminal and respiratory bronchioles and alveolar ducts with pigment deposition than did unexposed controls matched for age and smoking history (Wright and Churg, 1984, 1985). The functional significance of such changes remains to be determined, but current evidence indicates that such changes are of little clinical consequence (Becklake, 1984). Becklake and co-workers (Becklake et al., 1972) studied Quebec asbestos workers and found that the FEV_1/FVC in the nonsmokers with the highest dust exposure was slightly lower (78.3%) than in the other asbestos exposure categories (84–81%). Other investigators have also presented evidence of small airway abnormalities in asbestos-exposed workers (Jodoin et al., 1971; Rodriguez-Roisin et al., 1980; Fournier-Massey and Becklake, 1975; Begin et al., 1983).

Table 2 Ventilatory Function According to Occupational Exposure for Paris Area Workers Exposed to Dusts

Occupation exposure	N	FEV$_1$ Slope (ml/yr) Adjusted for FEV$_1$ Level (FEV$_1$/HEIGHT^3), age and smoking
None	177	42
At least 1 hazard	379	50[a]
Dust	273	51[a]
Mineral dust	178	52[a]
Silica	55	57[a]
Abrasives	11	58[b]
Coal	27	60[a]
Iron	34	63[c]
Other metals	32	43
Other mineral dusts	91	53[a]
Plant dust	58	58[c]
Grain dust	36	65[c]
Maize powder	20	47

Source: After Kauffmann et al., 1982.
[a]p - 0.01.
[b]p - 0.10.
[c]p - 0.001.

E. Grain Dust

Grain dust is a mixture of various types of grain as well as insect parts, molds, spores, fungi, mites, pigeon excreta, and pesticide residues. Exposure to grain dust may cause acute reversible airflow obstruction or grain fever (Chan-Yeung et al., 1985). Exposure to grain dust can also cause changes in FEV$_1$ over a work shift and changes that persist over a harvest season (James et al., 1986; El Karim et al., 1986; Broder et al., 1984). Lung function and respiratory symptoms can improve during layoffs, and abnormalities return when workers are rehired (Broder et al., 1980). New employees in the industry commonly develop increased cough and phlegm soon after being hired (Broder et al., 1984). These factors suggest that healthier workers tend to remain on the job and are available for study (Broder et al., 1985).

Cross-sectional surveys of workers have demonstrated an increase in the prevalence of chronic bronchitis and generally mild abnormalities in pulmonary function compared to reference groups. In a survey of 300 grain elevator workers in the Superior–Duluth area, abnormal expiratory flow rates were more common among workers who reacted cutaneously to common antigens (DoPico et al., 1977). Thirty percent of the nonsmokers had chronic bronchitis. Years of employment were not related to FEV_1 in this and another study of grain elevator workers (Broder et al., 1979).

Dosman found that smoking (expressed as pack-years) was a greater cause of bronchitis than was grain dust exposure, with the effects roughly additive (Dosman et al., 1979). There was a slightly more than the expected decrement in FEF_{25-75} in smoking grain workers with 30 years of service relative to nonsmoking workers and unexposed smokers (Dosman, 1977). In 90 lifetime nonsmoking grain workers matched by age to a nonsmoking, control group, the prevalence of chronic bronchitis was 23% compared to 3% of the controls (Dosman et al., 1980). The grain workers had more cough, wheezing, and shortness of breath, slightly lower FEV_1/FVC (1–2% difference), and reduced FEF_{25-75}. In a larger cross-sectional study (Cotton et al., 1983) of the same population, the combined effects of grain dust and smoking on lung function were additive, with only mild abnormalities seen.

Chan-Yeung and co-workers (1980) have published a series of studies on grain workers in Vancouver. Cough and phlegm were less in a control group of saw mill workers than in grain workers. The mean FEV_1 in nonsmoking civic and grain workers was 104% and 100% of predicted, respectively. Among smokers, these values were reduced to 99.6% (civic workers) and 97.5% of predicted (grain workers). In a 2-½ and 6 year follow-up study, it was found that the decline in FEV_1 increased with age, but was independent of initial lung function level, respiratory symptoms, or atopy (Tabona et al., 1984; Chan-Yeung et al., 1981). Workers with a large (7100ml/year) significant decline in FEV_1 were more likely to have a decline in FEV_1 over a work week and later nonspecific bronchial hyperreactivity. They also had the greatest odds of having highly dust-exposed jobs (Enarson et al., 1985).

In summary, grain dust exposure is associated with both acute and chronic respiratory symptoms and with a mild decrement in pulmonary function. The effects of dust exposure and smoking appear to be additive. A minority of workers who stay on the job have more rapid declines in pulmonary function that are related to dust exposure, and host factors such as bronchial reactivity may be important but need to be studied prospectively.

F. Cotton Dust

Exposure to the dust of cotton, hemp, and flax has been associated with byssinosis, a clinical syndrome characterized initially by Monday morning chest tightness (Tockman and Baser, 1984). Exposure to these dusts also is associated with bronchitis (Morgan et al., 1982; Bouhuys et al., 1969; Molyneux and Tombleson, 1970). Cigarette smoking increases the risk of byssinosis (Molyneux and Tombleson, 1970; Berry et al., 1974; Merchant et al., 1972). In Lancashire cotton mill workers, once bronchitis was considered, smoking did not result in an additional risk for byssinosis (U.S.D.H.S.S., 1985). The combined effect on bronchitis of work in a cotton mill and smoking was not more than additive. It has been suggested that smoking mediates the development of byssinosis by causing chronic bronchitis (airway inflammation) (U.S.D.H.S.S., 1985); byssinosis and chronic bronchitis tend to coexist (Merchant et al., 1972; Imbus and Suh, 1973). However, when cotton dust exposure was measured in North Carolina cotton mills, at the highest dust levels, cigarette smoking resulted in more byssinosis than expected if the effect was additive. At lower cotton dust exposure levels, cigarette smoking did not affect byssinosis prevalence (Merchant et al., 1973a).

Byssinosis may be associated with a drop in FEV_1 over a work shift. In a cross-sectional survey of 10,133 active textile workers, workers with coexisting bronchitis had the greatest change in FEV_1 (Imbus and Suh, 1973). Byssinosis and bronchitis also influenced level of function. Workers without bronchitis who also did not have byssinosis had the highest FEV_1. Both byssinosis and bronchitis were associated with a lower FEV_1, with a slightly greater decrement attributable to byssinosis. When bronchitis and byssinosis coexisted, the decrement in FEV_1 as a percentage of predicted was roughly additive but the FEV_1 was still greater than 70% of predicted in these active workers. Merchant and co-workers (1973b) developed dose–response curves for byssinosis and dust level, and also found a relationship between cotton dust level and change in FEV_1 over a shift. There are only a few studies, however, that suggest that cotton dust exposure is associated with chronic clinical effects and a long-term decline in lung function.

Bouhuys and co-workers (Bouhuys et al., 1977) studied a group of active, retired, and former South Carolina textile workers aged 45 years and older with an average 35 years of employment, and established a comparison group without a history of work in a textile mill recruited from two towns in Connecticut and one town in South Carolina. Dust levels in the South Carolina mills were not measured and job title was used as a surrogate for cotton dust exposure. In nonsmokers, current, and exsmokers, both FVC and FEV_1 were decreased in comparison to the control group in textile workers with the most potential for significant dust exposure in their jobs. Retired workers had lowest level of function (both FVC and FEV_1). Beck and co-workers (1984a) reanalyzed these data including only current and nonsmokers and found that the effects of job title (for weavers and carders) and smoking (with pack-years considered) were additive in predicting both a reduced FVC and FEV_1. The effects of cotton dust (i.e., work as a textile worker) and approximately a 50 pack-year history of smoking were similar. In males, the average decrement in FEV_1 and FVC relative to the comparison group was 300–400 ml, with FEV_1 generally affected more than FVC. In females, the differences were 100–200 ml. In retired workers aged 45–64, the mean decrement in FEV_1 and FVC was slightly greater. A relationship was also found between smoking, textile work, and decrement in FEF_{50}. Beck and co-workers (1982) completed a follow-up study on the original population of textile workers and controls. Over 6 years, the average FEV_1 loss in the textile workers was greatest among current and nonsmokers relative to the comparison group, and appeared roughly additive with smoking. Workers with respiratory symptoms such as byssinosis and bronchitis had lower levels of FEV_1 (Beck et al., 1984b). Further work also suggested a greater prevalence of obstructive disease among textile workers than control subjects. (Schachter et al., 1984). These studies initiated by Bouhuys, although including retired workers, have been criticized due to the crudeness of the cotton dust exposure assessment and noncomparability of the comparison groups, who came from different geographical areas (Tockman and Baser, 1984). Years of exposure were not considered as an exposure assessment in the absence of measured data.

Merchant and co-workers (1973a), using measured level of dust to indicate exposure category, found no effect of cotton dust exposure on FEV_1 in nonsmoking or exsmoking workers. Current smokers with cotton dust exposure had lower pulmonary function compared to unexposed smoking workers, but there was no trend toward a greater than expected drop in function with heavier smoking. In a more recent cross-sectional study of ex-cotton-workers in Lancashire, workers had an FEV_1 2–8% less than predicted in nonsmoking subjects who were never exposed to dust, which was comparable to the effect of currently smoking 1–14 cigarettes/day (Elwood et al., 1986).

Berry measured lung function repeatedly over 3 years in Lancashire cotton workers and a comparison group of workers in mills producing synthetic fabrics (Berry et al., 1973). After the exclusion of workers with less than three FEV_1 measurements, the mean decline in FEV_1 among cotton workers was 54 ml/year, adjusted for sex, smoking, and age (and was not related to level of FEV_1). In the synthetic fiber mills, the rate of decline was 32 ml/year, nearly all accounted for by one mill. Nonsmokers lost function at the rate of 40 ml/year, and smokers of one pack/day or more had a loss of 61 ml/year. There was no relationship in decline in FEV_1 to byssinosis grade, current dust concentration, years in the mills, or Monday fall in FEV_1, despite the observed decline in FEV_1 among cotton workers in this short longitudinal study.

Fox and co-workers (1973) studied 886 Lancashire cotton workers over 2 years and Jones (1984) estimated an average annual decline in FEV_1 of 23 ml/year based on these data, without consideration of dust level or smoking. In contrast, in India 1241 textile workers in three mills were studied over 5 years (Kamat et al., 1981) and a □ 100 ml/year decline in FEV_1 was found. Smoking also was not specifically assessed.

There are few data correlating pathological changes in the lung with cotton dust exposure. Pratt and co-workers (1980) studied lungs from 565 patients with known smoking histories; occupation was available as major type of work only. There was a relationship between centrilobular emphysema and smoking, but not with a history of cotton dust exposure. In nonsmokers there was a relationship between cotton dust exposure and mucus gland volume and goblet cell hyperplasia.

In summary, limited longitudinal and some cross-sectional studies suggest a loss of FEV_1 due to cotton and related dust exposure that may be of similar magnitude to the effect of smoking. The size of the specific effect depends on the study and population. Further longitudinal studies without methodological problems (adequate smoking assessment, longer follow-up) are needed to demonstrate conclusively that a permanent loss of lung function can occur from cotton dust exposure (Diem, 1983). Further pathological studies are also needed to correlate structure with better estimation of occupational cotton dust exposure.

IV. Summary and Conclusion

As first described in the 1959 Ciba symposium, and later in the 1984 Surgeon General's report (U.S.D.H.S.S., 1984), the spectrum of COPD includes three disease processes: chronic mucus hypersecretion, characterized by cough and phlegm; expiratory airflow limitation; and emphysema, defined anatomically by abnormal dilatation of the distal airspaces with alveolar wall destruction. It is well established that occupational exposure to dust will result in chronic mucus hypersecretion. In addition, evidence has accumulated that occupational exposure to a variety of dusts and perhaps other occupational exposures results in an increased decline in FEV_1 and decrement in FEV_1/FVC as indices of air flow obstruction (Table 3). The best evidence is in the coal mining industry, where studies begun in the 1950s with adequate estimation of past respirable dust exposure have been completed. The magnitude of the effect of coal dust exposure on function is, on average, less than the effect attributable to smoking, and the combined effects of smoking and coal dust appears additive. Pathological evidence of emphysema exists in coal miners that appears related to dust exposure.

Table 3 Summary of Effects of Occupational Exposure in Selected Occupational Groups

Occupational Group	Bronchitis	Pulmonary Function	Comments	Selected References
Coal miners	Related to dust exposure. Additive with smoking	Decline in FEV_1 related to lifetime respirable dust exposure. Smoking effect is additive. Dust effect is less than that of smoking, but may be similar in a minority of workers.	Best-studied industry. Pathological evidence of excess of emphysema observed.	Kibelstis et al., 1973 Rogan et al., 1973 Lowe and Khosla, 1972 Love and Miller, 1982 Attfield, 1985 Soutar and Hurley, 1986 Marine et al., 1988
Gold miners	Related to dust exposure; effect harder to see in nonsmokers in one study. Additive with smoking in study with dust measurements available	Decline in FEF_{25-75} and FEV_1 with lifetime respirable dust. No accelerated loss of FEF_{25-75} in smokers compared to nonsmokers	Longitudinal data not available. Relationship between emphysema at autopsy and respirable dust	Sluis-Cremer, et al., 1967a,b Wiles and Faure, 1977 Becklakey et al., 1987
Grain-dust exposed workers	Related to dust exposure. Additive with smoking	Cross-sectional studies suggest a mild decrease in function, and an additive effect with smoking. A minority of workers have an accelerated decline in FEV_1	More longitudinal data needed. Difficult to study due to migration out of the industry	Broder et al., 1984 DoPico et al., 1977. Dosman et al., 1979 Chan-Yeung et al., 1980 Enarson et al., 1985

Cotton-dust-exposed workers	Related to dust, exposure; possibly additive with smoking. Byssinosis related to bronchitis	Cross-sectional data indicate a lower FEV$_1$ in cotton workers with (?) additive effects of exposure and smoking. Effects of exposure and smoking may be similar. Scanty longitudinal data	Beck, et al., 1982, 1984a; Bouhuys et al., 1977; Merchant et al., 1973a,b; Molyneux and Tombleson, 1970; Berry et al., 1973; Imbus and Suh, 1973
Paris area workers (silica and other dust exposed)	Increased mortality, in workers with bronchitis	Exposed workers lost FEV$_1$ 10–20 ml/year faster than unexposed workers. Additive effect of smoking. / Longitudinal study limited by lack of quantitative exposure data. Pathological evidence of small airway lesions in other workers with mineral dust exposure. Functional significance needs to be established	Kauffmann et al., 1979, 1982; Annesi and Kauffman 1986; Churg et al., 1985
General population	Increased cough, phlegm, wheeze, breathlessness, as a result of exposure to dust or fumes. Additive with smoking	Exposure to dust a predictor of FEV$_1$/FVC of less than 60% in a cross-sectional study. Longitudinally, a small but significant decline noted in FEV$_1$. Additive effect with smoking. Significant clinical COPD related to occupation in a case–control study / Lack of actual exposure data and possible recall bias limit interpretation, but when considered with industry specific studies, are consistent	Kjuus et al., 1981; Krzyanoski et al, 1986; Korn et al., 1987

Few longitudinal studies have been completed in other miners. Based on cross-sectional data, the effect of exposure on pulmonary function is mild, but results are subject to the limitations of study design. In one case–control study in goldminers that identified subjects with postmortem emphysema as cases, a relationship between dust exposure and emphysema was found. Workers exposed to a variety of other mineral dusts also have had a decrement in FEV_1 noted due to occupational exposure. These latter studies, although indicating an effect of occupation, generally lack specific exposure measurements. Although microscopic small airway lesions have been observed both in mineral-dust- and asbestos-exposed workers, the clinical significance of these changes need to be correlated with function measurement.

Exposure to grain dust noted in cross-sectional studies results in a mild decrement in pulmonary function that is additive with smoking. However, in one longitudinal study (Tabona et al., 1984; Enarson et al., 1985), workers with a large excess loss of function were identified. In cotton-dust-exposed workers, past studies have not demonstrated a consistent exposure-related decline in FEV_1.

Does dust exposure result in clinically significant airflow obstruction? On the basis of the studies done in coalminers (Rogan et al., 1973; Love and Miller, 1982; Attfield, 1985; Soutar and Hurley, 1986; Hurley and Soutar, 1986) and other mainly mineral-dust-exposed workers (Kauffmann et al., 1979, 1982), excess rate of loss of FEV_1 have ranged from roughly 10 ml/year or less to approximately 20 ml/year. In a population-based survey, the odds of having an FEV_1/FVC of less than 60% was increased by nearly 70% in dust-exposed subjects (Korn et al., 1987). Marine and co-workers (1988) found roughly twice the prevalence (7.7%) of an FEV_1 of 65% of predicted in nonsmoking workers with the highest dust exposure, compared to workers without exposure (3.2%). On average, the rate of decline of function is less than that attributable to aging and cigarette smoking, generally leading to a mild decrement in pulmonary function that is unlikely to be clinically significant by itself. However, these data also suggest that a minority of workers could have experienced more clinically significant changes in pulmonary function due to dust exposure alone (Hurley and Soutar, 1986; Marine et al., 1988). When considered together with the effects of cigarette smoking, the effect of occupational exposure is additive and could further contribute to disability.

Similar studies have not been done in grain- and cotton-dust-exposed workers, and there is a need for further longitudinal studies in these industries to study the relationship between exposure and decrement in lung function. Additional studies of occupationally exposed workers are also required to allow us to understand better host susceptibility factors, and better quantitate dose–response relationships.

References

Annesi, I., and Kauffmann, F. (1986). Is respiratory mucus hypersecretion really an innocent disorder? *Am. Rev. Respir. Dis.* **134**:688–693.

Attfield, M. D. (1985). Longitudinal decline in FEV$_1$ in United States coal miners. *Thorax* **40**:132–137.

Beck, G. J., Doyle, C. A., and Schachter, E. N. (1981). Smoking and lung function. *Am. Rev. Respir. Dis.* **123**:149–155.

Beck, G. J., Schachter, E. N., Maunder, L. R., and Schilling, R. S. F. (1982). Prospective study of chronic lung disease in cotton textile workers. *Ann. Intern. Med.* **97**:645–651.

Beck, G. J., Maunder, L. R., and Schachter, E. N. (1984a). Cotton dust and smoking effects on lung function in cotton textile workers. *Am. J. Epidemiol.* **119**:33–43.

Beck, G. J., Schachter, E. N., and Maunder, L. R. (1984b). The relationship of respiratory symptoms and lung function loss in cotton textile workers. *Am. Rev. Respir. Dis.* **130**:6–11.

Becklake, M. R. (1984). Asbestos exposure and airway response. In *Occupational Lung Disease*. Edited by J. B. L. Gee. New York, Churchill Livingstone, pp. 25–50.

Becklake, M. R. (1985). Chronic airflow limitation: its relationship to work in dusty occupations. *Chest* **88**:608–617.

Becklake, M. R., Irwig, L., Kielkowski, D., Webster, I., DeBeer, M., and Landau, S. (1987). The predictors of emphysema in South African goldminers. *Am. Rev. Respir. Dis.* **135**:1234–1241.

Becklake, M. R., Fournier-Massey, G., Rossiter, C. E., and McDonald, J. C. (1972). Lung function in chrysotile asbestos mine and mill workers of Quebec. *Arch. Environ. Health* **24**:401–409.

Begin, R., Masse, S., and Bureau, M. A. (1982). Morphologic features and function of the airways in early asbestosis in the sheep model. *Am. Rev. Respir. Dis.* **120**:870–876.

Begin, R., Cantin, A., Berthiaume, Y., Boileau, R., Peloquin, S., and Masse, S. (1983). Airway function in lifetime-non smoking older asbestos workers. *Am. J. Med.* **75**:631–638.

Berry, G., McKerrow, C. B., Molyneux, M. K. B., Rossiter, C. E., and Tombleson, J. B. L. (1973). A study of the acute and chronic changes in ventilatory capacity of workers in Lancashire cotton mills. *Br. J. Ind. Med.* **30**:25–36.

Berry, G., Molyneux, M. K. B., and Tombleson, J. B. L. (1974). Relationship between dust level and byssinosis and bronchitis in Lancashire cotton mills. *Br. J. Ind. Med.* **31**:18–27.

Bouhuys, A., Barbero, A., Schilling, R. S. F., Van de Woestijne, K. P.,
Kalavsky, S., Kane, G., Toren, M., and Van Wayenburg, J. (1969).
Chronic respiratory disease in hemp workers. *Am. J. Med.* **46**:526-537.

Bouhuys, A., Schoenberg, J. B., Beck, G. J., and Schilling, R. S. F. (1977).
Epidemiology of chronic lung disease in a cotton mill community. *Lung*
154:167-186.

Broder, I., Mintz, S., Hutcheon, M., Corey, P., Silverman, F., Davies, G.,
Leznoff, A., Peress, L., and Thomas, P. (1979). Comparison of
respiratory variables in grain elevator workers and civic outside workers
of Thunder Bay, Canada. *Am. Rev. Respir. Dis.* **119**:193-203.

Broder, I., Mintz, S., Hutcheon, M. A., Corey, P. N., and Kuzyk, J.
(1980). Effect of layoff and rehire on respiratory variables of grain
elevator workers. *Am. Rev. Respir. Dis.* **122**:601-608.

Broder, I., Hutcheon, M. A., Mintz, S., Davies, G., Leznoff, A., Thomas,
P., and Corey, P. (1984). Changes in respiratory variables of grain
handlers and civic workers during their initial month of employment. *Br.
J. Ind. Med.* **41**:94-99.

Broder, I., Corey, P., Davies, G., Hutcheon, M., Mintz, S., Inouye, T.,
Hyland, R., Leznoff, A., and Thomas, P. (1985). Longitudinal study of
grain elevator and control workers with demonstration of healthy worker
effect. *J. Occup. Med.* **27**:873-880.

Brunekreef, B., Noy, D., and Clausing, P. (1987). Variability of exposure
measurements in environmental epidemiology. *Am. J. Epidemiol.*
125:892-898.

Burrows, B., Knudson, R. J., Cline, M. G., and Lebowitz, M. D. (1977).
Quantitative relationships between cigarette smoking and ventilatory
function. *Am. Rev. Respir. Dis.* **115**:195-205.

Burrows, B., Knudson, R. J., Camilli, A. E., Lyle, S. K., and Lebowitz, M. D.
(1987). The horse-racing effect and predicting decline in forced expiratory
volume from screening spirometry. *Am. Rev. Respir. Dis.* **135**:788-793.

Burrows, B., Lebowitz, M. D., Camilli, A. E., and Knudson, R. J. (1986).
Longitudinal changes in forced expiratory volume in one second in adults.
Methodologic considerations and findings in healthy nonsmokers. *Am.
Rev. Respir. Dis.* **133**:974-980.

Chan-Yeung, M., Schulzer, M., MacLean, L., Dorkin, E., and Gryzbowski,
S. (1980). Epidemiologic health survey of grain elevator workers in British
Columbia. *Am. Rev. Respir. Dis.* **121**:329-338.

Chan-Yeung, M., Schulzer, M., MacLean, L., Dorken, E., Tan, F., Lam, S.,
Enarson, D., and Gryzbowski, S. (1981). A follow-up study of the grain elevator workers in the port of Vancouver. *Arch. Environ. Health* **36**:75-81.

Chan-Yeung, M., Enarson, M., and Grzybowski, S. (1985). Grain dust and
respiratory health. *Can. Med. Assoc. J.* **133**:969-973.

Churg, A., and Wright, J. L. (1983). Small-airway lesions in patients exposed to nonasbestos mineral dusts. *Hum. Pathol.* **14**:688–693.

Churg, A., and Wright, J. L. (1984). Small airways disease induced by asbestos and nonasbestos mineral dust. *Chest* **85**:36S–38S.

Churg, A., Wright, J. L., Wiggs, B., Pare, P. D., and Lazar, N. (1985). Small airways disease and mineral dust exposure. *Am. Rev. Respir. Dis.* **131**:139–143.

Ciba Guest Symposium (1959). Terminology, definitions and classifications of chronic pulmonary emphysema and related conditions. *Thorax* **14**:286–299.

Cockcroft, A., Wagner, J. C., Ryder, R., Seal, R. M. E., Lyons, J. P., and Anderson, N. (1982). Post-mortem study of emphysema in coalworkers and non-coalworkers. *Lancet* **2**:600–603.

Cotton, D. J., Graham, B. L., Li, K. Y. R., Froh, F., Barnett, G. D., and Dosman, J. A. (1983). Effect of grain dust exposure and smoking on respiratory symptoms and lung function. *J. Occup. Med.* **25**:131–141.

Diem, J. E. (1983). A statistical assessment of the scientific evidence relating cotton dust exposure to chronic lung disease. *Am. Stat.* **37**:395–403.

Dodgson, J. (1984). The measurement of dust and fumes. In *Occupational Lung Diseases*, second edition. Edited by W. K. C. Morgan and A. Seaton. W. B. Saunders, Philadelphia, pp. 212–238.

Dosman, J. A. (1977). Chronic obstructive pulmonary disease and smoking in grain workers. *Ann. Intern. Med.* **87**:784–786.

Dosman, J. A., Graham, B. L., and Cotton, D. J. (1979). Chronic bronchitis and exposure to cereal grain dust (editorial). *Am. Rev. Respir. Dis.* **120**:477–480.

Dosman, J. A., Cotton, D. J., Graham, B. L., Li, R. K. Y., Froh, F., and Barnett, G. D. (1980). Chronic bronchitis and decreased forced expiratory flow rates in lifetime nonsmoking grain workers. *Am. Rev. Respir. Dis.* **121**:11–16.

DoPico, G. A., Reddan, W., Flaherty, D., Tsiatis, A., Peters, M. E., Rao, P., and Rankin, J. (1977). Respiratory abnormalities among grain handlers. *Am. Rev. Respir. Dis.* **115**:915–927.

El Karim, M. A. A., El Rab, M. O. G., Omer, A. A., and El Haimi, Y. A. A. (1986). Respiratory and allergic disorder in workers exposed to grain and flour dusts. *Arch. Environ. Health* **41**:297–301.

Elwood, P. C., Sweetnam, P. M., Bevan, C., and Saunders, M. J. (1986). Respiratory disability in ex-cotton workers. *Br. J. Ind. Med.* **43**:580–586.

Enarson, D. A., Vedal, S., and Chan-Yeung, M. (1985). Rapid decline in FEV_1 in grain handlers. Relation to level of dust exposure. *Am. Rev. Respir. Dis.* **132**:814–817.

Fletcher, C., and Peto, R. (1977). The natural history of chronic airflow obstruction. *Br. Med. J.* **1**:1645–1648.

Fletcher, C. M., Peto, R., Tinker, C. M., and Speizer, F. E. (1976). *The Natural History of Chronic Bronchitis and Emphysema. An Eight Year Study of Early Chronic Obstructive Lung Disease in Working Men in London.* New York, Oxford University Press.

Fournier-Massey, G., and Becklake, M. R. (1975). Pulmonary function profiles in Quebec asbestos workers. *Bull. Physiopathol. Respir.* **11**:429–445.

Foxman, B., Higgins, I. T. T., and Oh, M. S. (1986). The effects of occupation and smoking on respiratory disease mortality. *Am. Rev. Respir. Dis.* **134**:649–652.

Fox, A. J., Tombleson, J. B. L., Watt, A., and Wilkie, A. G. (1973). A survey of respiratory disease in cotton operatives. *Br. J. Ind. Med.* **30**:42–47.

Garshick, E., Schenker, M. B., Munoz, A., Smith, T. J., Woskie, S. R., Hammond, S. K., and Speizer, F. E. (1987). A case-control study of lung cancer and diesel exhaust exposure in railroad workers. *Am. Rev. Respir. Dis.* **135**:1242–1248.

Gilson, J. C. (1970). Occupational bronchitis? *Proc. R. Soc. Med.* **63**: 857–864.

Glindmeyer, H. W., Diem, J. E., Jones, R. N., and Weill, H. (1982). Non-comparability of longitudinally and cross-sectionally determined annual change in spirometry. *Am. Rev. Respir. Dis.* **125**:544–548.

Glindmeyer, H. W., Jones, R. N., Diem, J. E., and Weill, H. (1987). Useful and extraneous variability in longitudinal assessment of lung function. *Chest* **92**:877–882.

Greaves, I. A., and Schenker, M. B. (1987). Smoking and susceptibility to non-neoplastic lung disease. In *Variations in Susceptibility to the Agents in the Air: Identification, Mechanisms, and Policy Implications.* Edited by J. D. Brain, J. Warren, and R. Shaikh. Baltimore, Johns Hopkins University Press.

Graham, B. L., Dosman, J. A., Cotton, D. J., Weisstock, S. R., Lappi, V. G., and Froh, F. (1984). Pulmonary function and respiratory symptoms in potash workers. *J. Occup. Med.* **26**:209–214.

Graham, W. G. B., O'Grady, R. V., and Dubuc, B. (1981). Pulmonary function loss in Vermont granite workers. A long term follow-up and critical reappraisal. *Am. Rev. Respir. Dis.* **123**:25–28.

Hankinson, J. L., Reger, R. B., and Morgan, W. K. C. (1977). Maximal expiratory flows in coal miners. *Am. Rev. Respir. Dis.* **116**:175–180.

Higgins, I. T. T. (1973). The epidemiology of chronic respiratory disease. *Prev. Med.* **2**:14–33.

Hurley, J. F., and Soutar, C. A. (1986). Can exposure to coalmine dust cause a severe impairment of lung function? *Br. J. Ind. Med.* **43**:150–157.

Imbus, H. R., and Suh, M. W. (1973). Byssinosis. A study of 10,133 textile workers. *Arch. Environ. Health* **26**:183–191.

James, A. L., Cookson, W. O. C. M., Buters, G., Lewis, S., Ryan, G., Hickey, R., and Musk, A. W. (1986). Symptoms and longitudinal changes in lung function in young seasonal grain handlers. *Br. J. Ind. Med.* **43**:587–591.

Jodoin, G., Gibbs, G. W., Macklem, P. T., McDonald, J. C., and Becklake, M. R. (1971). Early effects of asbestos exposure on lung function. *Am. Rev. Respir. Dis.* **104**:525–535.

Johnson, E. S. (1986). Duration of exposure as a surrogate for dose in the examination and dose response relations. *Br. J. Ind. Med.* **43**:427–429.

Jain, B. L., and Patrick, J. M. (1981). Ventilatory function in Nigerian coal miners. *Br. J. Ind. Med.* **38**:275–280.

Jones, R. H. (1984). Cotton and chronic lung disease. *Chest* **85**:587–589.

Kamat, S. R., Kamat, G. R., Salpekar, V. Y., and Lobo, E. (1981). Distinguishing byssinosis from chronic obstructive pulmonary disease. Results of a prospective five-year study of cotton mill workers in India. *Am. Rev. Respir. Dis.* **124**:31–40.

Kauffmann, F., Drouet, D., Lellouch, J., and Brille, D. (1979). Twelve years spirometric changes among Paris area workers. *Int. J. Epidemiol.* **8**:201–211.

Kauffmann, F., Drouet, D., Lellouch, J., and Brille, D. (1982). Occupational exposure and 12-year spirometric changes among Paris area workers. *Br. J. Ind. Med.* **39**:221–232.

Karava, R., Hernberg, S., Koskela, R. S., and Kalevi, L. (1976). Prevalence of pneumoconiosis and chronic bronchitis in foundry workers. *Scand. J. Work Environ. Health* **2**(Suppl):64–72.

Kennedy, S. M., Wright, J. L., Muller, J. B., Pare, P. D., and Hogg, J. C. C. (1985). Pulmonary function and peripheral airway disease in patients with mineral dust or fume exposure. *Am. Rev. Respir. Dis.* **132**:1294–1299.

Kibelstis, J. A., Morgan, E. J., Reger, R., Lapp, N. L., Seaton, A., and Morgan, W. K. C. (1973). Prevalence of bronchitis and airway obstruction in American bituminous coal miners. *Am. Rev. Respir. Dis.* **108**:886–893.

Kjuus, H., Istad, H., and Langard, S. (1981). Emphysema and occupational exposure to industrial pollutants. *Scand. J. Work Environ. Health* **7**:290–297.

Korn, R. J., Dockery, D. W., Speizer, F. E., Ware, J. H., and Ferris, B. G. Jr. (1987). Occupational exposure and chronic respiratory symptoms. A population based study. *Am. Rev. Respir. Dis.* **136**:298–304.

Krzyzanowski, M., Jedrychowski, W., and Wysocki, M. (1986). Factors associated with the change in ventilatory function and the development of chronic obstructive pulmonary disease in a 13 year follow-up of the Cracow Study. *Am. Rev. Respir. Dis.* **134**:1011–1019.

Lebowitz, M. D. (1977). Occupational exposure in relation to symptomatology and lung function in a community population. *Environ. Res.* **14**:59–67, 1977.

Love, R. G., and Miller, B. G. (1982). Longitudinal study of lung function in coal miners. *Thorax* **37**:193–197.

Lowe, C. R. (1969). Industrial bronchitis. *Br. Med. J.* **1**:463–486.

Lowe, C. R., and Khosla, T. (1972). Chronic bronchitis in ex-coal miners working in the steel industry. *Br. J. Ind. Med.* **29**:45–49.

Lowe, C. R., Campbell, H., and Khosla, T. (1970). Bronchitis in two integrated steel works. III. Respiratory symptoms and ventilatory capacity related to atmospheric pollution. *Br. J. Ind. Med.* **27**:121–129.

Madison, R., Afifi, A. A., and Mittman, C. (1984). Respiratory impairment in coke oven workers: relationship to work exposure and bronchial inflammation detected by sputum cytology. *J. Chron. Dis.* **37**:167–176.

Manfreda, J., and Johnston, B. (1987). Occupational factors in the etiology of airflow obstruction. *Am. Rev. Respir. Dis.* **135**:A341.

Manfreda, J., Sidwall, G., Maini, K., West, P., and Cherniak, R. M. (1982). Respiratory abnormalities in employees of the hard rock mining industry. *Am. Rev. Respir. Dis.* **126**:629–634.

Marine, W. M., Gurr, D., and Jacobsen, M. (1988). Clinically important effects of dust exposure and smoking in British coal miners. *Am. Rev. Respir. Dis.* **137**:106–112.

Merchant, J. A., Kilburn, K. H., O'Fallon, W. M., Hamilton, J. D., and Lumsden, J. C. (1972). Byssinosis and chronic bronchitis among cotton textile workers. *Ann. Intern. Med.* **76**:423–433.

Merchant, J. A., Lumsden, J. C., Kilburn, K. H., O'Fallon, W. M., Ujda, J. R., Germino, V. H., and Hamilton, J. D. (1973a). An industrial study of the biological effects of cotton dust and cigarette smoke exposure. *J. Occup. Med.* **15**:212–221.

Merchant, J. A., Lumsden, J. C., Kilburn, K. H., O'Fallon, W. M., Ujda, J. R., Germino, V. H., and Hamilton, J. D. (1973b). Dose–response studies in cotton textile workers. *J. Occup. Med.* **15**:222–230.

Molyneux, M. K. B., and Tombleson, J. B. L. (1970). An epidemiologic study of respiratory symptoms in Lancashire mills, 1963–66. *Br. J. Ind. Med.* **27**:225–234.

Morgan, W. K. C. (1978). Industrial bronchitis. *Br. J. Ind. Med.* **35**:285–291.

Morgan, W. K. C. (1984). Industrial bronchitis and other nonspecific conditions affecting the airways. In *Occupational Lung Diseases*, second edition. Edited by W. K. C. Morgan and A. Seaton. Philadelphia, W. B. Saunders, pp. 521–540.

Morgan, W. K. C., Vesterlund, J., Burrell, R., Gee, J. B. L., and Willoughby, W. F. (1982). Byssinosis: some unanswered questions. *Am. Rev. Respir. Dis.* **126**:354–357.

Pham, Q. T., Mastrangelo, G., Chau, N., and Haluszka, J. (1979). Five year longitudinal comparison of respiratory symptoms and function in steelworkers and unexposed workers. *Bull. Europ. Physiopathol. Respir.* **15**:469–480.

Pratt, P. C., Vollmer, R. T., and Miller, J. A. (1980). Epidemiology of pulmonary lesions in nontextile and cotton textile workers. A retrospective autopsy analysis. *Arch. Environ. Health* **35**:133–138.

Rodriguez-Roisin, R., Merchant, J. E. M., Cochrane, G. M., Hickey, P. H., Turner-Worwick, M., and Clark, T. J. H. (1980). Maximal expiratory flow volume curves in workers exposed to asbestos. *Respiration* **39**:158–165.

Rogan, J. M., Attfield, M. D., Jacobsen, M., Rae, S., Walker, D. D., and Walton, W. H. (1973). Role of dust in the working environment in the development of chronic bronchitis in British coal miners. *Br. J. Ind. Med.* **30**:217–226.

Rom, W. N., Kanner, R. E., Renzetti, A. D., Shigeoka, J. W., Barkman, H. W., Nichols, M., Turner, W. A., Coleman, M., and Wright, W. E. (1981). Respiratory disease in Utah coal miners. *Am. Rev. Respir. Dis.* **123**:372–377.

Ruckley, V. A., Gauld, S. J., Chapman, J. S., Davis, J. M. G., Douglas, A. N., Fernie, J. M., Jacobsen, M., and Lamb, D. (1984). Emphysema and dust exposure in a group of coal workers. *Am. Rev. Respir. Dis.* **129**:528–532.

Schacter, E. N., Maunder, L. R., and Beck, G. J. (1984). The pattern of lung function in abnormalities in cotton textile workers. *Am. Rev. Respir. Dis.* **129**:523–527.

Sluis-Cremer, G. K., Walters, L. G., and Sichel, H. S. (1967a). Chronic bronchitis in miners and non-miners: an epidemiological survey of a community in the gold-mining area in the Transvaal. *Br. J. Ind. Med.* **24**:1–12.

Sluis-Cremer, G. K., Walters, L. G., and Sichel, H. S. (1967b). Ventilatory function in relation to mining experience and smoking in a random sample of miners and non-miners in a Witvatersrand town. *Br. J. Ind. Med.* **24**:13–25.

Soutar, C. A. (1987). Update on lung disease in coalminers. *Br. J. Ind. Med.* **44**:145–148.

Soutar, C. A., and Hurley, J. F. (1986). Relation between dust exposure and lung function in miners and ex-miners. *Br. J. Ind. Med.* **43**:307–320.

Speizer, F. E. (1981). Epidemiology of environmentally induced chronic respiratory disease. *Chest* **80**:21S–23S.

Tabona, M., Chan-Yeung, M., Enarson, D., MacLean, L., Dorken, E., and Schulzer, M. (1984). Host factor affecting longitudinal decline in lung spirometry among grain elevator workers. *Chest* **85**:782–786.

Tockman, M. S. (1982). Epidemiology in the workplace: the problem of misclassification. *J. Occup. Med.* **124**:21–24.

Tockman, M. S., and Baser, M. (1984). Is cotton dust exposure associated with chronic effects? *Am. Rev. Respir. Dis.* **130**:1–3.

U.S. Department of Health and Human Services. (1984). The health consequences of smoking. Chronic obstructive lung disease. A Report of the Surgeon General. DHHS (PHS) 84-50205.

U.S. Department of Health and Human Services. (1985). The health consequences of smoking. Cancer and chronic lung disease in the workplace. A Report of the Surgeon General. DHHS (PHS) 85-50207.

Walker, D. D., Archibald, R. M., and Attfield, M. D. (1971). Bronchitis in men employed in the coke industry. *Br. J. Ind. Med.* **28**:358–363.

Wang, J. D., and Miettinen, O. S. (1982). Occupational mortality studies. Principles of validity. *Scand. J. Work Environ. Health* **8**:153–158.

Wegman, D. H., Peters, J. M., Boundy, M. G., and Smith, T. J. (1982). Evaluation of respiratory effects in miners and millers exposed to talc free of asbestos and silica. *Br. J. Ind. Med.* **39**:233–238.

Wiles, F. J., Faure, M. H. (1977). Chronic obstructive lung disease in gold miners. In *Inhaled Particles* IV, part 2. Edited by W. H. Walton and B. McGowan. Oxford, Pergamon Press, pp. 727–735.

Woskie, S. R., Smith, T. J., Hammond, S. K., Schenker, M. B., Garshick, E., Speizer, F. E. (1988). Estimation of the diesel exhaust exposure of railroad workers. I. Current exposures. *Am. J. Ind. Med.* **13**:381–394.

Wright, J. L., and Churg, A. (1984). Morphology of small-airway lesions in patients with asbestos exposure. *Hum. Pathol.* **15**:68–74.

Wright, J. L., and Churg, A. (1985). Severe diffuse small airways abnormalities in long term chrysotile asbestos miners. *Br. J. Ind. Med.* **42**:556–559.

12

Smoking Cessation

SYDNEY R. PARKER and JOHN W. KUSEK

National Heart, Lung and Blood Institute
National Institutes of Health
Bethesda, Maryland

I. Overview

Tobacco smoking remains by far the most important cause of premature, preventable death among developed countries of the world, despite a massive amount of scientific evidence published and a vast array of information disseminated to the general public about the health hazards of cigarette smoking, especially its relationship to coronary heart disease and lung cancer. As discussed elsewhere in this volume and previously reviewed in detail in the 1984 U.S. Surgeon General's Report (U.S. DHHS, 1984), cigarette smoking is the major cause of chronic obstructive pulmonary disease (COPD) in the United States and other industrialized countries of the world.

Only a minority of cigarette smokers—perhaps 10–20%—develop significant airway obstruction (Buist, 1979). However, tobacco smoking is responsible for over 85% of the deaths due to COPD (Kronebusch, 1985). A number of risk factors other than cigarette smoking have been implicated in the development of COPD but there is no question that elimination of cigarette smoking is the single most effective measure for decreasing the morbidity and mortality associated with these lung diseases.

Because of the overwhelming importance of cigarette smoking as a public health problem, it is not surprising that approaches to changing smoking behavior are numerous and diverse. Some of these measures include prevention programs, cessation programs, legislative action (taxation, labeling requirements, advertising restrictions), and tobacco product changes (Cullen et al., 1986). There is no question that these activities have been effective in reducing cigarette consumption and modifying smoking practices in the United States. Since publication of the first Surgeon General's Report in 1964 (U.S. DHEW, 1964), it has been estimated that 33 million Americans have stopped smoking, resulting in a significant decline in the percentage of current smokers, especially among men (U.S. DHHS, 1986b). Moreover, there has been a significant decrease in tar and nicotine content of manufactured cigarettes consumed. However, approximately one-third of the adult U.S. population continues to smoke resulting in at least 350,000 premature deaths annually (Kronebusch, 1985). Thus, cigarette smoking remains an extremely important public health problem in the United States and indeed, throughout the world (World Health Organization, 1986).

It has become increasingly obvious in the last few years that eradication of cigarette smoking will take the combined and aggressive efforts of public health and voluntary agencies, physicians, dentists, and other health care providers, as well as the general public. In particular, physicians are able to make a major contribution in reducing illness associated with tobacco use by counseling patients to quit smoking. It is not surprising that many people identify the physician as a highly creditable source of health-related information. Moreover, when this fact is considered together with estimates that about three-fourths of the smoking population, at least in the United States, visit a physician at least once a year (U.S. DHHS, 1984), even physician counseling among patients resulting in relatively low smoking quit rates could have a substantial impact on smoking prevalence.

The role of physicians in smoking intervention has become increasingly apparent (Ockene, 1987a,b) and encompasses the identification, evaluation, treatment, follow-up, and possible referral of smokers. To set the stage for a discussion of physician counseling of patients, the magnitude of and changes in cigarette smoking within the United States will be discussed as well as a perspective on the global consumption of tobacco. Within the context of encouraging smoking cessation among patients, the effects of quitting smoking on lung health as it relates to reduction in respiratory symptoms and decline of lung function will be reviewed briefly. This chapter will focus on the simple yet effective ways by which physicians can promote smoking cessation among their patients. Finally, with an eye to the future, the impact of public policy on cigarette smoking in the United States and its potential importance as a deterrent to smoking worldwide will be examined.

II. Prevalence of and Trends in Cigarette Smoking

A. United States

Since the first Surgeon General's Report (U.S. DHEW, 1964) was published, profound changes have taken place in the prevalence of cigarette smoking and the type of cigarettes consumed in the United States. There has been a substantial decline in the prevalence of cigarette smoking among men; from 52% in 1965 to 33% in 1985. In contrast, little change occurred in male smoking rates in the period between 1955 and 1964. For women, the change in smoking prevalence was more modest; decreasing from 34% in 1965 to 28% in 1985 (U.S. DHHS, 1986a). The greater decline in the rate of smoking among men compared to women can be attributed to two factors: higher rates of cessation and lower rates of starting among the young. The trend of decreasing prevalence among men is similar among blacks and whites. This is encouraging since the smoking-related disease burden among black Americans is substantial (Cooper and Simmons, 1985). The smoking prevalence in white males decreased from 51.3% in 1965 to 31.8% in 1985, whereas among black males the decrease during the same 20 year period was from 59.6% to 40.6%. However, the decrease in prevalence for white women has been more substantial when compared to that of black women. The smoking prevalence among white women decreased from 34.5% to 28.3% during 1965 to 1985; for black women the overall prevalence rate essentially remained stable: 32.7% in 1965 and 31.6% in 1985. Hispanic men smoke at about the same rate (31%) as white men, while Hispanic women have a much lower smoking rate (21%) than white and black women (Centers for Disease Control, 1987).

Results of a recent behavioral risk factor survey conducted by the U.S. Centers for Disease Control (Remington et al., 1985) indicated that the highest prevalence rate of cigarette smoking for both black and white men and women was in the 30–44 years age group, with rates for black males, black females, white males, and white females of 43%, 35.5%, 39.4%, and 35.9%, respectively. Among Hispanic men, however, the highest smoking prevalence was observed in those over 45 years (42.2%) of age; for Hispanic women, the highest smoking rates were found in the age group 18–29 years (22.7%).

The rate at which young people take up cigarette smoking can tell us, with some certainty, the future smoking trends in adults. Surveys indicate that the prevalence of cigarette smokers among high school seniors declined to its lowest point in 1984, with 18.7% of all seniors surveyed defined as daily smokers (Shopland and Brown, 1985). This is in contrast to the peak prevalence rate of 28.2% in 1977. Despite these encouraging trends, individuals who smoke only occasionally in their senior year have been observed to increase their amount of smoking sharply in their first year or two after high school. For example, one recent survey noted that white women aged 18–24 had the highest rates of smoking (around 40%), suggesting that the decreasing trend of smoking at the time of high school graduation may be offset by an increase in the proportion of women who begin to smoke following graduation (Remington et al., 1985). If the initiation of smoking in this age group continues at the current rate, it is likely that in the near future the overall smoking prevalence rate among women will exceed that of men.

The trends in smoking during the past 25 years have had a significant impact on the per capita cigarette consumption in the United States. Annual per capita consumption (the number of cigarettes consumed divided by the population, including smokers and nonsmokers 18 years of age and older) increased steadily from 1955, reaching its peak in 1963, as shown in Figure 1. Since the mid-1970s, per capita consumption has declined steadily (Shopland and Brown, 1985). This decline does not reflect the greater decline in the prevalence of cigarette smoking. This can be explained in part by the increase in the proportion of heavy smokers among the smoking population. Among male and female smokers, there is now a greater percentage of heavier smokers than there was in the mid-1960s and 1970s. The percentage of male smokers who consumed 25 cigarettes or more per day (heavy smokers) in 1965 was 24%; today the figure is 31%. For females the increase is even greater; the proportion of heavy smokers increased from 13% in 1965 to 23% in 1985 (U.S. DHHS, 1986a). In general, white men and women are heavier smokers than their black counterparts. For example, in 1980, 45.1% of white males aged 35–44 who were current smokers smoked at least 25 cigarettes per day, compared to only 13.2% of the currently smoking black males in the same age group. Today the greatest proportion of heavy smokers is among white men aged 45–64 (45.3%) and white women aged 35–44 (35.5%) (U.S. DHHS, 1983).

The type of cigarettes that Americans smoke has also changed markedly over the past several decades. In 1984, 94% of total cigarette sales were for filter-tipped cigarettes, up from 60% in 1963. Low-tar, low-nicotine cigarettes have been heavily promoted by manufacturers, resulting in their gaining a 60% share of the market in 1980. The sales-weighted average of tar and nicotine per cigarette consumed in the United States has declined steadily since 1968, the first year these data were collected, and is

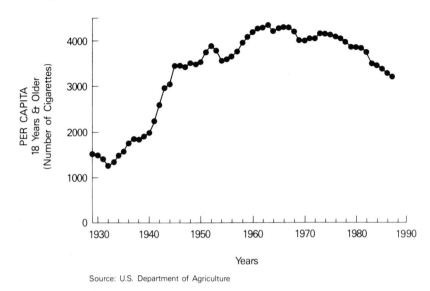

Figure 1 U.S. per capita cigarette consumption: 1955–1984 (adapted from Shopland and Brown, 1985).

currently averaging 12–13 mg tar and less than 1 mg nicotine. In 1954 the average cigarette contained approximately 38 mg tar and 2.3 mg nicotine (U.S. DHHS, 1983). Unfortunately, the trend towards increasing use of low-tar and low-nicotine cigarettes reflects, in part, the belief among smokers and health care professionals that smoking these cigarettes is "safer" than smoking higher-yield brands. Recent controlled studies (Benowitz et al., 1983, 1986) indicate, however, that "low-yield" cigarettes do not contain less nicotine than high-yield cigarettes. Moreover, smokers of "low-yield" cigarettes, by altering their smoking techniques, do not consume less nicotine than users of high-yield brands. These studies have been substantiated in at least one population-based study: smokers who self-select lower-yield cigarettes tend to smoke more cigarettes and, therefore, have a similar degree of exposure to tobacco smoke compared to smokers of higher-yield brands (Maron and Fortmann, 1987).

B. Worldwide Consumption

Compared to the situation in the United States, cigarette consumption is increasing dramatically worldwide, with most of the increase occurring in developing countries and in eastern Europe. Over the past 20 years, tobacco

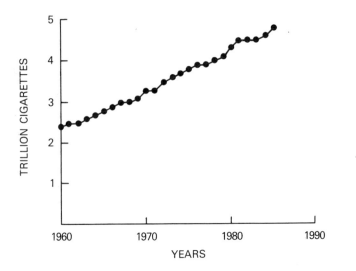

Figure 2 Cigarette consumption worldwide: 1960–1985 (courtesy of Chandler, 1986).

production has increased by 37% and consumption has increased 38%, with similar rates of increase projected for the next decade (Cullen et al., 1986). Over a billion people now smoke, consuming almost five trillion cigarettes each year (Fig. 2), an average of more than half a pack a day. Half the global increase in tobacco use in the last decade has occurred in China, though the Chinese represent only one-fifth of the world's people (Chandler, 1986). The greatest increases in tobacco consumption during the past decade have been in the developing countries. These increases are paralleled by the increase in U.S. cigarette exports which have shifted to most Asian and African countries. In general, among countries (United Kingdom, United States, Canada, and Australia) that have initiated either public health campaigns to publicize the hazards of smoking or passed legislation restricting smoking in certain locations (hospitals, public elevators, etc.) the *overall* smoking prevalence rates have decreased. Still troubling, however, is the increasing prevalence of smoking among women in many countries. Table 1 presents data on male and female smoking rates as an overview of adult smoking habits worldwide (World Health Organization, 1986). International data must be interpreted with care because there is no uniform classification of smokers among countries, the quality of the data is variable, and smoking status is derived from self-reports (Cullen et al., 1986). However, in a number of countries about a

Table 1 Prevalence of Smoking Among Men and Women in Selected Countries

Country	Percentage of Total Who Smoke		National Survey	Year of Survey
	Male	Female		
Australia	37	30	Yes	1983
Bangladesh	70	20	No	1984
Brazil	52	37	No	1983
Canada	41	32	Yes	1983
China	56	1	No	1981
Egypt	40	1	Yes	1982
France	47	20	Yes	1978
Federal Republic of Germany	40	29	Yes	1980
Hong Kong	33	4	Yes	1984
India	61	7	No	1984
Indonesia	6–75	5–10	No	1984
Ireland	49	36	Yes	1980
Italy	54	32	Yes	1981
Japan	70	14	Yes	1980
Pakistan	44	6	No	1982
Poland	63	29	Yes	1980
Romania	52	9	No	1970
Singapore	51	8	Yes	1975
Sweden	30	30	Yes	1982
Thailand	51	4	Yes	1976–1981
United Kingdom	38	33	Yes	1982
U.S.A.	34	29	Yes	1981–1983
U.S.S.R.	44	10	No	1981

Source: Adapted from World Health Organization, 1986. Data for the U.S. derived from Remington et al., 1985.

third of the women smoke, but women in the Soviet Union, China, and Japan smoke very little, with rates ranging from 1 to 14%. Among developed countries, male smoking rates generally fall between a third and a half, with unusually high rates of two-thirds recorded in Japan.

III. Smoking Cessation: Effect on Respiratory Symptoms and Lung Function

Among the most noticeable benefits of smoking cessation is a reduction in respiratory symptoms. A number of epidemiological studies have observed that stopping cigarette smoking results in a significant decrease in cough and phlegm (Buist et al., 1976; Comstock et al., 1970; Huhti and Ikkala, 1980). Many people who stop smoking report a rapid reduction in both of these symptoms. The physician should capitalize on this fact and utilize these tangible and immediate benefits to lung health during the early stages of smoking cessation counseling.

Not as obvious, but in the long run likely to be important to the health of the patient who smokes, are the benefits of smoking cessation on decline of lung function. To date, no randomized controlled studies have shown the effects of quitting smoking on decline of lung function. A recent report from the Multiple Risk Factor Intervention Trial (MRFIT), which intervened on high levels of cholesterol, cigarette smoking, and high blood pressure in over 12,000 men at high risk for coronary heart disease, found that among continuing smokers at three of the participating clinics with good quality control of pulmonary function measurements, the rate of decline of lung function was 60.4 ml/year compared to 49.5 ml/year among those who quit smoking over the course of the 8-year period of follow-up (Townsend, 1987). Based on this subset of the MRFIT cohort, if a middle-aged, healthy smoker stopped smoking permanently, he could expect his forced expiratory volume in 1 sec (FEV_1) to deteriorate at the same rate as a nonsmoker's. A recent report from a population-based longitudinal study (Camilli et al., 1987) actually observed an increase in the (FEV_1) among men and women younger than 35 years of age who quit smoking, suggesting that the earliest effects of cigarette smoking are relatively rapidly reversible and could represent, at least in part, a bronchoconstrictive effect. Among subjects older than 35 years who quit smoking, the rates of decline were intermediate between those of smokers and nonsmokers. However, in a small number of male subjects aged 50–69 who quit early enough to allow calculation of change in FEV_1 from the time of quitting, the rates of decline were very similar to those in nonsmokers suggesting that smoking cessation may reduce the rate of FEV_1 decline relatively promptly even in late middle age. This information can be used to motivate older persons to quit smoking. The use of appropriate visual aids relating effects of smoking on lung function (as shown in Fig. 3) can be used as an important component of physician counseling to show explicitly the benefits of quitting smoking and the hazards of continuing to smoke on the decline of lung function over time and its health consequences (Fletcher and Peto, 1977).

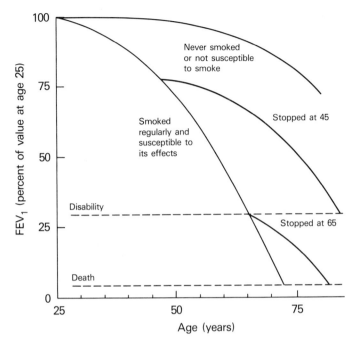

Figure 3   Risks for men with varying "susceptibility to cigarette smoke and consequences of smoking cessation" (reprinted from Fletcher and Peto, 1977).

To address the question of whether COPD can be prevented, the National Heart, Lung, and Blood Institute of the U.S. Public Health Service is supporting a multicenter study on early intervention for chronic obstructive pulmonary disease, called the Lung Health Study (Division of Lung Diseases, 1985). The primary purpose of this study is to determine whether an intervention program incorporating smoking cessation (including a physician-delivered smoking cessation message based on results of pulmonary function testing) and use of an inhaled bronchodilator (ipratropium bromide) in persons at high risk for COPD, can slow down the decline in pulmonary function (FEV_1) and reduce the incidence of pulmonary morbidity over the 5 year period of follow-up. A total of 5,886 cigarette smokers aged 35–59 who demonstrate evidence of early airway obstruction have been recruited at 10 clinical centers throughout the United States and Canada. Participants were randomly assigned to receive (1) usual care (no intervention), (2) smoking intervention plus placebo inhaler, or (3) smoking intervention plus active bronchodilator. Inhaler assignment is double-blind. All participants will have their pulmonary function tested yearly; the intervention participants will be seen at the clinics every 4 months to promote and maintain smoking cessation and inhaler use compliance. The follow-up period will end in 1994.

The results of the Lung Health Study should establish: whether screening spirometry is useful to identify early airflow limitation; whether physicians can play a vital role in helping their patients quit smoking; whether quitting smoking even when early airflow limitation is present has substantial benefits to lung function and respiratory morbidity; and whether control of airways hyperreactivity by long-term bronchodilator drug treatment produces a clinically significant effect in curtailing the premature loss of pulmonary function among persons at high risk for COPD.

IV. Physician Interventions

Physicians have the potential for effecting major changes in the smoking behavior of patients. This influence can be exerted in at least four different ways:

1. Acting as a nonsmoking role model for patients and the community

2. Advising patients to quit and providing guidance on how to quit

3. Referring patients to formal smoking-cessation courses

4. Becoming active in the community for public policy initiatives, discouraging smoking in public places and worksites, and creating smoking prevention programs in schools

A. Nonsmoking Role Model

The first method of influencing smokers is by acting as a nonsmoking role model and adopting a healthy lifestyle. The nonsmoking status of physicians is essential to ensure credibility with patients in discussing the hazards of smoking. If a physician smokes, he or she is less likely to counsel his or her patients to quit. Similarly, the greater the number of poor health habits the physician possesses, the smaller the likelihood of his or taking an active role in encouraging healthy habits in patients (Wells et al., 1984). Physicians in the United States have already quit smoking at a greater rate than the rest of the population. Between 1959 and 1972 physicians' smoking rates decreased from 39% to 20% (Garfinkel, 1976). A 1975 survey of health professionals showed that 21% of physicians smoked (U.S. DHEW,

1976); however, by 1984 this smoking rate had decreased to 10–15% (Wells et al., 1984).

Physicians may underscore their role as nonsmokers by posting no smoking signs in the office and by providing literature on smoking cessation in the waiting room. It should be absolutely clear to their patients that the office is a nonsmoking environment and that this decision is based on physicians' concern for the health of their patients and staff.

B. Advice on Quitting

Potential for Influencing Patients' Smoking Behavior

The second method by which physicians can influence patients' smoking behavior is by direct discussion of the harmful habit, provision of a clear recommendation to quit, and advice on methods of quitting. Techniques derived from behavioral science have been shown in recent years to help the physician become more effective in motivating patients to quit and assisting them in the process. Such advice is seen by the public as the most effective means of prompting cessation or reduction in smoking, ranking as more effective than prohibitions of smoking at work or in public places; urging of children, spouse, and relatives; higher taxes; antismoking campaigns at work; or televised antismoking advertisements (Louis Harris and Associates, 1984). If physicians actively counseled smokers to quit smoking, even a modest success rate in this endeavor could have an important impact on public health. Physicians have contact with at least 70% of all smokers each year, and with 61% of smokers who consider themselves to be "in excellent health" (Ockene, 1987b). Thus, approximately 38 million of the 53 million adult smokers in the United States could potentially be reached by physicians during the course of medical care. If only 5% of these quit, almost two million smokers would enjoy the benefits of a more healthy lifestyle.

There is a discrepancy between patients' and physicians' perceptions of how frequently physicians advise patients to quit. Only 44% of smokers who have seen a doctor in the past year report having *ever* been advised to quit by a physician. Smokers who are hypertensive, obese, diabetic, sedentary, or users of oral contraceptives are no more likely to have been told to quit than those without these additional risks (Anda et al., 1987). Yet a high proportion of physicians report advising patients to quit. Most physicians report asking questions about smoking, and virtually all report providing antismoking advice to at least some smoking patients. In a survey of Massachusetts physicians, 90% reported asking questions about smoking (Wechsler et al., 1983), however, few of them had any confidence in their ability actually to help patients quit. Only 58% of the physicians felt prepared to counsel patients regarding smoking, and only 3% believed themselves to be successful in helping patients quit. A similar survey of California physicians indicated that 85% believed smoking is dangerous and counseling is important, but only 21% thought they knew how to counsel patients. Moreover, only 12% judged themselves to be personally effective (Wells et al., 1984). These differences in perceptions may be due to several factors. Smokers may selectively forget antismoking advice. Also physicians may equate asking questions about smoking with giving antismoking advice. The smoking cessation message may have been less than forceful and not accompanied by written material on cessation. The physician's lack of confidence in his or ability to influence patients' smoking behavior may be due to lack of skills to recommend to the patient about specific methods to quit, which may be more likely to be remembered by the patient.

Several randomized controlled studies have shown that physicians can have a significant impact on the smoking habits of their patients, even with a minimal intervention. If the intervention is more intensive, more frequent, and includes the use of follow-up appointments, self-help materials, and nicotine gum, the physician's intervention can be even more effective. For a comprehensive review of studies of physician advice for smoking cessation, see the 1984 Report of the Surgeon General (U.S. DHHS, 1984).

The largest study to date on the effect of physicians' antismoking advice (Russell et al., 1979) showed a significant effect of advice and the provision of educational materials over no advice after a year. During a period of 4 weeks, all 2138 cigarette smokers attending the offices of 28 general practitioners in 5 group practices were randomized to 1 of 4 groups: (1) nonintervention control, (2) questionnaire-only control, (3) advice to stop by the general practitioner, or (4) advice plus a leaflet and a warning of follow-up. Antismoking advice was delivered in the physician's own style over 1–2 min during a routine consultation. After 1 year, the smoking quit rates of these groups were 10.3%, 14.0%, 16.7%, and 19.1%, respectively.

Even minimal intervention can produce a higher quit rate in patients than in controls, although in absolute terms the effect is small. Folsom and Grimm (1987) noted that patients who received only a 1–2 min message to quit showed a quit rate of 8.8% after 3 months, compared to a 6.8% quit rate in the controls. In this minimum intervention study, the number of patients who attempted to quit was small in both groups; however, those in the intervention group showed twice as many quit attempts as did controls.

Distribution of written material to accompany antismoking advice can increase success. A recent study (Janz et al., 1987) comparing physician advice plus a tested self-help booklet to advice alone or to no advice showed that physician's advice plus a booklet including several modern self-help methods increased both the number of smokers who attempted to quit and the number of those who were successful. In fact, patients receiving advice plus the booklet were more than twice as likely to quit as those in the other two groups.

One of the risks of a minimal intervention is that it may not be strong enough to be remembered and acted upon by the patient. As mentioned previously, the smoker may not perceive a brief discussion on smoking to be a recommendation to quit, or may selectively forget the advice after a period of time. In one recent study (Folsom and Grimm, 1987), only 60% of those in the smoking intervention group recalled receiving any advice 3 months later. Moreover, 15% of these did not perceive the advice as a message to quit smoking.

Follow-up appointments to discuss progress in quitting can significantly increase the effectiveness of physicians' advice to quit. In a study of 234 smokers, all were given 3–5 min of counseling including review of their history of smoking; health risks; review of strategies for quitting, such as cold turkey, self-management, aversion, acupuncture, hypnosis, group therapy, nicotine gum, confrontation about smoking; and a recommendation to quit. The controls received no further counseling while the experimental group received follow-up appointments at 1, 3, and 6 months to review progress and identify and solve problems. Six to 14 months later, 23% of the experimental group had quit compared with only 12% of the control group (Wilson et al., 1982).

Men at risk for medical complications of smoking may be more receptive to antismoking advice. In a study of 1445 male smokers aged 40–59 who were identified as at high risk for cardiopulmonary disease, 51% of those who were given 15 min counseling with a physician regarding the hazards of smoking, and advice to quit, were nonsmokers after a year (Rose and Hamilton, 1978). This is compared to a quit rate of 10% in the control group whose medical examination results were sent to their physician. Relapse remained a problem, however, in the experimental group; by 3 years, the 51% quit rate in the experimental group had declined to 36%, while the control group quitters had increased from 10% to 14%. This indicates a clear need for follow-up and the discussion of relapse prevention skills, a topic that has been addressed in recent behavioral research, and is discussed below.

The prescription of nicotine gum can be a useful adjunct to the physician's counseling of the patient regarding smoking, when it is provided along with counseling on ways to use the gum and to quit smoking. Nicotine gum, by replacing the nicotine absorbed from a cigarette, can enable the smoker to break the smoking habit without at the same time having to overcome nicotine dependence, which is faced at a later time by gradual withdrawal of the gum (Russell et al., 1980). The gum has been shown to decrease significantly withdrawal symptoms such as irritability, hostility, and restlessness faced by smokers in the process of quitting (Schneider and Jarvik, 1984; Jarvis et al., 1982). Nicotine gum does show some minor side effects such as bad taste; irritation of the gums, mouth, throat; and occasional nausea. Less common side effects may include ulceration of the tongue, aching jaw, flatulence, hiccups, and epigastric discomfort (Russell et al., 1980). Patients may become dependent on the gum itself. One study has observed that 7% of the patients receiving the gum used it for more than 6 months (Jarvis et al., 1982).

Evaluation studies of the usefulness of nicotine gum have shown that when it is the major treatment, the median nonsmoking rate after 6 months is 23%, and 11% at the end of 12 months of follow-up (Schwartz, 1987). When nicotine gum is part of another treatment, median quit rates are better: about 35% at 6 months and 29% after 1 year. For example, when used along with group therapy, nicotine gum has been shown to have a significant effect over the effect of a placebo gum. In one study (Hjalmarson, 1984), 29% of participants in a 6-week smoking therapy group who used nicotine gum were nonsmokers throughout the follow-up year, while 16% of those who used placebo gum were nonsmokers. Similarly, when smokers were instructed to return to the clinic for follow-up every day for a week, then once a week for 4 weeks, 30% of the nicotine gum users were nonsmokers at 1 year, while 20% of the placebo gum users were nonsmokers (Schneider et al., 1983).

Physicians who prescribe nicotine gum for their patients can expect approximately 10% of these patients to quit, which is a number greater than that obtained if gum is not prescribed. However, counseling on ways to quit and instructions on the use of the gum are essential. One large study of physicians' advice to quit showed that of patients who received advice to quit, plus a brochure and nicotine gum, 8.8% were not smoking at the end of 1 year. Of those who received only advice and a brochure, 4.1% were not smoking, while 3.9% of controls were abstinent (Russell et al., 1983). This study shows a clear advantage of the gum when combined with advice to quit, although the absolute percentage of quitters is still small. Another larger study of advice to quit has not shown these differences between experimental groups (British Thoracic Society, 1983). This large "real world" study involving 150 physicians and 1550 of their patients with smoking-related diseases did not show an advantage of nicotine gum over verbal advice to quit; verbal advice plus a brochure; or verbal advice, brochure, plus nicotine gum. This study was conducted during routine clinical care, and smokers were not self-selected to participate in smoking cessation. These results confirm that physicians' advice to quit, by itself, can have a modest but important effect, since the widespread application of a small effect can have an important impact on public health. However, this study indicates that the positive effects of gum use may not always be found when it is used in the course of regular medical care with patients who are not initially seeking help with quitting smoking.

It is clear that the prescription of the gum must be accompanied by instructions on its use in smoking cessation. When simply prescribed with no instructions or help with quitting, the effects of nicotine gum are no different from that of a placebo (Schneider et al., 1983). For a comprehensive review of nicotine gum and its impact on smoking quit rates, see Schwartz (1987).

Nicotine gum is probably most useful in the early stages of quitting, when physiological withdrawal symptoms are greatest. After that time, the withdrawal symptoms diminish while the psychological factors influencing relapse or maintenance become more important. Smokers particularly need to learn how to cope with temptations to relapse, such as conditions of interpersonal frustration or negative affect.

Guidelines for Assisting a Patient in Quitting

Smoking History

The first step in motivating a patient to quit is to elicit a complete smoking history. This information should include number of cigarettes smoked per day, type of cigarette smoked, age at onset of smoking, patterns of inhaling, past efforts at quitting, length of time off cigarettes in the past, problems encountered with past smoking-cessation efforts, and social factors mitigating for and against smoking such as the smoking habits and attitudes of a spouse, friends, and children (Pechacek and Grimm, 1983). The smoking history may include questioning about smoking-related symptoms such as morning cough, shortness of breath, or frequent upper respiratory tract infections. This provides the physician with background information to use in advising the patient to quit and legitimizes the topic as a normal part of the physician interview. The physician should ask the patient how willing he or she is to quit, and for the patient's own reasons for wanting to quit. The physician might find it useful to place a reminder sticker in the patient's chart to prompt a discussion of smoking at subsequent visits (Cohen et al., 1987).

Motivating the Patient to Quit

To begin the process of encouragement to quit, the physician should discuss with the patient the serious health risks of cigarette smoking. First, the general risks of the many diseases caused by smoking should be discussed.

Patients may be aware of the risk of lung cancer, but may not be aware of the risk of other forms of cancer, heart disease, or emphysema. More importantly, risk information should be personalized as much as possible, and the interactions of other risk factors should be discussed. The patient may have additional risk factors that are synergistic with the risk of smoking, such as occupational exposure, use of birth control pills, or a family history of heart disease or cancer. The patient should be made aware of his or her personal susceptibility to smoking-related disease. During the physical examination may be a useful time to introduce the topic of individual risk, especially during examination of the lungs and heart. Linking the smoking habit to patient's symptoms such as cough and shortness of breath may be useful (Pechacek and Grimm, 1983). Laboratory and radiographic data may be helpful in pointing to the risk of smoking. One helpful aid in providing simple risk information to the patient is the booklet "Clinical Opportunities for Smoking Intervention: A Guide for the Busy Physician" (NHLBI, 1986). The booklet provides risk information that may be used in counseling, as well as answers to questions frequently asked by patients who are interested in quitting.

Two tests may be performed in the physician's office that may be especially useful in pointing out the harmful effects of smoking for the individual. First, simple spirometry can provide a tool to assess the damage smoking has already caused to the patient's lungs and to calculate the individual's personal risk of developing chronic obstructive pulmonary disease, by the Tecumsah Index of Risk (Higgins et al., 1982; Higgins and Keller, 1983). By knowing the patients' age, sex, current smoking habits, and height, the physician can calculate the patient's risk of developing COPD in the next 10 years. For example, a 51-year old man who smokes two packs a day and has an FEV_1 of 85% predicted would have a one in 4 chance of developing COPD in the next 15 years if he continued to smoke. If he quits, he reduces his risk to one in 30. The use of the Tecumsah Index of Risk may be especially helpful when one is working with older smokers who have some impairment in lung function.

The second test that may be useful in dramatizing the harmful effects of smoking is the measurement of expired carbon monoxide (CO). The physician can point out that the CO value found in the smoker's expired air is an indicator of "the amount of your blood that is being taken up with CO, and is, therefore, not carrying oxygen" (Pechacek and Grimm, 1983). However, during smoking-cessation efforts, care should be taken in measuring CO levels. If the smoker is reducing his or her amount of smoking or is smoking sporadically, the CO level may not show much change. However, if the smoker has stopped completely, the CO level will almost certainly show a dramatic decrease.

When motivating a patient to quit, the physician should not use scare tactics, since these may produce counterproductive anxiety in the patient. Even if the physician uses spirometry or expired CO to point out the harmful impact of smoking on the patients' body, he or she should emphasize the positive benefits of quitting, and that many of the deleterious effects of smoking are potentially reversible, so it is not too late to quit. Physicians should encourage patients to make a list of their own reasons for quitting and to review these periodically.

The physician should give the patient a clear and unmistakable recommendation to quit and ask the patient if he or she is willing to make a contract to do so on a certain date. Asking the patient to sign a contract to quit on a certain date formalizes the commitment to quit and provides the smoker with a period of preparation. The physician should keep a copy of the signed agreement and inform the patient that he or she plans to follow-up on the contract agreement at the next visit, or ask the patient to call in weekly for a few weeks to report progress. Some form of follow-up, such as three to four physician–patient contacts, is important in increasing the patient's perceptions that the physician takes the issue of smoking cessation seriously.

The physician should discuss the problem of withdrawal symptoms such as irritability, anxiety, depression, and impaired ability to concentrate, emphasizing that these symptoms are temporary and will subside within 2 weeks of quitting. These symptoms can be alleviated by decreasing nicotine intake through switching brands of cigarettes prior to quitting, quitting abruptly, then using techniques such as deep breathing or another substitute behavior for smoking, or by use of nicotine gum. In counseling women of childbearing age, the physician might consider suggesting quitting in the last half of the menstrual cycle, since withdrawal symptoms may be greater if the women quits in the first half of the cycle (Russell and Portser, 1987). The smoker should know that a cigarette craving lasts only 3–5 min whether or not he smokes, and craving becomes less frequent after 7–10 days. The physician may discuss the patient's concerns about weight gain, pointing out that only one-third of quitters may gain weight, and even so, the gain is not great. However, the patient must be careful not to substitute sweets for cigarettes, but to find other substitutes such as carrots or celery sticks, if the urge to snack is great.

The physician should emphasize the importance of social support from family and friends. The patient might enlist the aid of these to encourage, but not nag, the smoker in his or her process of cessation. Finally, the physician should express confidence in the patients' ability to quit, acknowledging that the process may be difficult. Printed self-help materials can be useful in reinforcing the physician's advice and providing additional information on ways to quit.

Self-Monitoring

Once the patient has made the commitment to quit, the physician can encourage the patient to use the time before the quit date as a period of self-monitoring. This strategy is commonly used in smoking-cessation clinics and self-help programs in conjunction with other strategies. It has been helpful to many smokers attempting to quit. This includes noting situations in which they find themselves smoking, and the rewards they receive from the process. The use of a smoking diary for 1–2 weeks can be a powerful tool for helping the patient become aware of his or her smoking patterns (Lichtenstein and Danaher, 1978). The patient should record each cigarette smoked, the circumstances surrounding the smoking, and the importance of each cigarette. The process will yield useful information to the smoker and may help to reduce the smoking rate.

Breaking Situational Associations

After the self-monitoring period, the smoker should try to break the association of the smoking behavior with a variety of situations that normally stimulate lighting up. Drinking coffee or alcohol, or talking on the telephone, or the time after dinner are examples of situations that often cue smoking behavior. The smoker might narrow the range of places to smoke to one inconvenient spot, such as the garage or bathroom (Glasgow, 1985). During this period the smoker may cut in half the number of cigarettes he or she smokes, or switch to a low-tar and low-nicotine brand.

Quitting

On the target quit day, the patient is to throw away all cigarettes and remove all smoking-related objects such as ashtrays and matches from the home, office, and car (Lichtenstein and Danaher, 1978) and he or she should review the personal reasons for quitting. He or she should be prepared to take an action when feeling tempted to smoke, since it has been found that taking any action is helpful to the exsmoker in avoiding relapse (Shiffman, 1982). Practicing deep breathing for a few minutes or taking a walk may help to overcome the urge to smoke.

Preventing Relapse

Relapse remains a major problem in the process of quitting smoking. Relapse occurs most often in situations involving negative emotional states. Moreover, 80% of all relapse episodes have been found to fall into one of three categories: coping with negative emotional states, social pressure to smoke, and interpersonal conflict (Marlatt and Gordon, 1980).

The reasons exsmokers relapse in the early stages of cessation may not always be the same as those governing later relapse. In a study of 837 participants in smoking-cessation programs, O'Connell (1985) found that predictors of short-term success are either not related or inversely related to long-term success. Those who have the most trouble in the early phases of cessation may be those who are the least vulnerable to later relapse. For example, high nicotine intake prior to cessation is related to early, or 3-month, relapse. However, high nicotine intake is negatively related to relapse between 3 and 12 months, suggesting that persons who are highly addicted to nicotine are more likely to relapse in the early stages. However, if they succeed in remaining abstinent for 3 months, they may be more reluctant to return to smoking, not wishing to give up their hard-won gains or to go through the process of quitting again.

Those smokers who report that they tend to smoke in situations involving negative emotions seem to have a more difficult time in the later stages of cessation than in the early ones. Negative-affect smokers may make it through the cessation program because of the strong support offered and because of initial motivation. However, if they do not develop other methods of coping with stressful situations, a stressful situation may bring about a return to smoking. In fact, 42% of those subjects who were considered high-negative-affect smokers and who experienced stressful situations relapsed between months 3 and 12 after cessation, while none of the high-stress/low-negative-affect group relapsed (O'Connell, 1985).

The important aspect of coping with an urge to relapse may be the act of performing a coping response, regardless of the response chosen. In a study of exsmokers who called a telephone hotline when they experienced a temptation to smoke, it was found that if the quitter used any coping strategy, he or she was less likely to relapse. The number of strategies used had no effect, and almost all the strategies were equally effective (Shiffman, 1984). Coping strategies, such as talking one's self out of the cigarette or thinking about the positive consequences of not succumbing versus the negative consequences of succumbing, were often used, while behavioral strategies such as eating or drinking, doing a distracting activity, or relaxing were also mentioned. Two specific strategies—exerting will power and punishing one's self—were found to be ineffective in coping with the urge to smoke.

The physician should discuss with the patient that relapse can be a problem after the initial quitting; however, there are ways to prevent relapse. The following may be helpful strategies in relapse prevention and may be useful in discussing relapse prevention with patients (Brownell et al., 1986).

Early Maintenance

Social Support. In the early stages of quitting, social support can encourage the quitter and help to sustain him or her in the presence of withdrawal symptoms and potential situations conducive to relapse. It must be noted, however, that the presence of a smoker in the home decreases success, so the smoker in this situation must be vigilant in anticipating urges to smoke cued by the smoking of others.

Reinforcement. The quitter should find ways of rewarding himself or herself in the early stages of quitting. These rewards should continue through the process, must be realistic, and should be easily accessible to the patient.

Coping. The smoker should choose a few powerful strategies for coping with urges to smoke. The strategies should be personally relevant and should include cognitive strategies for the patient's discussions with himself or herself on the topic. For example, in the face of withdrawal symptoms, the patient could practice deep breathing, escape from the situation by taking a walk, or imagine that he or she is "riding a wave" until the urge is over.

Pharmacologic Agents. Nicotine gum, as discussed previously, may be useful in preventing relapse at this stage of quitting. When prescribing nicotine gum, the physician should provide instructions to the patient on the use of the gum (Russell et al., 1980). The physician should emphasize to the smoker that the gum will not, in and of itself, cure the smoking habit. The smoker should stop smoking completely on his or her target day, and use the gum when necessary. If the urge is expected, he or she should begin chewing early, since it takes 15–20 min for the nicotine to reach its peak level. The smoker should use the gum for 3–6 months and carry a supply of gum for emergencies for up to a year. The patient should not continue to smoke while using the gum. Smokers with peptic ulcers should not use the gum, and caution is advised in those who are pregnant or who have muscular disease. It is contraindicated immediately following myocardial infarction and in patients with life-threatening arrhythmias or severe or worsening angina pectoris. More detailed instructions on the use of the gum, its side effects, and contraindications may be found on the manufacturers' package insert.

Late Maintenance

Since relapses can occur at any time, even after years of nonsmoking, the exsmoker must be continually vigilant to avoid relapse. He or she should be prepared for the fact that maintenance of nonsmoking may be as difficult as quitting. Self-help printed material kept on hand may be useful in reinforcing earlier messages. Late stages of quitting are also times when the exsmoker should create lifestyle changes that replace smoking as a reinforcer, such as initiating exercise and improving nutritional habits to prevent weight gain.

The smoker must continue to anticipate situations in which he or she will be tempted to smoke, such as cues in the environment or times of frustration. Stress management may be important in late maintenance. Dealing with negative affect, particularly that associated with interpersonal conflict, may be helpful in preventing relapse.

C. Referral

The third way of helping patients to quit is to refer them to a formal smoking-cessation program. However, physicians may not know the effectiveness of smoking programs in the local area and may be hesitant to make referrals to an unknown program. This section will review some of the programs generally available, discuss components of successful programs, and provide guidelines for judging the usefulness of a program.

Self-Help Materials

Most smokers prefer to quit on their own rather than join a smoking-cessation program (Schwartz and Dubitsky, 1967). Therefore, a wide variety of self-help materials are available to assist smokers in quitting. Most of these have not been evaluated to determine their impact on long-term abstinence rates. A recent comprehensive review (Schwartz, 1987) of published and non-published evaluations of self-help trials has determined that the median abstinence rate after 1 year is 18%. Guides that are not complex appear to be the most useful. Moreover, people who self-select to quit on their own appear to succeed 16–20% of the time in being abstinent after 1 year. Noticeably lacking in the published literature is information on the variety of aids to quitting available over-the-counter. Therefore, no conclusions can be drawn regarding the majority of these aids.

Two self-help kits that may be recommended to smokers attempting to quit are the booklets "Freedom from Smoking in 20 Days," produced by the American Lung Association (1980), and the "I Quit Kit," produced by the American Cancer Society (1977). Both of these are readily available and have been evaluated. The "Freedom from Smoking" program consists of a manual on how to stop smoking, and another on how to maintain abstinence. An evaluation (Davis et al., 1984) of 1237 smokers who received the books revealed that of those who used the combination of both manuals, or who received an antismoking leaflet plus the maintenance manual, 18% were abstinent after 1 year. The cessation manual alone produced a 15% cessation rate and the leaflets alone 12% cessation.

An evaluation of the American Cancer Society's "I Quit Kit," showed a 27% success rate at the end of one year, compared to 15% and 0% for two other self-help guides. The easy-to-follow program was read by 80% of the subjects who received it (Glasgow et al., 1981).

If a physician is working with a patient to create a smoking-cessation effort, and the patient is using self-help materials, the physician should seek feedback from the patient on the usefulness of the materials. This not only assists in future recommendations to patients, but also provides an opportunity to discuss particular problems the smoker is having in the process of quitting.

Single-Component Programs: Hypnosis and Acupuncture

Hypnosis has proven to be a popular choice for smokers who are attempting to quit. It is also the most frequently advertised method of smoking cessation, as measured by frequency of telephone book listings (Schwartz, 1987). It may be conducted in individual or group sessions once or over several sessions. However, it is very difficult to assess the effectiveness of hypnosis as a cessation method. Many hypnotherapists claim high success rates, but solid scientific evaluations of the technique with adequate 1-year follow-up and numbers of subjects are not frequently conducted. A review of those reported indicate quit rates of 0–68% for individual hypnosis and 8–88% for group hypnosis (Schwartz, 1987). Overall success rates were slightly higher for group programs. Since hypnosis is frequently combined with other methods to encourage cessation, it is difficult to attribute results to hypnosis alone. It appears that hypnosis itself produces only modest quit rates, but these are improved by the addition of other methods. As with any method, counseling and follow-up are needed to maintain abstinence.

Similarly, acupuncture is gaining popularity in the United States as an aid to smoking cessation. However, as with evaluation of hypnosis, evaluation of acupuncture is fraught with poorly designed studies. Studies in which the "correct" site is compared to the "incorrect" site have not shown an advantage of the correct acupuncture site over the placebo site. However, results of 1-year follow-up range from 8 to 32% with a median of 30%, and almost all of these studies fail to validate self-reported cessation. The one study that objectively validated the self-reported quit rate observed only an 8% success rate at 15 months (Clavel et al., 1985). Review of the studies on acupuncture has not demonstrated its efficacy as a smoking-cessation aid beyond its placebo effect. Counseling and support are necessary to produce greater success in stopping smoking.

Regardless of the evaluation studies of many available cessation approaches, some patients will choose these methods of attempting to quit. If so, the physician should recognize that there is some benefit to a good placebo, but that the motivation of the patient is critical. Moreover, counseling and support from the physician can increase the patient's chances of becoming successful. Follow-up of the patient's progress toward long-term abstinence will assist the patient in working toward his or her goal.

Group Smoking Cessation Programs

Many types of smoking programs have been developed to assist smokers in quitting. Reviews in the early 1970s revealed that most of these were effective in the short run, but after a year, only 20–30% of the participants were abstinent (Hunt and Bespalec, 1974). It seems, however, that any type of treatment or attention placebo offered at a group cessation clinic will produce 40–60% posttreatment success but only 15–25% long-term abstinence (U.S. DHEW 1979). More recently developed programs have often showed abstinence rates of 30–40% or greater.

One may generally categorize the most common group-oriented programs into three categories: those primarily educational in nature, those emphasizing group process and discussion, and those containing multiple components derived from behavioral science technologies.

Educational cessation methods generally consist of lectures by a variety of professionals, films, keeping a record of smoking, literature, instructions on how to quit, direct information, and answers to questions. There may be some discussion, but the approach is didactic, and the conversation is between a participant and a leader. Such programs were more popular before 1978. Review of the 12 educational trials conducted between 1962 and 1984 that included 1-year follow-up indicated that approximately 25% of participants in these programs are abstinent after 1 year, and 25% of the programs reported success rates greater than 33% (Schwartz, 1987).

Group cessation programs that emphasize group counseling and support from other participants have been more popular in recent years. These include a wide variety of approaches, however, and may also include printed materials, films to trigger discussion, buddy systems, follow-up meetings or contacts, and occasionally aversive techniques or other behavioral techniques. Review of the 31 trials published between 1962 and 1984 with 1-year follow-up indicate that a median of 28% of participants in these programs are abstinent after 1 year. Of the eleven programs published between 1978 and 1984, 36% of the participants were abstinent. Moreover, almost two-thirds of these programs achieved abstinence rates over 33%. These cessation rates do not include studies of the effectiveness of proprietary programs, which often claim greater success rates. If a physician is considering referral to a smoking program, whether it be for profit or not for profit, he or she should request information on success rates experienced. Estimates of success rates should be based on the number of participants who entered the program rather than upon the number who completed it and self-reports of abstinence should be verified objectively.

Multicomponent programs are generally the most successful smoking programs today (Orleans et al., 1981). Although it is difficult to determine the most effective components of the programs, several components are found in most state-of-the-art programs. Glasgow (1985), in a review of self-management strategies, has described five that are the most often used in modern quitting programs. Many of these have been developed and refined through behavioral science research.

Self-monitoring: Smokers are asked to observe their own behavior to increase awareness of the smoking behavior and provide information about smoking patterns.

Goal setting/contracting: Programs often have participants set a target date for quitting in the near future and establish weekly goals for progressive reductions in nicotine content of brand, or number of cigarettes smoked, prior to cessation. Contracts for quitting may be written and may include a monetary component.

Stimulus control/alternative behaviors: Smokers are encouraged to break the situational associations of smoking by progressively narrowing the range of situations in which they smoke. They are also encouraged to develop alternative behaviors to cope with the urge to smoke.

Aversion: One of the most successful additions to smoking programs has been the process of making cigarette smoking an aversive act. Rapid smoking is the most effective of these methods (Lichtenstein et al., 1973). Subjects are instructed to take a puff of a cigarette every 6 sec until they cannot tolerate any more. Subjects often became nauseated by the procedure, although not usually to the point of vomiting. Trials that have used rapid smoking have reported abstinence rates of 50–60% at 6 months or a year (Lichtenstein et al., 1973; Powell and McCann, 1981; Best et al., 1977). Although concerns have been raised about the safety of this procedure, because of the possibility of nicotine poisoning and cardiovascular stress, it appears that rapid smoking is safe and effective for healthy subjects. Moreover, patients with mild to moderate cardiac and pulmonary disease may use the technique under certain conditions (Sachs et al., 1979), although there are some contraindications (Hall et al., 1984).

Maintenance strategies: Most smoking programs are now incorporating components to teach the participants skills to overcome the temptation to smoke and prevent relapse. For example, they might include role-playing of situations in which they expect to be tempted to smoke or situations of interpersonal frustration or social pressure to smoke. Relaxation training may be incorporated so that subjects are trained to pair a particular word with relaxation.

If a physician is considering referring patients to smoking cessation programs in the local area, he or she should request information regarding the experience of the program's leaders, history of the program, and past success rates. Although available programs may not contain all the elements from behavioral science previously discussed, those that include at least some of these are more likely to produce long-term abstinence. It must be remembered that patients have individual needs and preferences for particular approaches. The physician should be familiar with the range of programs available in the local area, so that he or she can assist the patient in finding a program that suits the patient's individual needs and preferences. Regardless of the program the smoker attends, the physician should follow up the patient's progress in quitting, and ensure the patient that he or she is taking a positive step toward better health.

V. Public Policy

The fourth way that physicians may make changes in the behavior of patients is by taking an active part in national, state, and community antismoking activities. Likewise, physician organizations that deal with the tobacco issue, such as "Doctors Ought to Care," are appropriate forums for promoting change in attitudes about cigarette smoking and other forms of tobacco use. In the United States, physicians, voluntary organizations, and government agencies have become active in recent years in promoting legislation to limit smoking in public places. A comprehensive review of the current status of U.S. public policy approaches restricting smoking is found in the 1986 Surgeon General's Report on Involuntary Smoking (U.S. DHHS, 1986c). Highlights from this report follow.

After the First Report of the Surgeon General on the Health Consequences of Smoking (U.S. DHEW, 1964), the public became much more aware of the hazards of smoking and the medical reasons for quitting. As a result, public policy initiatives were developed to encourage the smoker to quit. By the early 1970s, however, public attitudes toward smoking became more negative and were bolstered by the growing evidence regarding both the harmfulness of active smoking and the health risks to nonsmokers of exposure to involuntary smoke. Thus, a movement known as the non-smokers' rights movement led the efforts, in many cases, to pass legislation to protect the nonsmoker by limiting smoking in public places, and more recently, in private worksites.

As of 1986, 41 states and the District of Columbia have enacted laws regulating smoking in at least one public place. Although the restrictiveness of these state laws vary widely, they most often restrict smoking on public transportation, in hospitals, elevators, indoor cultural or recreational facilities, schools, public meeting rooms, and libraries. Many states now restrict smoking in restaurants and retail stores.

Smoking at the workplace is restricted for public sector employees in 22 states and for private sector employees in 9 states. In addition, local communities across the country have enacted smoking ordinances, many of which affect private worksites and restaurants. Most restrictive laws prohibit smoking except in designated areas, making nonsmoking the norm rather than smoking.

In addition, many employers are implementing policies regarding smoking in the absence of legislation requiring it. About one-half of all U.S. companies now have workplace smoking restrictions that generally limit smoking to designated areas (Bureau of National Affairs, 1987). Total workplace smoking bans are rare. The practice of preferentially hiring nonsmokers is also rare but is likely to be considered more often in the future.

Although it is difficult to determine the impact of restricting smoking policies in public and in the workplace, these policies appear to be a product of changing public opinion about smoking as well as confirming nonsmoking as the societal norm. They may reduce the total number of daily cigarettes smoked, since smokers have to postpone smoking to other times and places. They may be of assistance to those who are in the process of quitting by limiting the number of cues in the environment that would normally stimulate them to light up a cigarette. In addition, they may be the additional inconvenience that motivates the smoker to consider giving up the habit.

Physicians are in a unique position to take a leadership role in encouraging nonsmoking. By their individual relationships with patients, they can be a motivator for action for better health among individual patients. As members of the community, they are credible sources of health information on the harmful effects of smoking. As activists for nonsmoking policies, they can encourage the establishment of nonsmoking as the community norm.

In summary, physicians should expand their sphere of influence regarding health issues to include community action concerning the limitation of tobacco consumption. Such involvement is likely to have a major impact on public health in the decades ahead.

References

American Cancer Society (1977). *I Quit Kit.* New York, American Cancer Society.

American Lung Association (1980). *Freedom from Smoking in 20 Days, and a Lifetime of Freedom from Smoking.* New York, American Lung Association.

Anda, R. F., Remington, P. L., Sienko, D. G., and Davis, R. M. (1987). Are physicians advising smokers to quit? The patient's perspective. *JAMA* **257**:1916–1919.

Benowitz, N. L., Hall, S. M., Herning, R. I., Jacob, P., Jones, R. T., and Osman, A. L. (1983). Smokers of low-yield cigarettes do not consume less nicotine. *N. Engl. J. Med.* **309**:139–142.

Benowitz, N. L., Jacob, P., Kozlowski, L. T., and Yu, L. (1986). Influence of smoking fewer cigarettes on exposure to tar, nicotine, and carbon monoxide. *N. Engl. J. Med.* **315**:1310–1313.

Best, J. A., Bass, F., and Owen, L. E. (1977). Mode of service delivery in a smoking-cessation program for public health. *Can. J. Public Health* **68**:469–473.

British Thoracic Society (1983). Comparison of four methods of smoking withdrawal in patients with smoking-related disease. *Br. Med. J.* **286**:595–597.

Brownell, K. D., Glynn, T. J., Glasgow, R., Lando, H., Rand, C., Gottlieb, A., and Pinney, J. M. (1986). Interventions to prevent relapse. *Health Psychol.* **5**(Suppl):53–68.

Buist, A. S. (1979). The relative contribution of nature and nurture in chronic obstructive pulmonary disease. *West. J. Med.* **131**:114–121.

Buist, A. S., Sexton, G. J., Nagy, J. M., and Ross, B. B. (1976). The effect of smoking cessation and modification on lung function. *Am. Rev. Respir. Dis.* **114**:115–122.

Bureau of National Affairs (1987). *Where There's Smoke,* second edition. Washington, D.C., Bureau of National Affairs.

Camilli, A. E., Burrows, B., Knudson, R. J., Lyle, S. K., and Lebowitz, M. D. (1987). Longitudinal changes in forced expiratory volume in one second in adults. *Am. Rev. Respir. Dis.* **135**:797–799.

Centers for Disease Control (1987). Cigarette smoking among blacks and other minority populations. *Morbid. Mortal. Weekly Rep.* **36**:404–407.

Chandler, W. U. (1986). Banishing tobacco. *Worldwatch Paper 68.* Washington, D.C., Worldwatch Institute.

Clavel, F., Benhamou, S., Company-Heurtas, A., and Flamant, R. (1985). Helping people to stop smoking: randomized comparison of groups being treated with acupuncture and nicotine gum with control group. *Br. Med. J.* **291**:1538–1539.

Cohen, S. J., Christen, A. G., Katz, B. P., Drook, C. A., Davis, B. J., Smith, D. M., and Stookey, G. K. (1987). Counseling medical and dental patients about cigarette smoking: the impact of nicotine gum and chart reminders. *Am. J. Public Health* **77**:313–316.

Comstock, G. W., Brownlow, W. J., Stone, R. W., and Sartwell, P. E. (1970). Cigarette smoking and changes in respiratory findings. *Arch. Environ. Health* **21**:50–57.

Cooper, R., and Simmons, B. E. (1985). Cigarette smoking and ill health among black Americans. *N. Y. State J. Med.* **85**:344–349.

Cullen, J. W., McKenna, J. W., Massey, N. M. (1986). International control of smoking and the U.S. experience. *Chest* **89**(Suppl):206S–218S.

Davis, A. L., Faust, R., and Ordentlich, M. (1984). Self-help smoking-cessation programs: a comparative study with 12-month follow-up by the American Lung Association. *Am. J. Public Health* **74**:1212–1217.

Division of Lung Diseases, National Heart, Lung, and Blood Institute (1985). Protocol for the study on early intervention for chronic obstructive pulmonary disease-the lung health study. Washington, D.C., U.S. Department of Health and Human Services.

Fletcher, C., and Peto, R. (1977). The natural history of chronic airflow limitation. *Br. Med. J.* **1**:1645–1648.

Folsom, A. R., and Grimm, R. H. (1987). Stop smoking advice by physicians: a feasible approach? *Am. J. Public Health* **77**:849–850.

Garfinkel, L. (1976). Cigarette smoking among physicians and other health professionals 1959–1972. *CA* **26**:373–375.

Glasgow, R. E. (1985). Smoking. Self-management of chronic disease. In *Handbook of Clinical Interventions and Research*. Edited by K. Holroyd and T. Creer. London, Academic Press, pp. 99–126.

Glasgow, R. E., Shafer, L., and O'Neil, H. K. (1981). Self-help books and amount of therapist contact in smoking-cessation programs. *J. Consult. Clin. Psychol.* **49**:659–667.

Hall, R. G., Sachs, D. P. L., Hall, S. M., and Benowitz, N. L. (1984). Two-year efficacy and safety of rapid smoking therapy on patients with cardiac and pulmonary disease. *J. Consult. Clin. Psychol.* **52**:574–581.

Higgins, M. W., Keller, J. B., Becker, M., Howatt, W., Landis, J. R., Rotman, H., Weg, J., and Higgins, I. (1982). An index of risk for obstructive airways disease. *Am. Rev. Respir. Dis.* **125**:144–151.

Higgins, M. W., and Keller, J. B. (1983). Estimating your patient's risk of COPD: how to target your preventive efforts at high-risk patients. *J. Respir. Dis.* **4**:97–108.

Hjalmarsen, A. I. M. (1984). Effect of nicotine chewing gum in smoking cessation: a randomized, placebo-controlled double blind study. *JAMA* **252**:2835–2838.

Huhti, E., and Ikkala, J. (1980). A 10-year follow-up study of respiratory symptoms and ventilatory function in a middle-aged rural population. *Eur. J. Respir. Dis.* **61**:33–45.

Hunt, W. A., and Bespalec, D. A. (1974). An evaluation of current methods of modifying smoking behavior. *J. Clin. Psychol.* **30**:431–438.

Janz, N. K., Becker, M. H., Kirscht, J. P., Eraker, S. A., Billi, J. E., and Woolliscroft, J. O. (1987). Evaluation of a minimal contact smoking-cessation intervention in an outpatient setting. *Am. J. Public Health* **77**:805–809.

Jarvis, M. J., Raw, M., Russell, M. A. H., and Feyerabend, C. (1982). Randomized controlled trial of nicotine chewing gum. *Br. Med. J.* **285**:537–540.

Kronebusch, K. (1985). *Smoking-related deaths and financial costs.* Washington, Office of Technology Assessment, U.S. Congress.

Lichtenstein, E., and Danaher, B. G. (1978). What can the physician do to assist the patient to stop smoking? In *Chronic Obstructive Lung Disease: Clinical Treatment and Management.* Edited by R. E. Brashers and M. L. Rhoades. St. Louis, C. V. Mosby, pp. 227–241.

Lichtenstein, E., Harris, D. E., Birchler, G. R., Wahl, J. M., and Schmahl, D. P. (1973). Comparison of rapid smoking, warm, smoky air and attention placebo in the modification of smoking behavior. *J. Consult. Clin. Psychol.* **40**:92–98.

Louis Harris and Associates, Inc. (1984). *Healthy Lifestyles, Unhealthy Lifestyles: A National Research Report of Behavior, Knowledge, Motivations, and Opinions Concerning Individual Health Practices.* New York, Garland Publishing.

Marlatt, G. A., and Gordon, J. R. (1980). Determinants of relapse: implications for the maintenance of behavior change. In *Behavioral Medicine: Changing Health Lifestyles.* Edited by P. O. Davidson and S. M. Davidson. New York, Brunner Mazel, pp. 410–452.

Maron, D. J., and Fortmann, S. P. (1987). Nicotine yield and measures of cigarette smoke exposure in a large population: are lower-yield cigarettes safer? *Am. J. Public Health* **77**:546–549.

National Heart, Lung, and Blood Institute (1986). *Clinical Opportunities for Smoking Intervention: A Guide for the Busy Physician.* NIH Publication No. 86-2178. Bethesda, MD, U.S. Department of Health and Human Services, National Institutes of Health.

Ockene, J. K. (1987a). Physician-delivered intervention for smoking cessation: strategies for increasing effectiveness. *Prev. Med.* **17**:723–737.

Ockene, J. K. (1987b). Smoking intervention: the expanding role of the physician. *Am. J. Public Health* **77**:782–783.

O'Connell, K. (1985). Identification of variables associated with maintenance of nonsmoking in ex-smokers. Paper presented at the American Psychological Association Annual Meeting, Los Angeles, California.

Orleans, C. T., Shipley, R. H., Williams, C., and Haac, L. A. (1981). Behavioral approaches to smoking cessation I: a decade of research progress: 1969–1979. *J. Behav. Ther. Exp. Psychol.* **12**:125–129.

Pechacek, T. F., and Grimm, R. H. (1983). Cigarette smoking and the prevention of coronary heart disease. In *Primary Prevention of Coronary Heart Disease: A Practical Guide for the Clinician.* Edited by R. Podell and M. Stewart. Menlo Park, CA, Addison-Wesley, pp. 34–77.

Powell, D., and McCann, L. (1981). The effects of a multiple component treatment program and maintenance procedures on smoking cessation. *Prev. Med.* **10**:94–104.

Remington, P. L., Forman, M. R., Gentry, E. M., Marks, J. S., Hogelin, G. C., and Trowbridge, F. L. (1985). Current smoking trends in the United States. The 1981–1983 behavioral risk factor surveys. *JAMA* **253**:2975–2978.

Rose, G., and Hamilton, P. J. S. (1978). A randomized controlled trial of the effect on middle-aged men of advice to stop smoking. *J. Epidemiol. Commun. Health* **32**:275–281.

Russell, M. A. H., Wilson, C., Taylor, C., and Baker, C. D. (1979). Effects of general practitioners' advice against smoking. *Br. Med. J.* **2**:231–235.

Russell, M. A. H., Raw, M., and Jarvis, M. J. (1980). Clinical use of nicotine chewing gum. *Br. Med. J.* **280**:1599–1602.

Russell, M. A. H., Merriman, R., Stapleton, J., and Taylor, W. (1983). Effect of nicotine chewing gum as an adjunct to general practitioners' advice against smoking. *Br. Med. J.* **287**:1782–1785.

Russell, P., and Portser, S. A. (1987). Reports of menstrual distress and tobacco withdrawal symptoms in a smoking-cessation program for women. Paper presented at the 1987 Annual Meeting of the Society of Behavioral Medicine, Washington, D.C.

Sachs, D. P. L., Pechacek, T. F., Hall, R. G., and Fitzgerald, J. (1979). Clarification of risk-benefit issues in rapid smoking. *J. Consult. Clin. Psychol.* **47**:1053–1060.

Schneider, N. G., Jarvik, M. E., Forsythe, A. B., Read, L. L., Elliott, M. L., and Schweizer, A. (1983). Nicotine gum in smoking cessation: a placebo controlled, double blind trial. *Addict. Behav.* **8**:253–261.

Schneider, N. G., and Jarvik, M. E. (1984). Time course of smoking withdrawal symptoms as a function of nicotine replacement. *Psychopharmacology* **8**:143–144.

Schwartz, J. L., and Dubitsky, M. (1967). Expressed willingness of smokers to try 10 smoking withdrawal methods. *Public Health Rep.* **82**:855–861.

Schwartz, J. L. (1987). *Review and Evaluation of Smoking Cessation Meth-*

ods: *The United States and Canada, 1978-1985.* NIH Pub. No. 87-294. United States Department of Health and Human Services, Public Health Service, National Institutes of Health.

Shiffman, S. (1982). Relapse following smoking cessation: a situational analysis. *J. Consult. Clin. Psychol.* **50**:71–86.

Shiffman, S. (1984). Coping with temptations to smoke. *J. Consult. Clin. Psychol.* **52**:261–267.

Shopland, D. R., and Brown, C. (1985). Area review: current trends in smoking control. Changes in cigarette smoking prevalence in the U.S.: 1955 to 1983. *Ann. Behav. Med.* **7**:5–8.

Townsend, M. C. (1987). Effects of smoking and smoking cessation on FEV_1 decline at three MRFIT centers. *Am. Rev. Respir. Dis.* **135**:A342.

United States Department of Health, Education, and Welfare (1964). *Smoking and Health Report of the Advisory Committee to the Surgeon General of the Public Health Service.* Washington, D.C., U.S. Government Printing Office.

United States Department of Health, Education, and Welfare (1976). *Survey of Health Professionals.* Publication No. (CDC)21-74-552(P). Department of Health, Education, and Welfare, Public Health Service, Office of Smoking and Health, National Clearinghouse for Smoking and Health.

United States Department of Health, Education, and Welfare (1979). Smoking and health. *A Report of the Surgeon General.* DHEW Publication No. (PHS)79-50066. Washington, D.C., Government Printing Office.

United States Department of Health and Human Services (1983). The health consequences of smoking. Cardiovascular disease. *A Report of the Surgeon General.* DHHS Publication No. (PHS)84-50204. Washington, D.C., Government Printing Office.

United States Department of Health and Human Services (1984). The health consequences of smoking. Chronic obstructive lung disease. *A Report of the Surgeon General.* DHHS Publication No. (PHS)84-50205. Washington, D.C., Government Printing Office.

United States Department of Health and Human Services (1986a). Smoking and health. *A National Status Report.* DHHS Publication No. (CDC)87-8396. Washington, D.C., Government Printing Office.

United States Department of Health and Human Services (1986b). The 1990 health objectives for the nation: a midcourse review. Washington, D.C., Office of Disease Prevention and Health Promotion.

United States Department of Health and Human Services (1986c). The health consequences of involuntary smoking. *A Report of the Surgeon General.* DHHS Publication No. (CDC)87-8398. Washington, D.C., Government Printing Office.

Wechsler, H., Levine, S., Idelson, R. K., Robinson, M., and Taylor, J. O.

(1983). The physician's role in health promotion—a survey of primary care practitioners. *N. Engl. J. Med.* **308**:97–100.

Wells, K. B., Lewis, C., Leake, B., and Ware, J. E. (1984). Do physicians preach what they practice? *JAMA* **252**:2846–2848.

Wilson, D., Wood, G., Johnston, N., and Sicurella, J. (1982). Randomized clinical trial of supportive follow-up for cigarette smokers in a family practice. *Can. Med. Assoc. J.* **126**:127–129.

World Health Organization (1986). IARC monographs on the evaluation of the carcinogenic risk of chemicals to humans tobacco smoking. *IARC* **38**:47–81.

World Health Organization (1986). Worldwide Use of Smoking Tobacco 1. Production of and trade in tobacco. In IARC monographs of the evaluation of the carcinogenic risk of chemicals to humans. Tobacco Smoking. Lyon, France, Volume **38**:47–81.

13

Economics of Smoking Reduction

GRAHAM A. COLDITZ

Harvard Medical School
Brigham and Women's Hospital
Boston, Massachussetts

I. Introduction

Although an extensive body of literature describes the detrimental physical effects of smoking, relatively little has been published on its economic implications. The economic consequences of smoking can be calculated using techniques developed for estimating the economic costs of illness. Cost-of-illness studies have traditionally been classified into two types: prevalence-based and incidence-based analyses. Most cost-of-illness studies have used a prevalence-based approach that identifies the cost incurred during a given year by persons with a particular illness, regardless of the stage of that illness. Such prevalence-based estimates are particularly suited for highlighting the magnitudes of direct costs on an annual basis and the economic burden of medical conditions. These costs include outlays for medical care (direct costs) as well as the costs associated with illness-related work loss and the cost of future earnings for those who died prematurely during the year (indirect costs).

We have undertaken a study that has used an incidence-based approach, which focuses on the present value of future costs of morbidity and mortality (Oster et al., 1984). This analysis estimates the magnitude of future economic costs to society for smokers who are currently disease-free and the potential economic benefits to society that are accrued from their quitting. In this chapter the methods and results of the expected costs of smoking and benefits of quitting are presented as they relate to chronic obstructive pulmonary disease (COPD).

II. The Costs of COPD

Incidence-based analyses focus on the lifetime costs of a given disease in persons who contract the disease during a particular period, regardless of when these costs will be incurred. An incidence-based analysis may be used to develop estimates for the direct and indirect costs of illness, but these costs are estimated for the lifetime of an affected individual rather than for a cross-section of affected individuals in a given year. This approach is therefore ideal for assessing the total expected lifetime costs that the average smoker will incur as a consequence of his or her smoking. Likewise, this approach is well suited to assessing the economic benefits to society of having smokers quit, since most of these benefits arise not immediately but over the subsequent lifetime in the form of improved health and decreased demand for health care services.

Previous studies of the costs of smoking have used prevalence-based approaches. Such studies aggregate all medical conditions attributable to smoking, the value of foregone productivity, and often other items such as the cost of fire property damage caused by smoking. These estimates have been presented as the total dollar cost of smoking each year. Such estimates reflect only current year economic costs and do have a national perspective rather than the perspective of the individual smoker. Thus, although individuals who currently smoke may be aware of the potential health-related consequences (e.g., heart disease, lung cancer, or COPD), they may not be aware of the economic consequences to society. Translation of the health consequences of smoking into dollar costs may be used to increase awareness of the burden of smoking on society and ultimately stimulate greater efforts to modify the behavior of cigarette smokers.

In estimating the lifetime costs of COPD, we viewed every smoker as engaged in a lifetime series of gambles with his or her health, each gamble occurring in a successive future year of life. For each future year, the economic costs, including treatment expenses and lost earnings, were averaged over all those at risk of disease to calculate the average or expected value of those costs. This expected value is equal to the probability of COPD multiplied by the costs for disease. The costs of smoking for a current smoker are equal to the sum of these expected annual losses, each discounted to reflect its appropriate present value. Costs that do not accrue in the same year should not be directly summed, since they are expressed in different units of value (i.e., different years' dollars). Discounting is a technique that expresses these costs in terms of their value in a common metric for each year. Calculation of the costs of smoking therefore depends on estimation of the lifetime costs of COPD at every possible age of onset.

Just as there are expected costs of smoking resulting from the higher probability of COPD, so there are expected economic benefits associated with reductions in the risk of disease. By definition, these benefits are equal to the losses likely to be avoided when individuals quit smoking. Hence, the benefits of smoking cessation may be represented by a series of annual cost savings. As with the calculation of smoking costs, summation of these expected annual savings, each appropriately discounted to reflect the year to which it corresponds, yields an estimate of the economic benefits of quitting.

A. Smokers' Risk of COPD

In our analyses we regarded COPD as exclusively a smoker's disease. This assumption was based on work reported by Fletcher and co-workers, who indicated that among the patients they observed in their 8 year study of British workers, the lung destruction that characterizes COPD was not present among any of the nonsmokers (Fletcher et al., 1976). Therefore, we assume the incidence of COPD among nonsmokers would be zero. Unfortunately, almost no data are available on the incidence of COPD among smokers in the general population. Therefore, we estimated COPD incidence for smokers on the basis of prevalence data from the U.S. population for sex and age, and cigarette smoking (National Center for Health Statistics, 1974) (Table 1). Incidence rates were generated assuming a mean survival time of 5 years past diagnosis (Diener and Burrows, 1975). Separate incidence rates for light, moderate, and heavy smokers were estimated using these overall average rates and data on relative risks of COPD reported by Ferris and associates (1976) (Tables 2, 3).

B. Mortality and Life Expectancy

Although the survival pattern of COPD patients is closely related to their initial level of lung function and the rate at which it continues to decline, there are only sparse data on survival probabilities for patients after the COPD is diagnosed. In our analyses, we used data from a 14 year prospective study of 200 COPD patients (Diener and Burrows, 1975). This is the most extensive study of survival patterns among COPD patients completed to date and suggests that a 5 year probability of survival is just greater than 50%.

Table 1 Prevalence of COPD in the United States, By Age and Sex, 1976 (per 100,000 Persons)

Age Group (years)	Men	Women
17–44	120	80
45–64	2,210	650
65 +	5,880	1,160

Source: National Center for Health Statistics (1974).

Table 2 Effect of Levels of Cigarette Consumption on a Smoker's Relative Risk of COPD, by Sex

Number of Cigarettes per Day	Men	Women
1–14	0.68	0.63
15–35	1.00	1.00
36 +	1.80	2.30

Source: Ferris et al. (1976).

C. Cost of Care for COPD

Incidence-based estimates of costs of care for an illness require information on utilization patterns over the years after disease onset. There are almost no data on the progressive need for medical intervention or the actual pattern of medical care use for COPD. As a result, we used available data on utilization patterns on an entire COPD population to estimate the expected lifetime costs of care for COPD. Using data from the National Center for Health Statistics (1977) on the number of physician visits for which COPD was the first, second, or third listed diagnosis, and a population of 2.1 million persons with COPD (National Center for Health Statistics, 1979), we estimated that the typical patient saw an office-based physician for treatment approximately 4.6 times per year. We then extrapolated the number of physician visits from one visit in the first year to diagnose the condition using the assumption that at the mean time past onset (4.5 years) a patient would see a physician an average number of times (4.6 office visits annually). We estimated that the first visit each year would cost $75, which would include the costs of all diagnostic tests, and that each additional visit would cost $30. These rates were determined through consultation with private physicians in the United States who regularly saw COPD patients in their practices.

Table 3 Annual Incidence Rates of COPD, by Level of Cigarette Consumption, Age, and Sex (per 100,000 Persons)

Age–Sex Group	Nonsmokers	Daily Cigarette Smoking		
		1–14	15–35	36+
Men				
35–39	0	122	180	324
40–44	0	252	370	666
45–49	0	394	580	1,044
50–54	0	537	790	1,422
55–59	0	673	990	1,782
60–64	0	809	1,190	2,142
65–69	0	1,278	1,880	3,384
70–74	0	1,476	2,170	3,906
75–79	0	1,673	2,460	4,428
80+	0	1,673	2,460	4,428
Women				
35–39	0	63	100	230
40–44	0	95	150	345
45–49	0	164	260	598
50–54	0	214	340	782
55–59	0	252	400	920
60–64	0	296	470	1,081
65–69	0	914	1,450	3,335
70–74	0	1,084	1,720	3,956
75–79	0	1,216	1,930	4,439
80+	0	1,216	1,930	4,439

Source: Oster et al. (1984).

Using National Center for Health Statistics data (1983) on hospital discharges, we estimated the probability of a hospitalization for COPD for each year past onset. The average length of stay for patients with a primary diagnosis of COPD was 9.5 days (National Center for Health Statistics, 1978). We estimated the cost of each COPD hospital episode at $2,708 by multiplying the average length of stay by the estimated cost of a COPD hospital day. The cost of each hospital day for COPD was taken from the results of an extensive study of chronic lung disease patients in California

(State of California 1982), in which average costs of $335 per day were reported for 1978. These costs were adjusted to the U.S. average and inflated to reflect 1980 costs, giving the average cost of a hospital day for a COPD patient of $285.

D. Nursing Home Care

A similar approach to that used for estimating hospitalization for COPD was used to estimate the probability of admission to a nursing home. We assume half the residents with a primary diagnosis of respiratory disease were in nursing homes as a direct result of COPD. To these we added the number of residents with a primary diagnosis of emphysema. By this technique we estimated that the COPD nursing home population was equal to 47,250 in 1977 (National Center for Health Statistics, 1981). Dividing this by the estimated number of persons with COPD, we determined that the annual likelihood of nursing health care for the average COPD patient was 0.022.

We assume that no nursing home care would be required at the time of onset, and that 2.2% of COPD patients would require this care at 4.5 years after onset, corresponding to the mean time of onset for the COPD population. Using these two points, we then estimated the likelihood of nursing home care in each year past onset using simple linear regression. The average monthly charge for nursing home care in 1977 was $689 (National Center for Health Statistics, 1980), or $932 when inflated to 1980 dollars. Thus, the average annual cost of nursing home care in 1980 was $11,844.

E. Drugs and Oxygen

Drug costs were estimated on maintenance therapy with a bronchodilator from the time of diagnosis forward. We also assumed that steroids would be used by half the patients who survived 5 years past onset. The retail costs of these drugs were determined through an informal survey of Boston area pharmacies, and the resultant costs were adjusted to reflect the difference in prices between 1983 and 1980. While many COPD patients require regular oxygen therapy, we were unable to find a reliable source of information on the frequency or prevalence of its use. Hence this oxygen therapy was not included in our estimates of annual costs of care. As a result, our estimates for this direct cost category are conservative.

F. Direct Costs for COPD

The present value of expected total direct costs per patient was calculated by discounting, to the year of onset or diagnosis, the average cost of care in each year past onset, adjusting each years' discounted total to reflect the likelihood of patient survival, and then summing the result of the present value stream of prospective cost. The technique of calculating the present value of the direct cost of illness has been described in detail (Oster et al., 1984). Our estimates of the present value of the total direct cost for COPD are $5,689 per patient. This value is the same for all age and sex groups because data limitations require average values for utilization and mortality to be assigned to all COPD patients.

G. Productivity Losses

In accordance with results reported by Fletcher, and associates (1976), we assume that a COPD patient would experience no significant disability at the time of onset and for disability to increase to complete withdrawal from all forms of productive activity approximately 7.5 years later. Disability levels for the first 7 years past onset of COPD were estimated using least squares regression fitted to these two points. The relative activity rate for COPD patients for each year past onset was assumed to equal 100 minus the disability level. A relative activity of 100 indicates a complete functional status and a rate in between indicates the proportion of full activity in which a COPD patient is able to engage. The relative activity rates were multiplied by the labor force participation and housekeeping rates for age- and sex-matched peers to estimate postonset participation rates for COPD patients. We assume the relative productivity of COPD patients was equal to their relative participation rate; whatever work COPD patients were able to perform, they performed at a level of productivity equivalent to their age- and sex-matched peers. The present value of indirect costs to COPD patients was calculated by discounting to the year or onset of diagnosis the average productivity or earnings losses that would be expected in each year from onset and then summing the present value stream of expected costs. The present value of the indirect costs for COPD are shown in Table 4.

Individual productivity is frequently valued on the basis of market place earnings, which assumes that the economy reflects economic productivity. The estimates of market place productivity we have used are based on U.S. Census Bureau estimates of average employee earnings. Although housekeepers have no earnings, their responsibilities are numerous and their productivity is typically quite high. We have used Brody's (1975) estimates of the value of household productivity (inflated to 1980 dollars). The present value of COPD indirect costs is much greater for men than women until about age 60. This is a reflection of the higher earning levels and work force participation by men than women until about the age of

Table 4   The Present Value of Indirect Costs for Patients with COPD, by Sex and Age of Onset, in U.S. Dollars[a]

Age of Onset	Men	Women
35–39	$399,519	$185,832
40–44	325,802	154,451
45–49	245,048	121,875
50–54	163,659	88,758
55–59	88,409	59,008
60–64	35,511	35,476
65–69	14,537	20,412
70–74	7,993	11,445
75–79	5,057	6,097

[a]Discounted at a 3% annual rate, assuming a 1% annual rate of growth in labor productivity.
Source: Oster et al. (1984).

retirement. After the age 60, however, women's greater participation in housekeeping activities throughout the rest of their lives causes the productivity losses they experience to outweigh the indirect costs incurred among men. The total costs of COPD (the sum of the direct and indirect costs) are presented in Table 5.

Combining the data on incidence of COPD and the cost for patients with COPD, we estimated the economic costs of smoking due to increased risks of COPD. These data are presented in Table 6.

III.   The Benefits of Quitting

In our analysis of the benefits of quitting cigarette smoking that accrue due to reductions in the risk of COPD, we assume that smokers quit voluntarily not because they are experiencing clinical symptoms. Second, we assume the incidence of COPD among exsmokers in the year immediately following smoking cessation would be equal to the rate experienced by those continuing to smoke. Finally, in the second and all later years past cessation, we assume that the risk of COPD would be reduced by an amount proportionately equal to the relative improvement in the rate of decline in lung function. In assessing the relative improvement on the rate of decline of lung function we assessed the following rates: nonsmoker, 30 ml/year; light (1–14 cigarettes per day), 60 ml/year; moderate (15–35 cigarettes per day), 80 ml/year; heavy (36 or more cigarettes per day), 100 ml/year.

Table 5 Present Value of Total Costs for Patients with COPD, by Sex and Age on Onset, in 1980 U.S. Dollars, Discounted at 3% Annual Rate, Assuming a 1% Rate of Growth in Labor Productivity

Age of Onset	Men	Women
35–39	$405,207	$191,522
40–44	331,491	160,139
45–49	250,737	127,564
50–54	169,348	94,446
55–59	94,098	64,697
60–64	41,199	41,165
65–69	20,226	26,101
70–74	13,682	17,134
75–79	10,746	11,786

Source: Oster et al. (1984).

These rates reflect average values, since it is known that the effect of smoking on lung function is not uniform (Fletcher et al., 1976; Beck et al., 1981). The effect of smoking on lung function was used to estimate the risk reduction by cessation from smoking, since incidence data for exsmokers by level of cigarette consumption are not available.

In estimating the cost of smoking, we assume that no change will occur in the smokers' lifetime smoking habits. Similarly, in generating our estimates of the benefits of quitting, we measured these benefits against the costs that would be incurred if there were no change in smoking habits. Our benefit estimates are thus based on the assumption that if an individual is currently a two-pack a day smoker, his or her benefits of quitting should be measured against the expected costs of those who continue to smoke two packs a day for life. In addition, our benefit estimates reflect the gains for a smoker who quits for life. The benefits of quitting in terms of decreased direct and indirect costs due to chronic obstructive pulmonary disease are provided in five year age groups for men and women (Table 7).

In conclusion, costs presented in this chapter reflect the costs to society of COPD that may be attributed to cigarette smoking. These costs are greater than the costs of coronary heart disease or lung cancer that may be attributed to smoking (Oster et al., 1984), principally due to the chronic nature of the disease. Our estimates of the cost of smoking and benefits of quitting are probably conservative, since they do not take into account economic costs other than those directly related to disease (e.g., the cost of residential and commercial fires), noneconomic costs, or the cost of

Table 6 Costs of COPD Attributable to Cigarette Smoking, Estimated in 1980 U.S. Dollars

Age–Sex	Cigarettes/Day		
	1–114	15–35	36 +
Men			
35–39	$14,753[a]	$21,695	$39,051
40–44	13,348	19,692	35,333
45–49	10,530	15,486	27,875
50–54	7,188	10,571	19,028
55–59	4,313	6,343	11,417
60–64	2,607	3,834	6,901
65–59	1,850	2,720	4,896
70–74	1,318	1,939	3,490
75–79	946	1,392	2,505
Women			
35–39	4,261	6,763	15,555
40–44	4,075	6,468	14,877
45–49	3,680	5,841	13,434
50–54	3,106	4,930	11,340
55–59	2,606	4,136	9,513
60–64	2,298	3,647	8,389
65–69	1,921	3,050	7,014
70–74	1,296	2,057	4,731
75–79	836	1,328	3,054

[a]Dollar value represents average economic cost to every smoker in an age and smoking group.
Source: Oster et al. (1984).

smoking-related diseases among nonsmokers (U.S. Surgeon General, 1986). In addition, our estimates of the cost of smoking and the benefits of quitting do not include the cost of cigarettes. One major aspect of the impact of COPD that was omitted from this analysis is pain and suffering, since this dimension of illness has not yet been quantified.

Two other costs excluded from the cost-of-illness approach are transfer payments (pensions) and taxes. When income loss is used as a measure of indirect costs, adding pensions or relief payments would be double counting. As with tax payments it would be double counting to add income tax loss to

Table 7 Economic Benefits Due to Reduced Expenditures on COPD and Increased Productivity Among Smokers who Quit, by Level of Smoking, Age and Sex.

Age–Sex	Cigarettes/Day		
	1–114	15–35	36 +
Men			
35–39	$6,882	$12,654	$25,861
40–44	6,032	11,095	22,679
45–49	4,588	8,445	17,269
50–54	3,010	5,546	11,351
55–59	1,741	3,217	6,596
60–64	1,060	1,965	4,040
65–59	739	1,372	2,823
70–74	522	968	1,990
75–79	364	673	1,381
Women			
35–39	1,999	3,967	10,359
40–44	1,889	3,751	9,800
45–49	1,663	3,307	8,645
50–54	1,383	2,753	7,205
55–59	1,155	2,302	6,034
60–64	1,023	2,043	5,357
65–69	791	1,580	4,145
70–74	524	1,046	2,743
75–79	330	648	1,724

Source: Oster et al. (1984).

loss of earnings, and triple counting if the tax receipts were used to pay for medical care.

We used a 3% discount rate. This was chosen because we estimated all future direct and indirect costs of illnesses in constant dollars and used a real rate of discount to impose comparability between different years' costs. All estimates of future treatment expenses and forgone earnings were projected at 1980 prices and were then discounted at an annual rate of 3%. The use of a 3% real rate of discount should result in conservative cost and benefit estimates, since it is substantially higher than historical real rates of return (that is, the rate of return that can be earned over the rate of inflation).

Although incidence rates for smoking-related diseases have been rising, our estimates are conservatively based on a projection of incidence continuing at its current rate.

An overriding concern in developing the economic costs of COPD attributable to cigarette smoking, and the economic benefits of quitting, was the lack of specific data on the incidence of COPD by levels of cigarette smoking. This necessitated approximations of incidence rates for levels of cigarette smoking and of the incidence of COPD among former smokers who had by necessity undergone some prior increase in their rate of deterioration in lung function as a consequence of their cigarette smoking (Fletcher et al., 1976). More recent data suggest that the height-adjusted rate of decline in lung function for women who smoke cigarettes is less than that for men, hence making our estimates of incidence among women higher than may be observed (Dockery et al., 1988).

For even light smokers of cigarettes (1–14 cigarettes per day), direct costs range from $410 for women aged 35–39 to $750 for men aged 60–64. These direct costs contrast with the costs of smoking cessation programs. We have recently estimated that the costs of physician's time in offering advice plus nicotine gum in a primary care setting amounts to $4.00 per patient (Oster et al., 1986). When nicotine gum is added to physicians' advice, cessation rates increased from 4.5% of smokers quitting on physicians' advice and counseling to 6.1% of patients who used nicotine gum and quit cigarette smoking. Among a group of 250 patients, we estimate that four patients will give up cigarette smoking when a prescription for nicotine gum is given along with a physicians' advice against smoking. If we assume that a quarter of patients comply with the use of nicotine gum and the remaining patients purchase the gum but do not use it, the total cost of the intervention is $4,069. This represents $340 per patient who quits or $16.30 per patient who is offered the advice together with the nicotine gum. These costs are considerably less than the direct costs that society will bear as a consequence of COPD due to smoking.

Although coronary heart disease and lung cancer have been the principal focus on the majority of studies addressing the health consequences of smoking, the economic data presented in this chapter suggest that COPD is as important from the vantage point of society as these other illnesses.

References

Beck, G. J., Doyle, C. A., and Schachter, E. N. (1981). Smoking and lung function. *Am. Rev. Respir. Dis.* **123**:149–155.

Brody, W. H. (1975). The economic value of a housewife. Research and statistics, Note 9, DHEW Pub No (35A) 75-11701. Washington, D.C.

Diener, C. F., and Burrows, B. (1975). Further observation on the course and prognosis of chronic obstructive lung disease. *Am. Rev. Respir. Dis.* 11:719–724.

Dockery, D. W., Speizer, F. E., Ferris, B. G., Jr., Ware, J. H., Louis, T. A., and Spiro, A. (1988). Cumulative and reversible effects of lifetime smoking on simple tests of lung function in adults. *Am. Rev. Respir. Dis.* 137:286–296.

Ferris, B. G., Chen, S. P., and Murphy, L. H., Jr. (1976). Chronic non-specific respiratory disease in Berlin, New Hampshire: a further follow-up study. *Am. Rev. Respir. Dis.* 113:475–485.

Fletcher, D., Peto, R., Tinker, C., and Speizer, F. E. (1976). *The Natural History of Chronic Bronchitis and Emphysema. An Eight-Year Study of Early Chronic Obstructive Lung Disease in Working Men in London.* Oxford, Oxford University Press.

National Center for Health Statistics (1974). Prevalence of selected chronic respiratory conditions, United States, 1970. Vital and Health Statistics, Series 10, No. 84 DHEW Pub No. (HRA) 74-1511. Washington, D.C.

National Center for Health Statistics. (1977). Office visits for disease of the respiratory system, National Ambulatory Medical Care Survey, United States, 1975–1976. Vital and Health Statistics, Series 13, No. 42, DHEW Pub. No. (PHS) 70-1793. Washington, D.C.

National Center for Health Statistics. (1978). Inpatient utilization of short-stay hospitals by diagnosis, United States, 1975. Vital and Health Statistics, Series 13, No. 35, DHEW (PHS) 78-1786. Washington, D.C.

National Center for Health Statistics. (1979). Prevalence of selected chronic respiratory conditions reported in Health Interviews, rates by sex and age, and per cent and rates for selected health related characteristics, United States. Washington, D.C. Unpublished data.

National Center for Health Statistics. (1980). Nursing home utilization in California, Illinois, Massachusetts, New York and Texas: 1977 National Nursing Home Survey. Vital and Health Statistics, Series 13, No. 48, DHHS Pub. No., (PHS) 80-1799. Washington, D.C.

National Center for Health Statistics. (1981). Characteristics of nursing home residents, health status and care received: National Nursing Home Survey. Vital and Health Statistics, Series 13, No. 51 DHHS Pub. No. (PHS) 81-1712. Washington, D.C.

National Center for Health Statistics. (1983). Washington, D.C. Unpublished data.

Oster, G., Colditz, G. A., and Kelly, N. L. (1984). *The Economic Costs of Smoking and Benefits of Quitting.* Lexington, MA, Lexington Books.

Oster, G., Huse, D. M., Delea, T. E., and Colditz, G. A. (1986). Cost-effectiveness of nicotine gum as an adjunct to Physician's advice against cigarette smoking. *J.A.M.A.* 256:1315–1318.

State of California, Department of Health Services (1982). Report of the 1982 California Legislative on the Chronic Obstructive Lung Disease Project. Sacramento.

U.S. Surgeon General. The Health Consequences of Involuntary Smoking. A report of the Surgeon General. U.S. Department of Health and Human Services, Public Health Service. Rockville, MD, 1986.

14

Efficacy of Current Therapy for Patients with Chronic Obstructive Pulmonary Disease

JAMES L. MCKEON

Royal Newcastle Hospital
Newcastle, New South Wales, Australia

MICHAEL J. HENSLEY
and NICHOLAS A. SAUNDERS

University of Newcastle
Newcastle, New South Wales, Australia

I. Introduction

Chronic obstructive pulmonary disease (COPD) becomes symptomatic late in its natural course, when the pathological processes are largely irreversible. At presentation, many patients with COPD have moderate to severe ventilatory impairment (FEV_1 = 1.0–1.5 L), marked exercise limitation, and poor quality of life. These patients make up most of the population receiving therapy for COPD and will be the group discussed in this chapter. We will discuss patients with chronic bronchitis and emphysema, but not those with chronic asthma. This latter group appears to have a much better prognosis than patients with COPD who are nonatopic smokers without a history of asthma (Burrows et al., 1987).

A. Definitions

This chapter will deal mainly with the efficacy of currently available therapy for COPD. *Efficacy* can be defined as the extent to which a maneuver, procedure, or service does more good than harm under optimal conditions. *Effectiveness* is the extent to which the intervention works "in the real world." *Efficiency* is expressed as the effects obtained in relationship to the effort expended in terms of money, resources, and time. The suggested protocol for the evaluation of a maneuver, procedure, or service is first to document efficacy under controlled circumstances and then effectiveness under the anticipated conditions of use. If there is documented effectiveness, an economic analysis should be undertaken to assess its value compared to other interventions for the same problem and possibly to interventions for another health problem.

It is important to know which treatments cause improvement in meaningful patient outcomes. The outcome variables that should be considered in the management of patients with COPD include survival, symptoms, quality of life, exercise tolerance, pulmonary function, prevention of complications, and side effects of treatment.

In many cases, information on the efficacy of treatments for patients with COPD is simply not available, presumably because the answers demand long-term, prospective clinical trials. Most studies reported to date assess the effectiveness of treatment by changes in pulmonary function over a short time. However, changes in physiological variables should be related to symptoms and to other outcome variables relevant to the patient's quality of life, and should be assessed in both the short and the long term. If we are to assess the "good" a particular therapy can achieve, we need to include practical patient outcomes in future clinical trials. An investigation of efficacy requires that "good" be balanced against "harm" being caused by therapy. Text books of pharmacology have long lists of potential side effects of drugs used in the treatment of patients with COPD, but there are very few thorough assessments of the frequency of side effects in such patients.

This is particularly true for steroid therapy, where the gains may be marginal, and the potential complications of therapy are serious. It is impossible to assess the risk–benefit ratio for any treatment if the frequency of side effects has not been carefully investigated.

B. Pulmonary Function Tests as the Outcome Variable

Therapy for COPD is often assessed in terms of improvement in lung function, with the assumption that this will lead to improvements in symptoms, exercise tolerance, and prognosis. Of the many pulmonary function tests available, which test is the most useful for assessing efficacy?

In patients with COPD, forced expiratory volume in 1 sec (FEV$_1$) declines on the average by 40-50 ml per year (Anthonisen et al., 1986; Barter and Campbell, 1976) and correlates with prognosis (Anthonisen et al., 1986) and exercise tolerance (McGavin et al., 1978). There is a diurnal variation in FEV$_1$ in patients with COPD with a coefficient of variation of 7-8% (Hruby and Butler, 1975; Pennock and Rogers, 1978). FEV$_1$ is less reproducible when repeated at 2-3 weekly intervals in patients with chronic bronchitis (coefficient of variation = 14.8%; Mungall and Hainsworth, 1979). Therefore, FEV$_1$ is an easily measured, fairly reproducible measure of pulmonary function that correlates with patient outcomes.

Vital capacity (VC) also correlates with exercise tolerance in patients with COPD (McGavin et al., 1978). Improvement in symptoms after use of salbutamol aerosol has been related to improvements in VC in patients with radiological evidence of pulmonary emphysema (Bellamy and Hutchison, 1981). In those patients, absolute change in VC after salbutamol was greater than change in FEV$_1$ and was shown to be due to reduction in RV without change in total lung capacity (TLC). Therefore, VC should also be measured when the effects of bronchodilator drugs are investigated in patients with COPD. Static lung volumes (RV, FRC, TLC) are not as useful as FEV$_1$ for predicting outcome (Anthonisen et al., 1986) or exercise tolerance (Pineda et al., 1984) and will not be referred to in this chapter.

The change in FEV$_1$ and VC after administration of bronchodilator drugs is used as a measure of airways responsiveness in patients with COPD and is expressed in either absolute terms (L) or as a percentage improvement over baseline values. In patients with COPD who have an FEV$_1$ less than 1 L, the use of percentage improvement may suggest significant airways responsiveness when only small absolute changes occur (e.g., a 25% improvement in FEV$_1$ from 0.4 to 0.5 L is an absolute change of only 100 ml). Thus, the conventional criterion for "reversibility" (15% improvement of the initial FEV$_1$) may be misleading. Eliasson and Degraff (1985) showed that use of "percentage improvement" could not be used to define disease (e.g., asthma versus emphysema) and when it was applied to a patient population it resulted in the most obstructed patients showing the greatest "reversibility." This is a contradiction of the very definition of reversibility. They suggested that percentage improvement was a poor way to define reversibility and that the absolute difference of the FEV$_1$ before and after bronchodilator was a more appropriate measure.

Tweeddale and associates (1987) recently studied 150 patients with airflow obstruction (FEV$_1$ range 0.5-4.7 L) and found that the variability in FEV$_1$ over a 20 min period was similar over the entire range of FEV$_1$ studied. The increases in FEV$_1$ and VC required to exclude natural variability with 95% confidence were 160 ml and 330 ml, respectively. In this chapter, changes in FEV_1 after bronchodilator drugs have been expressed in absolute terms rather than as percentage improvement over baseline.

In patients with COPD without hypoxemia, the mean annual rate of decline in FEV_1 (44 ml/year) varies greatly between patients (standard deviation of the mean = 129 ml/year) (Anthonisen et al., 1986a). Patients with low initial values of FEV_1 ($<30\%$ predicted) show relatively little further decline over 2 years, probably due to a survival effect: more of those surviving have a lower rate of decline. In treated patients with well-preserved initial FEV_1 ($>50\%$ predicted), the rate of decline correlates negatively with bronchodilator response, wheezing, and psychological disturbances (Anthonisen et al., 1986a,b). However, these three factors explain only about 11% of the variation in the rate of decline in FEV_1, which, thus, cannot be accurately predicted in any individual. Conversely, the rate of decline in FEV_1 in untreated patients is positively correlated with beta-adrenergic responsiveness (Barter et al., 1974; Postma et al., 1986) so that bronchodilator reversibility would appear to be an adverse factor in untreated patients but a favorable one in treated patients with COPD.

The decline in FEV_1 has also been demonstrated to be positively correlated with the degree of bronchial reactivity as measured by methacholine response (Barter and Campbell, 1976; Campbell et al., 1985) or by histamine response (Postma et al., 1986).

Burrows and associates (1987) recently showed that clinical classification of patients with COPD has useful prognostic implications. They classified patients according to a reported history of asthma, smoking history, and skin prick test evidence of atopy. Nonatopic smokers without a history of asthma had a 10 year survival of only 40%, compared with 75% for atopic subjects or nonsmokers with a history of asthma. The annual rates of decline in FEV_1 for these two groups were 70 ml/year and 5 ml/year, respectively. Thus, this simple classification offers useful prognostic information for counseling and treating patients with COPD.

II. Pharmacological Therapy

A. Introduction

We carried out a literature search spanning the last 10 years and selected 45 studies that assessed the use of bronchodilators in patients with COPD and 21 studies that involved corticosteroids. We excluded studies that deliberately enrolled patients with "reversible" airflow obstruction or asthma. Papers selected were written in English and dealt with the efficacy of commonly available treatment for chronic bronchitis and emphysema. Each paper was assessed according to criteria developed by Canadian clinical epidemiologists (Department of Clinical Epidemiology & Biostatistics, McMaster University, 1981). These criteria are summarized as a series of questions that should be addressed when assessing the results of clinical trials:

1. Was the assignment of patients to treatments really randomized? (Was similarity between groups documented? Was there prognostic stratification?)

2. Were all clinically relevant outcomes reported? (In the case of COPD, we chose symptoms, exercise tolerance, pulmonary function, quality of life, and survival as the relevant outcomes.)

3. Were the study patients recognizably similar to your own? (Was enough information given to identify the type of patient?)

4. Were both statistical and clinical significance considered? (Was the difference clinically important? If not significant, was the study big enough to show a clinically important difference if it had occurred?)

5. Is the therapeutic maneuver feasible in your practice? (Available? Affordable? Sensible? Was it "blind"? Was compliance measured?)

6. Were all patients who entered the study accounted for at its conclusion? (Were drop-outs, withdrawals, noncompliers, and those who crossed over handled appropriately?)

For each study examined, we scored the answer to each of these questions as follows: 2 for "yes," 1 for "unsure," and 0 for "no," giving a maximum possible trial design score of 12 for each study. Tables 1–4 list the studies by author and year of publication, in ascending order according to their trial design score. Only eight bronchodilator studies and three corticosteroid studies fulfilled all the criteria proposed by the McMaster group (1981). Most studies were properly randomized, involved patients with COPD similar to those likely to be encountered in everyday practice, used commonly available treatments, and accounted for all patients entered into the trials. The areas of deficiency were the reporting of clinically relevant outcomes and the consideration of clinical as well as statistical significance. Only 15 (23%) papers reported at least 3 relevant outcomes and only 28 (42%) papers adequately assessed the clinical significance of their findings. All papers assessed pulmonary function, 22 (33%) papers assessed patients' exercise tolerance, and 28 (42%) papers assessed the effect of therapy on patients' symptoms. No paper assessed the effect of treatment on prognosis because most trials were conducted over relatively short periods (e.g., 6–8 weeks). Only two papers (Guyatt et al., 1987a; Mitchell et al., 1984a) reported on quality of life and only two (Taylor et al., 1985; Postma et al., 1985) studied the effect of therapy on the prevention of complications. In general, sample sizes were small.

B. Beta-Adrenergic Agents

We examined 32 studies of beta-adrenergic agents in patients with COPD (Table 1). Every study reported the effect of therapy on pulmonary function, but only 11 (34%) reported on exercise tolerance or symptoms.

Many beta-adrenergic drugs have been evaluated in patients with COPD, including inhaled salbutamol (Bellamy and Hutchison, 1981), inhaled metaproterenol (Dullinger et al., 1986), inhaled fenoterol (Tobin et al., 1984), oral salbutamol (Leitch et al., 1981), and oral terbutaline (Marvin et al., 1983). These agents produced statistically significant improvements in FEV_1 that were of small magnitude (e.g., mean [SEM] change in FEV_1 = 0.14[0.03] L; Tobin et al., 1984) and that lie within the range of natural variability of the FEV_1 in patients with airways obstruction (Tweeddale et al., 1987). Changes in VC were generally greater than changes in FEV_1; (e.g., change in VC = 0.55[0.11] L; Tobin et al., 1984). In the study by Bellamy and Hutchinson (1981), improvement in VC was most closely associated with symptomatic improvement. Inhaled metaproterenol has also been shown to improve breathlessness rating (Dullinger et al., 1986) but oral terbutaline had no effect on daily symptom scores (Marvin et al., 1983). Beta-adrenergic treatment improved symptoms in 6 of the 12 studies that assessed this outcome (Table 1).

Seven of the 11 studies that assessed exercise tolerance showed improvement in exercise tolerance with beta-adrenergic agents. For example, Leitch et al. (1981) showed an improvement of 56 m in a 12 min walk after oral salbutamol. Although statistically significant, the clinical significance of this change is doubtful. Four well-designed studies have failed to show any improvement in exercise tolerance with beta-adrenergic agents (Marvin et al., 1983; Dullinger et al., 1986; Tobin et al., 1984; Lightbody et al., 1978).

In an excellent double-blind, controlled study in 19 patients with COPD, Guyatt and associates (1987) showed that salbutamol administered by metered-dose aerosol improved pulmonary function, exercise tolerance, breathlessness, and quality of life. This paper produced strong evidence that bronchodilator therapy is efficacious in patients with COPD.

It is unlikely that the small changes in FEV_1 produced by beta-adrenergic agents will alter the natural course of COPD. The study by Emirgil et al. (1969) of patients with COPD failed to show any improvement

Table 1 Beta-adrenergic Studies: Therapies, Trial Design Score, and Outcomes

Study	n	Therapy	Score[a]	PF	Ex	Symp
Curzone et al. (1983)	15	ABC	6	+	0	0
Petty et al. (1970)	109	BC	6	+	+	0
Chick and Jenne (1977)	39	AB	6	+	0	0
Chan et al. (1984)	20	AB	7	+	0	0
Easton et al. (1986)	11	AB	8	+	0	0
Filuk et al. (1985)	16	BT	8	+	0	0
Starke et al. (1982)	22	AB	8	+	0	0
Astin (1972)	25	AB	8	+	0	0
Dull et al. (1981)	38	BT	8	+	0	0
Easton et al. (1986)	11	AB	8	+	0	0
Shim and Williams (1983)	17	BT	8	+	0	0
Hughes et al. (1982)	12	AB	8	+	0	0
Crompton (1968)	18	ABT	8	+	0	0
Popius and Salorinne (1973)	20	AB	8	+	0	0
Petrie and Palmer (1975)	8	AB	8	+	0	0
Connellan and Gough (1982)	10	B	9	+	+	0
Emirgil et al. (1969)	31	B	9	=	0	=
Leitch et al. (1981)	24	BT	9	+	+	0
Leitch et al. (1978)	24	AB	9	+	+	0
Taylor et al. (1985)	25	BT	9	+	0	=
Douglas et al. (1979)	21	AB	9	+	0	+
Jenkins et al. (1981)	10	AB	9	+	0	+
Lightbody et al. (1978)	10	ABC	10	+	=	=
Lefcoe et al. (1982)	15	ABT	10	+	0	=
Klock et al. (1975)	15	AB	10	+	0	=
Corris et al. (1983)	8	B	11	+	+	0
Bellamy and Hutchinson (1981)	20	B	11	+	0	+
Tobin et al. (1984)	12	AB	11	+	=	0
Papiris et al. (1986)	12	B	12	+	+	+
Guyatt et al. (1987a)	19	BT	12	+	+	+
Dullinger et al. (1986)	10	BT	12	+	=	+
Marvin et al. (1983)	15	BT	12	+	=	=

n, No. of patients; A, anticholinergic agent; B, beta-adrenergic agent; C, Corticosteroid; T, theophylline; PF, pulmonary function; Symp, symptoms; Ex, exercise; +, improved; = unchanged; 0, not assessed.
[a]See text for details of calculation of trial design score.

in symptoms or lung function after 12 months of treatment with broncho-dilators. The addition of breathing exercises or intermittent positive pressure breathing did not improve upon bronchodilator therapy.

Treatment with beta-adrenergic agents is associated with dosage-dependent side-effects: sinus tachycardia, tremor, atrial tachyarrhythmias, exacerbation of angina pectoris. These effects are mainly due to stimulation of B_1 receptors and occur with most beta-2-agonists as the dosage is increased. In some patients these side effects are serious and potentially life threatening but in general beta-2-agonists given by inhalation are well tolerated by the vast majority of patients. Thus, beta-adrenergic agents produce only small changes in pulmonary function, dyspnea, and exercise tolerance and are unlikely to alter prognosis. Their usefulness may be limited by significant side effects in some patients.

C. Anticholinergic Agents

Twenty-five papers that assessed the efficacy of anticholinergic agents in patients with COPD were reviewed (Table 2). In patients with chronic bronchitis, atropine given intravenously (Astin, 1982) or orally (Chick and Jenne, 1977) produced improvements in airways resistance and expiratory flow at 50% VC. However, anticholinergic side effects have limited the use of atropine. Aerosol ipratropium bromide, a less potent bronchodilator than atropine (Trinquet et al., 1975; Pierce et al., 1982), improved pulmonary function in patients with COPD (Tobin et al., 1984; Hughes et al., 1982; Leich et al., 1978). In the study by Tobin et al., the mean change in FEV_1 [SEM] was 0.20 [0.04] L and 0.49 [0.13] L in VC. The peak effect occurred 90 min after administration (Hughes et al., 1982). Oxitropium bromide has effects similar to ipratropium (Frith et al., 1986).

Anticholinergic treatment did not improve exercise tolerance in any of the four studies listed in Table 2 that assessed this outcome. In particular, there was no improvement in 12 min walking distance (Leitch et al., 1978), maximal workload on cycle ergometer, oxygen uptake ($\dot{V}O_2$), or heart rate during submaximal or maximal exercise (Tobin et al., 1984).

Of the six studies that assessed the effect of treatment on symptoms, only two reported an improvement. Side effects include dry mouth, unpleasant taste, and bronchoconstriction related to hypotonicity of ipratropium bromide solution (Mann et al., 1984). Systemic side effects such as blurred vision, mydriasis, and prostatism were not frequently reported with the newer anticholinergic agents such as ipratropium.

Thus, the newer anticholinergic agents produce small changes in pulmonary function similar to beta-adrenergic agents, but have minimal effects on symptoms and no effect on exercise performance. Side effects

Table 2 Anticholinergic Studies: Therapies, Trial Design Scores, Outcomes

					Outcomes	
Study	n	Therapy	Score[a]	PF	Ex	Symp
Curzone et al. (1983)	15	ABC	6	+	0	0
Chick and Jenne (1977)	39	AB	6	+	0	0
Chan et al. (1984)	20	AB	7	+	0	0
Starke et al. (1982)	22	AB	8	+	0	0
Astin (1972)	25	AB	8	+	0	0
Easton et al. (1986)	11	AB	8	+	0	0
Hughes et al. (1982)	12	AB	8	+	0	0
Frith et al. (1986)	24	A	8	+	0	0
Gross and Skorodin (1984)	10	A	8	+	0	0
Crompton (1968)	18	ABT	8	+	0	0
Barber et al. (1977)	8	A	8	+	0	0
Poppius and Salorinne (1973)	20	AB	8	+	0	0
Petrie and Palmer (1975)	8	AB	8	+	0	0
Lulling et al. (1980)	10	A	9	+	0	=
Leitch et al. (1978)	24	AB	9	+	+	0[a]
Douglas et al. (1979)	21	AB	9	+	0	0
Jenkins et al. (1981)	10	AB	9	+	0	+
Brown et al. (1984a)	20	A	10	+	·0	0
Lightbody et al. (1978)	10	ABC	10	+	=	=
Lefcoe et al. (1982)	15	ABT	10	+	0	=
Klock et al. (1975)	15	AB	10	+	0	=
Chervinsky et al. (1977)	10	A	11	+	0	+
Brown et al. (1986)	18	A	11	+	=	0
Tobin et al. (1984)	12	AB	11	+	=	0

See Table 1 for abbreviations.
[a]Anticholinergic agent *alone* did not improve exercise tolerance.

may be troublesome but not serious. Overall, their efficacy in patients with stable COPD appears no better than beta-adrenergic agents, although one study by Gross and Skorodin (1984) using maximum doses of atropine methonitrate found that this produced better bronchodilation than salbutamol.

D. Combination Therapy

A number of studies have demonstrated that the combination of a beta-2-adrenergic agent and an anticholinergic agent produces additive effects on FEV_1 and VC (Hughes et al., 1982; Chan et al., 1984; Frith et al., 1986;

Lightbody et al., 1978). However, even with high dosages (e.g., 5 mg salbutamol plus 0.5 mg ipratropium by nebulizer), the improvement with combination therapy is not great. For example, in the study by Brown et al. (1984a), FEV_1 45 min after combination therapy was 120 ml greater than after salbutamol alone. Not all studies have demonstrated additive effects for the peak bronchodilation achieved by combination treatment (Petrie and Palmer, 1975; Pierce et al., 1982; Starke et al., 1982). However, Starke and associates (1982) demonstrated that anticholinergic therapy may prolong the bronchodilator effect achieved for up to 12 hr, even though they appear to have used submaximal dosages of atropine.

The use of submaximal dosages of drugs in combination can produce misleading results. This problem can be overcome by the use of individual dose–response curves during serial administrations of therapy. This method ensures that a "plateau" of bronchodilation is achieved before a second agent is administered. Gross and Skorodin (1984) used this method in 10 male patients with emphysema, in whom all achievable bronchodilation was obtained by a single agent (atropine methonitrate); no additional bronchodilation was obtained by the addition of salbutamol. Easton and associates (1986), in a similar study, demonstrated that albuterol and ipratropium were equipotent in serial maximal dosages and that combination therapy was no more effective than either agent used alone. These two studies have provided convincing evidence that the use of a single agent in maximal dosages can achieve maximal bronchodilation that is not improved by the addition of a second agent.

Combined fenoterol and ipratropium did not improve exercise tolerance in 12 patients with emphysema, in the study by Tobin et al. (1984). The effects of combined therapy on quality of life and survival have not been studied.

Thus, combined therapy is unlikely to be any more efficacious than either agent, used alone, in maximal dosages. It is possible that combination therapy reduces side effects that would be experienced if either agent was used singly in maximal dosage. However, this claim has not been rigorously tested.

E. Methylxanthine Derivatives

Nineteen papers that assessed theophylline derivatives in patients with COPD were reviewed (Table 3). Eight papers (42%) reported on exercise tolerance and 12 papers (63%) reported on symptoms. In stable patients with COPD, oral theophylline at therapeutic levels (10–20 mg/L) produces only small changes in pulmonary function, (e.g., change in FEV_1 on the order of 150 ml and change in VC on the order of 350 ml; Alexander et al.,

Table 3   Theophylline Studies: Therapies, Trial Design Score, Outcomes

Study	n	Therapy	Score[a]	Outcomes		
				PF	Ex	Symp
Murciano et al. (1984)	15	T	6	=	0	0
Filuk et al. (1985)	16	BT	8	+	0	0
Dull et al. (1981)	38	BT	8	+	0	0
Shim and Williams (1983)	17	BT	8	+	0	0
Crompton (1968)	18	ABT	8	+	0	0
Leitch et al. (1981)	24	BT	9	+	+	0
Taylor et al. (1985)	25	BT	9	+	0	=
Lefcoe et al. (1982)	15	ABT	10	+	0	=
Belman et al. (1985)	7	T	10	+	0	0
Dull et al. (1982)	40	T	11	+	0	=
Alexander et al. (1980)	40	T	11	+	0	=
Eaton et al. (1980)	10	T	11	+	0	=
Evans (1984)	20	T	12	=	=	=
Guyatt et al. (1987)	19	BT	12	+	+	+
Dullinger et al. (1986)	10	BT	12	+	=	+[a]
Marvin et al. (1983)	15	BT	12	+	=	=
Eaton et al.(1983)	14	T	12	+	=	=
Jenne (1984)	10	T	12	+	+	+
Mahler et al. (1985)	12	T	12	=	=	+

See Table 1 for abbreviations.
[a]Theophylline *alone* did not improve symptoms.

1980; Jenne et al., 1984). Two studies failed to show significant improvements over placebo (Mahler et al., 1985; Evans, 1984). In general, the changes in pulmonary function after theophylline administration correlate with, but are usually smaller than, improvements after use of beta-adrenergic agents (Jenne et al., 1984). These small changes in lung function are most unlikely to alter prognosis.

Of the 12 studies that evaluated the subjective benefits of oral theophylline therapy, 9 found no evidence of significant improvement over placebo. In one study in which some patients preferred theophylline over placebo, there was a correlation between their preference and improvement in FVC (Jenne et al., 1984). Using a sensitive dyspnea index in 12 male patients on oral theophylline, Mahler et al. (1985) showed small improvements in dyspnea compared to placebo. However, since these workers used a very sensitive method to document improvement in the laboratory, the results may not apply to the patients' usual activities at home. Our general impression is that theophylline is somewhat disappointing in the treatment of symptomatic patients with COPD.

Only three of eight studies reviewed showed an improvement in exercise tolerance with theophylline administration (Table 3). For example, 24 patients with chronic bronchitis using slow-release (oral) theophylline showed a small (54 m) but significant increase in 12 min walking distance (Leitch et al., 1981). However, other workers found no improvement in 12 min walking distance with oral theophylline (Eaton et al., 1982; Dullinger et al., 1986; Mahler et al., 1985). When exercise tolerance was assessed by progressive cycle ergometry (Eaton et al., 1982; Dullinger et al., 1986), and during steady-state cycle exercise (Marvin et al., 1983), there was also no improvement over placebo. However, the study by Guyatt et al. (1987a), in which oral theophylline was shown to improve symptoms, pulmonary function, exercise tolerance, and quality of life, provides evidence that oral theophylline is efficacious in selected patients with COPD.

The side effects of theophylline are common, distressing, and sometimes life-threatening. These include anorexia, nausea, vomiting, diarrhea, headache, tremulousness, and palpitations. More serious side effects include convulsions and cardiac arrhythmias (Gilman et al., 1980). Although theophylline assays are now widely available and should be used routinely, there is still potential for toxicity because of variable hepatic metabolism and drug interactions. Recently, a nomogram was developed that allowed prediction of maintenance doses from a single theophylline level (Goldstein et al., 1986). However, patients' dosage requirements may still vary from week to week and an individual is not protected from future toxicity, especially if given inappropriate intravenous treatment with theophylline upon admission to the hospital when acutely ill.

Murciano and associates (1984) have suggested that theophylline might be beneficial in preventing and treating diaphragmatic fatigue in patients with airways obstruction. However, other workers have shown that the improvement in diaphragm function is so small as to be inconsequential in a clinical setting (Belman et al., 1985). In the study by Davidson and associates (1984), aminophylline improved exercise tolerance but worsened breathlessness during exercise.

When combined with beta-adrenergic drugs, theophylline produces small additive effects on pulmonary function (Taylor et al., 1985; Leitch et al., 1981). However, there was no improvement in exercise tolerance in two of the four studies reviewed that assessed combined therapy (Leitch et al., 1981; Guyatt et al., 1987a). Furthermore, symptomatic improvement was reported in only one of the five papers dealing with this outcome (Guyatt et al., 1987a). Therefore, the advantages to be gained by combined therapy are small and probably do not apply to all patients with COPD.

In summary, in patients with COPD, oral methylxanthines produce minimal changes in pulmonary function that are not consistently accompanied by improvements in exercise tolerance or dyspnea. They are associated with considerable toxicity, variable drug levels, have potentially life-threatening side effects, and, if used, require careful monitoring.

F. Corticosteroids

Corticosteroids are efficacious in the treatment of chronic asthma (Report to MRC, 1956), where airways are narrowed by mucosal edema and an inflammatory infiltrate. In patients who have chronic bronchitis (mucus hypersecretion), airflow obstruction may also be present due to airway narrowing, particularly in small airways (Hogg et al., 1968), from mucosal edema, lymphocytic infiltrate, and bronchiolar fibrosis (Mitchell et al., 1976). Thus, corticosteroids might be anticipated to be efficacious in COPD. We reviewed 21 papers dealing with corticosteroid use in COPD (Table 4). Endpoints of these studies have included symptoms, pulmonary function, and exercise tolerance, but survival, quality of life, and long term side effects have not been studied in any detail.

Twelve (57%) trials showed significant improvements in pulmonary function with steroid therapy. Most studies used similar dosages of prednisone (30 mg) or methylprednisolone (32 mg) for 10–14 days. Shim et al. (1978) reported that 7 of 24 patients (29%) had an increase in FEV_1 greater than 30% of the baseline value on prednisone but not on placebo. However, the absolute changes in FEV_1 were small (mean [SEM] increase 0.14 [0.11] L). Even after a "steroid response" the mean FEV_1 of "responders" was only 41% of predicted. As the dosage of prednisone was reduced, pulmonary function in four of seven responders worsened despite treatment with beclomethasone metered aerosol.

Mendella and associates (1982) studied 46 patients with COPD in a 4 week randomized comparison of 32 mg methylprednisolone and 2 weeks of placebo. Eight patients (18%) showed improvements in FEV_1 of greater than 25% of baseline values (mean increase of 0.44 L). The improvement in FEV_1 was not maintained in four of seven responders who were treated with beclomethasone metered aerosol (dosages: 800–1600 mg/day).

Mitchell and associates (1984a), in a study of the efficacy of prednisolone, showed improvements in pulmonary function, exercise tolerance, and symptoms in 43 patients with COPD. In a later study, however, the same workers reported no significant improvements with corticosteroids in 21 patients studied at the same hospital by the same methods (Mitchell et al., 1984b).

Table 4 Corticosteroid Studies: Therapies, Trial Design Scores, Outcomes

				Outcomes		
Study	n	Therapy	Score[a]	PF	Ex	Symp
Postma et al. (1985)	65	C	5	=	0	0
Curzon et al. (1983)	15	ABC	6	+	0	0
Petty et al. (1970)	109	BC	6	+	+	0
Oppenhemimer et al. (1968)	26	C	6	=	0	0
Stokes et al. (1982)	31	C	6	=	0	0
Harding and Freedman (1978)	36	C	6	+	0	0
Shim et al. (1978)	24	C	8	+	0	0
Albert et al. (1980)	44	C	8	+	0	0
Mendella et al. (1982)	46	C	8	+	0	0
Shim and Williams (1985)	12	C	8	+	0	0
Blair and Light (1984)	44	C	8	+	0	0
Klein et al. (1969)	18	C	9	=	0	+
Evans et al. (1974)	10	C	9	=	0	0
Lightbody et al. (1978)	10	ABC	10	+	=	=
Strain et al. (1985)	13	C	10	=	=	=
Lam et al. (1983)	16	C	10	+	+	+
Williams and McGavin et al.						
(1980)	29	C	11	+	+	+
Eliasson et al. (1986)	16	C	11	=	0	=
O'Reilly et al. (1982)	10	C	12	=	=	=
Mitchell et al. (1984b)	21	C	12	=	=	=

See Table 1 for abbreviations.

It appears that when oral steroids are given to patients with COPD, a proportion of them (15–20%) will respond with a small improvement in FEV_1 that is difficult to maintain as dosage is reduced. Eliasson and Degraff (1986) showed that the percentage of "steroid responders" in any study was inversely related to baseline FEV_1; the more "obstructed" a patient is, the more likely he or she is to "respond" to corticosteroids. They argue that this is an artifact arising from the definition of "response" as a 15% improvement over baseline.

There is no evidence that treatment improves quality of life or survival. Exercise tolerance was improved in four of the eight studies that assessed this outcome and symptoms were improved in four of nine studies.

Can a response to steroids be predicted? Bronchial reactivity as defined by histamine challenge does not predict a response to steroids (Oppenheimer et al., 1968; Winter et al., 1985). Although sputum eosinophilia (Shim et al., 1978) and blood eosinophilia (Harding and Freedman, 1978) were reported to predict response to steroids, other workers did not confirm this (Mendella et al., 1982). No differences occur between responders and nonresponders in age, sex, smoking history, duration or intensity of symptoms, wheeze, and baseline lung function (Mendella et al., 1982). Thus, it is not currently possible to predict with confidence who will respond to steroids.

Measurements of lung mechanics to differentiate between airway narrowing and loss of elastic recoil as the predominant cause of the airflow obstruction in COPD patients ($\dot{V}$max/Pel and SGaw/Pel relationships) might be expected to have a theoretical place in predicting steroid responsiveness, but these measurements are tedious and have not yet been shown to be of predictive value.

On the other hand, it may be possible to predict those patients who will not respond to corticosteroids. Mendella and associates (1982) reported that there were no responders in the group of COPD patients with less than 10% increase in FEV_1 after use of inhaled bronchodilator. In Shim's study (1978), there were no responders among patients with less than 15% increase in FEV_1 after isoproterenol metered aerosol. Therefore, patients who are not acutely responsive to inhaled beta-adrenergic drugs might be spared a trial of oral steroids.

Are the benefits worth the side effects of long-term steroid therapy? It seems unlikely that the small physiological improvements documented in response to corticosteroids will improve the prognosis of patients with COPD. The frequency of side effects in patients on long-term oral steroids for COPD is largely unknown and it does not seem possible to predict which patients will experience complications of therapy.

Albert and co-workers (1980) examined the use of corticosteroids for acute exacerbations of COPD in' a double-blind, randomized, placebo-controlled study of the effects of methylprednisolone (0.5 mg/kg intravenously every 6 hr for 72 hr) in 22 patients with chronic bronchitis who were admitted with acute respiratory insufficiency. Twenty-two similar patients received placebo treatment. The steroid-treated group had a greater improvement in FEV_1 after 72 hr than the placebo-treated group. Although the difference was *statistically* significant, it was probably not *clinically* significant (FEV_1 in controls improved by approximately 0.1 L after 72 hr, compared to 0.2 L in steroid-treated patients). The authors did not report on mortality, duration of hospitalization, or symptoms. They stressed that their findings should *not* be interpreted to mean that corticosteroids were indicated in *every* patient with chronic bronchitis who presents with acute respiratory failure.

Overall, there is little evidence that corticosteroids are efficacious in the treatment of COPD. The use of percentage improvement over baseline is not an appropriate outcome by which to assess "steroid responders." Future steroid trials should include quality of life, exercise tolerance, and symptoms as outcome measures in addition to measurement of pulmonary function.

III. Supplemental Oxygen Therapy

A. Continuous Home Oxygen

The best predictors of survival in COPD are FEV_1 and age (Anthonisen et al., 1986). Although several studies have shown that PaO_2 correlates poorly with survival (Weitzenblum et al., 1981; Cooper et al., 1985a,b; Anthonisen et al., 1986), two large clinical trials have shown that relief of hypoxemia by domiciliary oxygen is associated with improved patient survival (Medical Research Council Working Party, 1981; Nocturnal Oxygen Therapy Trial Group, 1980).

The MRC study involved 87 patients with COPD (mean $FEV_1 = 0.71$ L) who had cor pulmonale and at least one documented episode of heart failure with ankle edema. Patients were hypoxemic (mean $PaO_2 = 51$ mmHg), hypercapnic (mean $PaCO_2 = 54$ mmHg), with raised hematocrit (mean hematocrit $= 0.53$), and elevated pulmonary artery pressure (mean pulmonary artery pressure $= 34.4$ mmHg). Forty-two patients (33 males) were randomly allocated to receive home oxygen from cylinders for at least 15 h/day. Oxygen flow rates were adjusted to achieve PaO_2 of 60 mmHg at rest. There were 45 control patients (33 males) who did not receive supplemental oxygen. The main finding was a reduction in mortality in male patients treated with domiciliary oxygen. After 500 days, the risk of death appeared to be a constant 12% annually in the treated group and 29% annually in the control group. Two and 5 year survivals can be estimated from the survival curve shown in Figure 1; 2 year survival was approximately 50% for controls and 60% for treated patients; 5 year survivals were approximately 20% and 40%, respectively. Median survival was improved by approximately 21 months in the group treated with oxygen. The number of female patients was too small for meaningful survival analysis.

There were some disappointing results from the MRC trial: there was no reduction in hospitalization, no improvement in work attendance, no change in pulmonary hypertension, and only small changes in hematocrit and red cell mass.

The Nocturnal Oxygen Therapy Trial (NOTT) involved patients similar to those studied in the MRC trial (mean $FEV_1 = 0.75$ L; mean

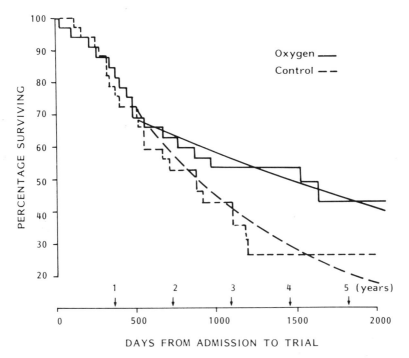

Figure 1 Medical Research Council Working Party, 1981: Comparison of percentage survival against time in the trial for those on 15 or more hr of oxygen per day (———) to controls (— — —).

PaO_2 = mmHg; mean hematocrit = 0.48; mean pulmonary artery pressure = 29.5 mmHg), but they were less hypercapnic (mean $PaCO_2$ = 44 mmHg). One hundred and two patients received nocturnal oxygen therapy (mean [SD] usage = 12.0 [2.5] hr/day) and 101 received continuous oxygen therapy (mean [SD] usage = 17.7 [4.8] hr/day). The main finding of the NOTT trial was a reduction in mortality in the group who received continuous oxygen therapy (Fig. 2). Two year survival was 78% (95% confidence interval = 68–87%) for the group who received continuous oxygen compared with 59% (95% confidence interval = 48–70%) for the group that received oxygen at night. Median survival was improved by approximately 18 months in the group receiving continuous home oxygen. There were improvements in neuropsychiatric functioning in both groups, but since there was no control group who did not receive oxygen, it is not possible to attribute this improvement to oxygen use and it may have been due to the increased attention the patients received. Disappointing

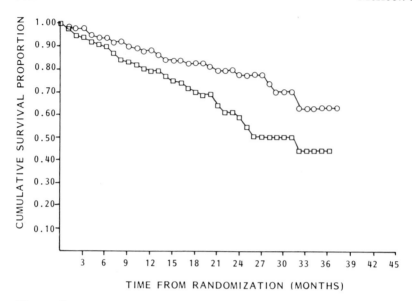

Figure 2 Nocturnal Oxygen Therapy Trial Group, 1980: Comparison of cumulative survival proportion of patients on continuous oxygen (o) to those on nocturnal oxygen (□). (Reproduced with permission from Nocturnal Oxygen Therapy Trial Group, 1980.)

results included a lack of improvement in exercise tolerance, hospital admissions, pulmonary hypertension, and cardiac index, and only a small change in hematocrit.

Neither the MRC nor the NOTT trial produced any very strong predictors as to which patients with hypoxic COPD are likely to do best with long-term oxygen therapy. A recent study (Ashutosh and Dunsky, 1987) suggests that an acute fall in pulmonary arterial pressure (PAP) on oxygen administration of >5 mmHg is predictive of a survival advantage. This evaluation requires right heart catheterization, however, and several groups are currently evaluating the use of noninvasive markers on acute hemodynamic response to oxygen to predict the survival advantage of long-term oxygen therapy in hypoxemic COPD (Ashutosh and Dunsky, 1987; Hunt et al., 1988).

What problems are associated with long-term oxygen therapy? The cost of providing this service is high. In New South Wales, Australia, the cost of renting an oxygen concentrator for 5 years is Aus$7,380 (July,

1986, figures). The cost is $6,866 if an oxygen concentrator is purchased, plus the cost of replacement parts. These costs are small compared to using continuous home oxygen from E-size cylinders at 2 L/min, which would cost Aus$25,000 per patient for 5 years. Portable cylinders are also expensive and cost approximately Aus$2,000/year when used for 2 hr per day at 4 L/min.

In Australia and the United Kindgom (Stretton, 1985), most of the cost of home oxygen is met by the government, with individual patients contributing only to the cost of electricity (approximately Aus$15.00 per month). There would appear to be no economic benefit since therapy does not improve work attendance (MRC, 1981). Domiciliary oxygen therapy needs to be carefully supervised for maximum cost-efficiency, which can best be achieved by a centralized, regional home oxygen service (McKeon et al., 1987; Crockett et al., 1986).

There are other problems besides cost. Oxygen cylinders are heavy, cumbersome, and must be delivered and refilled regularly. A potential fire hazard exists if patients smoke while receiving supplemental oxygen. There is also the danger of high-pressure accidents when smaller cylinders are filled from larger ones. Oxygen concentrators are more convenient than cylinders but they require regular maintenance and the cost of replacement parts, in particular the molecular sieve, can be quite high.

Long-term oxygen therapy restricts a patient's lifestyle considerably. It is hard to envisage that this system of increased dependency and continuing disability improves their quality of life. Long-term oxygen therapy may offer patients improved survival but at the cost of increased dependency.

B. Oxygen and Exercise

Patients with COPD often complain of exertional dyspnea that severely restricts their activities. Many of the treatments already discussed are not efficacious in improving exercise tolerance (see Tables 1–4). Digoxin has also been shown to be ineffective in improving exercise tolerance in patients with cor pulmonale (Brown et al., 1984b; Mathur et al., 1985).

Supplemental oxygen, used during exercise by patients with COPD, can improve exercise tolerance (Vyas et al., 1971b; Woodcock et al., 1981; Stein et al., 1982; Waterhouse and Howard 1983; McKeon et al., 1986b). Various methods of delivering oxygen have been used in laboratory studies. One method, which is potentially useful in the patient's home, involves lightweight (2.5 kg) portable cylinders of compressed gas that deliver supplemental oxygen at a rate of 4 L/min via nasal prongs. This method was used in the study by Woodcock et al. (1981), in which exercise tolerance was assessed by 6 min walking distance and maximal distance walked on a treadmill. Compared to placebo, there was an 8% improvement in 6 min distance and a 28% improvement in maximum treadmill distance. However, these improvements were small when expressed in absolute terms (24 m and 58 m, respectively). Oxygen reduced exertional dyspnea as assessed by a visual analog scale. Other workers noted similar changes in breathlessness when patients breathed supplemental oxygen during exercise (Waterhouse and Howard, 1983; McKeon et al., 1986b). However, it is difficult to extrapolate from small improvements in dyspnea on a treadmill to significant relief of breathlessness at home during activities of daily living. In the study by Bye and associates (1985), there was a 66% increase in endurance time when patients with COPD breathed oxygen compared to when they breathed compressed air (mean [SD] time on air = 5.9[1.3] min; on oxygen = 9.8[4.8] min). There was also a reduction in perceived exertion as measured by open magnitude scaling. In both normal persons and patients with COPD, oxygen leads to a reduction in minute ventilation at any given work load, which is due to a lower frequency of breathing (Bye et al., 1984; Stein et al., 1982; Vyas et al., 1971). Dyspnea on exercise is closely related to minute ventilation, irrespective of the inspired oxygen concentration (Swinburn et al., 1984). Hence, reduction in ventilation is associated with an improvement in breathlessness and allows higher work rates to be achieved while patients are breathing supplemental oxygen.

There are some problems associated with the use of portable oxygen: it is expensive, inconvenient, requires constant refilling of small cylinders, and poses some fire hazard. It would be easier if oxygen could be given before exercise as a "predose" with effect. This was suggested by Woodcock and associates (1981) to be effective in increasing exercise capacity and decreasing dyspnea, but these observations have not been confirmed by later studies (Rhind et al., 1986; McKeon et al., 1988a).

When used after exercise, supplemental oxygen improves recovery time by about 30 sec compared to recovery time in patients breathing compressed air (Rhind et al., 1986; Evans et al., 1986). However, this improvement is not reproducible when exercise is repeated on another day. Thus, pre or postexercise "doses" of supplemental oxygen are not likely to be beneficial for patients with COPD. Portable oxygen offers palliation of symptoms and a small improvement in exercise capacity, but it is inconvenient and expensive.

C. Nocturnal Oxygen Therapy

This is a controversial area in which a number of issues need to be considered. First, is nocturnal hypoxemia harmful in the absence of daytime hypoxemia? Only a prospective, long-term study, including outcomes such as survival, quality of life, hematocrit, and hemodynamic measurements, could answer this question. Such a study has yet to be performed. There is some evidence that the extent of nocturnal hypoxemia may not be clinically important (Stradling et al., 1987; Connaughton et al., 1987). On the other hand, Anthonisen (1985) and colleagues (1987a) state that although episodes of nocturnal hypoxemia have not been established to be harmful, it is probably unwise to assume that they are harmless. Thus, he and his co-workers believe that nocturnal oxygen therapy can be justified for episodes of nocturnal arterial oxygen desaturation below 75%. While this may be considered a common sense approach, it needs to be emphasized that there is no convincing evidence that this form of therapy will achieve significant benefits for the patient.

A second point is that daytime arterial oxygen saturation (SaO_2) is closely related to the lowest SaO_2 during sleep (Connaughton et al., 1986). Can nocturnal desaturation be predicted from awake SaO_2 with sufficient accuracy to be useful in making clinical decisions? It seems not. In one study of 24 patients, there was only a small difference between measured and predicted lowest SaO_2 asleep (3% SaO_2), but the standard deviation of that difference was sufficiently large (5% SaO_2) to make the prediction too imprecise to be useful clinically (McKeon et al., 1988b). Neither the nadir nor the duration of nocturnal desaturation can be accurately predicted from measurements of SaO_2 taken in patients with COPD while awake.

A third aspect of this question is if nocturnal desaturation cannot be predicted from awake SaO_2, which patients with COPD should be considered for a sleep study? Those with obesity, morning headaches, and daytime somnolence who are suspected of having obstructive sleep apnea syndrome may benefit from such a study (Flenley, 1985). Those with unexplained secondary polycythemia (Moore-Gillon et al., 1986) or right heart failure may also benefit from study during sleep. Patients who qualify for continuous home oxygen therapy on the basis of awake measurements do not require a formal sleep study, since nocturnal oxygen flow rates can be effectively prescribed in an empirical fashion in most cases (NOTT Study, 1980). Thus, only a minority of patients with COPD are likely to benefit from formal studies of oxygenation during sleep.

A last question is does supplemental oxygen improve quality of sleep in patients with COPD? This is controversial. There have been three studies in which nocturnal oxygen therapy was thought to have improved quality of sleep acutely (Calverly et al., 1982a; Goldstein et al., 1984; Kearley et al., 1980). However, the number of patients studied was small (n = 6, 10, and 11, respectively) and the finding of improvement with oxygen was not confirmed in two larger studies by Fleetham and associates (1982)

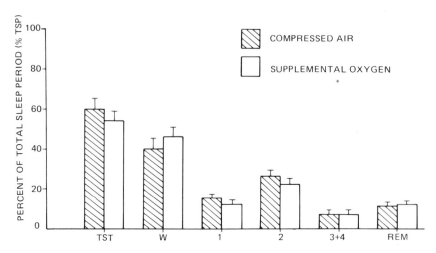

Figure 3 Quality of sleep in 24 patients with COPD on 2 consecutive nights randomized to receive either compressed air or supplemental oxygen on the first night.

and ourselves (Fig. 3). To our knowledge, there have been no long-term studies of the effect of oxygen on sleep quality.

Thus, nocturnal oxygen therapy may be indicated for a small proportion of patients with COPD, but the efficacy of such therapy has not been proven.

IV. Physical Training

A. Exercise Reconditioning

Even in patients with severe chronic airflow obstruction, exercise capacity can be improved by physical training (Petty et al., 1970). Two uncontrolled studies that used treadmill walking as a training technique for 3 weeks and 6 months, respectively, showed improvements in exercise tolerance (Nicholas et al., 1970; Paez et al., 1967). In another uncontrolled study, Vyas et al. (1971) showed that 4 weeks of training on a cycle ergometer produced an average improvement of 10% in maximal oxygen uptake in 11 patients with COPD. In all studies, the benefits were specific for the training technique and were not accompanied by improvements in pulmonary function.

Other controlled studies have since shown that these improvements were not due to a placebo effect (McGavin et al., 1977; Sinclair and Ingram,

1980; Cockcroft et al., 1981; Chester et al., 1977). Training techniques have included treadmill walking, stair climbing, bicycle training, and swimming. Greatest improvement (approximately 25%) occurred in 12 min walking distance, with smaller (approximately 10%) changes in maximal oxygen consumption. There were no significant changes in pulmonary function.

A recent study by Tydeman and associates (1984) examined a group of 24 patients with COPD who underwent exercise training over 2.5 years. There were significant improvements in 12 min walking distance (mean distance pretraining = 552; posttraining = 782 m). Before training, patients could walk a mean distance of 734 m at their own pace without stopping. After training, all but one patient could walk 1600 meters. The time to peak performance was 6–12 months. Improvements were maintained by regular exercise at home without the need for patients to return to the hospital for supervised training.

Outcomes such as survival, quality of life, and frequency of hospitalization have not been studied systematically. Exercise programs are inexpensive, especially if conducted at home without equipment. Patients need to be screened for ischemic heart disease and symptomatic arrhythmias before engaging in exercise training programs. With these safeguards, training can be undertaken safely in patients with COPD, and has the potential for improving patients' quality of life by increasing their mobility. There may even be an economic gain if patients are able to return to work, but this has not been established. General exercise training should be an integral part of any rehabilitation program for patients with COPD.

B. Inspiratory Muscle Training

Inspiratory resistance breathing improves maximum inspiratory pressure at the mouth (P_{Imax}) in some patients with COPD (Altose et al., 1986; Chen et al., 1985). Training by threshold resistance breathing also increases P_{Imax} (Larson et al., 1986). Improvement in inspiratory muscle endurance in patients with COPD occurs with isocapnic hyperventilation (Keens et al., 1977; Belman and Mittman, 1980). In contrast, general exercise training does not improve ventilatory muscle endurance (Belman and Kendregan, 1982).

Does Inspiratory Muscle Training Improve Exercise Tolerance?

Soon after two uncontrolled studies suggested that resistance breathing improved exercise tolerance in patients with COPD (Anderson et al., 1979; Belman and Mitman, 1980), several small controlled studies showed improvements in exercise tolerance using inspiratory resistance breathing as the training technique (Pardy et al., 1981; Sonne and Davis, 1982). Pardy and associates (1981) reported that 8 patients with COPD improved their 12 min walking distance from (mean [SD]) 671 [188] m to 760 [229] m after 8 weeks of inspiratory resistance breathing. However, there was no significant improvement in $\dot{V}O_2$ max on cycle ergometer. Sonne and Davis (1982) reported a 15% improvement of $\dot{V}O_2$ max in 6 patients with COPD after 6 weeks of inspiratory resistance breathing to a posttraining $\dot{V}O_2$ max of 0.83 ($\pm$ 0.14) L/min. However, there were only three control patients in this study.

Later studies have not been able to confirm these findings. McKeon and associates (1986a) studied 18 patients with COPD who had been treated with conventional bronchodilator and rehabilitation therapy. Eight patients used an inspiratory resistance breathing device and 10 patients used a placebo device for 6 weeks. There were no significant improvements in exercise performance in either group. Chen et al. (1985) reported similar negative results in 13 patients with COPD, despite improvements in inspiratory muscle strength and endurance. Bjerre-Jepson et al. (1981) compared 14 patients trained by inspiratory resistance breathing with 14 who used a placebo. Both groups improved exercise capacity but there was no significant difference between them.

Several of these studies have been open to criticism that as breathing through a small orifice was used to provide the inspiratory load, patients may still have been able to minimize the increase in respiratory work by altering their inspiratory flow rates and overall ventilation. A recent controlled study by Flynn et al. (1988) used a pressure threshold inspiratory valve, which overcomes these problems, to train the inspiratory muscles. Although clear improvement in P_{Imax} was obtained, no advantage was observed in either 12 min walking distance or any index of maximal incremental cycle exercise.

Breathing against an inspiratory threshold load was used in an uncontrolled study of 22 patients with COPD (Larson et al., 1986). There was a small improvement in 12 min walking distance in 10 patients who trained with a threshold load equal to 30% of their P_{Imax} (mean [SD] before exercise = 789 [144] m; after exercise = 850 [143] m). However, patients who used a load equal to 15% of P_{Imax} did not improve their exercise performance despite improvement in P_{Imax}. Furthermore, in neither group was there any improvement in patients' report of functional impairment, mood, health status, or pulmonary symptoms. The only patients who might achieve improvement in exercise performance from inspiratory muscle training are those demonstrated to develop inspiratory muscle fatigue during exercise (Pardy et al., 1981). The problems are how to identify such patients simply and whether the improvement in their exercise tolerance is clinically important.

How Does Inspiratory Muscle Training Compare with General Exercise Training in Improving Exercise Performance?

Cooper et al. (1985 a,b) compared a physiotherapy-trained group of seven COPD patients who undertook supervised walking and stair climbing for 8 weeks with nine patients who used inspiratory resistance breathing for the same time. The physiotherapy group improved their 6 min walking distance by 32 m and felt less breathless as measured by visual analog scales. The group using inspiratory resistance breathing also showed a small improvement in walking distance (23 m), but there was no change in breathlessness. Neither group improved their $\dot{V}O_2$ max on cycle ergometry.

Madsen et al. (1985) studied 10 patients with COPD who performed 6 weeks of general physical training (PT) followed by inspiratory muscle training (1 MT) for 6 weeks. After general training, there were improvements in 12 min walking distance (19%, range 1–28%), VO_{2max} (10%, range 2–33%), and breathlessness index (44%, range 3–86%). During inspiratory muscle training, there were no further improvements in any parameter.

Altose et al. (1986) compared the effects of IMT and general exercise training in 16 patients with COPD. Half the group used inspiratory resistance breathing and half trained on a treadmill for 6–12 months. In the inspiratory resistance breathing group, PI_{max} was significantly better after training, but there were no improvements in $\dot{V}O_{2max}$ or dyspnea. The group that trained on the treadmill did not show any change in PI_{max}, but improved in $\dot{V}_{Emax}$ (33.4 [4.2]–43.5 [6.6]L/min), $\dot{V}O_{2max}$ (0.90 [0.07]–1.24 [0.10]L/min), and breathlessness at end of exercise.

Thus, it seems that general exercise training consistently improves exercise performance in patients with COPD. Inspiratory muscle training improves inspiratory muscle strength in some patients, but does not improve exercise capacity to any practically significant degree. Inspiratory muscle training thus appears to have no advantage over standard rehabilitation programs that use general exercise training.

V.   Other Treatments

A.   Smoking Cessation

The most important way to prevent the progress and complications of COPD is to encourage people to stop smoking. With abstinence, there is an immediate improvement in pulmonary function and symptoms (Wilhelmsen, 1967; Peterson et al., 1968; Buist et al., 1976). The annual rate of decline in pulmonary function is also improved by cessation of smoking (Hughes et al., 1981). Secondary polycythemia improves with abstinence (Smith and Landaw, 1978; Sagone and Balcerzak, 1975). Cessation of smoking produces cost savings for the individual and has the potential to reduce health costs for the community by reducing the morbidity associated with the complications of COPD. Community-based interventions for cessation of cigarette smoking are discussed in Chapter 12.

B. Cor Pulmonale

Cor pulmonale is defined as "right ventricular enlargement (hypertrophy and/or dilatation) secondary to abnormal lungs, chest, bellows or control of breathing" (Fishman, 1980). Right heart failure, defined as peripheral edema with elevated jugular venous pressure, is not included in the definition of cor pulmonale, but commonly accompanies this condition. In patients with COPD, the development of cor pulmonale with right heart failure has serious prognostic implications. The median survival in this population is 2.4 years (MRC Trial, 1981). Three year survival is inversely related to pulmonary vascular resistance (Burrows et al., 1972). In assessing the efficacy of therapy for cor pulmonale, we also considered other important patient outcomes such as symptoms, exercise tolerance, pulmonary function, hemodynamics, and quality of life.

In acute exacerbations of COPD (Burrows, 1974; Whitaker, 1954) acute administration of supplemental oxygen reduces elevated pulmonary artery pressure. However, pulmonary artery pressure is not normalized acutely by oxygen treatment. Uncontrolled oxygen therapy may worsen hypercapnia (Campbell, 1960; Stradling, 1986). Therefore, the lowest flow rate that achieves an SaO_2 of 90% should be used and the $PaCO_2$ should be monitored by arterial blood gas analysis during therapy. The controlled use of supplemental oxygen in this fashion may be efficacious, although it has not been proven to improve outcomes such as mortality, duration of hospitalization, or patients' symptoms.

Although not curative, long-term home oxygen can prevent the relentless increase in pulmonary artery pressure usually associated with worsening right ventricular function (NOTT Trial, 1980; MRC Study, 1981; Weitzenblum et al., 1985). However, long-term home oxygen therapy does not improve exercise tolerance or pulmonary function and does not reduce hospitalization. Quality of life was improved by oxygen therapy in the NOTT study (1980), but the validity of this observation can be questioned because the study did not include a placebo-treated group. Thus, long-term oxygen improves prognosis and stabilizes abnormal hemodynamics in patients with cor pulmonale, but may not improve other outcomes.

Various vasodilators have been used in patients with COPD and cor pulmonale, including intravenous nitroglycerin (Fourrier et al., 1982; Morley et al., 1987), hydralazine (Lupi-Herrera et al., 1984), nifedipine (Sturani et al., 1983; Morley et al., 1987), captopril (Zielinski et al., 1986), and nitroprusside (MacNee et al., 1983). Beta-agonists have also been studied, including pirbuterol (MacNee et al., 1983; Peacock et al., 1983) and ter-butaline (Teule and Majid, 1980). In general, these agents produce similar effects on the pulmonary circulation, namely, falls in pulmonary vascular resistance and smaller falls in pulmonary artery pressure. The effect on cardiac output is variable. Pirbuterol did not improve exercise tolerance after 3 weeks of oral treatment (MacNee et al., 1983). The other studies listed above did not examine exercise tolerance or other important patient outcomes such as symptoms and quality of life. Only one study examined survival in a controlled, longitudinal fashion and found no improvement with vasodilator therapy (Morley et al., 1987). Hydralazine may have deleterious effects due to reduction of systemic vascular resistance (Packer et al., 1982) and nifedipine has been reported to have a deleterious effect on pulmonary gas exchange in patients with COPD (Melot et al., 1984). Thus, there is no evidence that vasodilators or beta-agonists are efficacious in the treatment of cor pulmonale.

Digoxin has been evaluated in patients with COPD and cor pulmonale and found to be lacking in efficacy (Mathur et al., 1981, 1985; Brown et al., 1984b). The studies by Mathur and Brown, in particular, were well-designed, randomized controlled trials that examined exercise capacity as well as hemodynamics, neither of which was improved by digoxin. Mathur and associates (1985) also reported no improvement in pulmonary function or general health status with digoxin therapy. Thus, digoxin has no place in the management of cor pulmonale due to COPD and should not be used since patients with COPD have been reported to have an an increased incidence of side effects due to digoxin (Hunter, 1967; Kirby et al., 1970).

Diuretics are commonly used to treat right heart failure when it ac-companies cor pulmonale. Pulmonary artery pressure may be lowered if there is a reduction in total blood volume caused by diuretic treatment (Gertz et al., 1979). Whether this treatment improves symptoms, mortality, or exercise tolerance has not been shown. The potential side effects of treatment include hypokalemic, hypochloremic alkalosis with worsening of ventilatory failure, hypotension, prerenal uremia, and exacerbation of gout and diabetes mellitus. Diuretics may be efficacious for acutely ill hospitalized patients, but this has not been established.

Overall, therapy for cor pulmonale is disappointing. Supplemental oxygen produces small improvements in pulmonary hemodynamics in acute exacerbations of COPD but not during long-term therapy. Vasodilators and digoxin are ineffective and sometimes dangerous.

Diuretics may be useful in the acute situation but have many potential side effects. Prevention of complications by cessation of cigarette smoking is a much more efficacious strategy than any of the therapies listed above.

C. Secondary Polycythemia

In patients with COPD, secondary polycythemia is associated with increased mortality (Mitchell et al., 1964) and considerable morbidity. There is an increased incidence of right heart failure in patients with a hematocrit higher than 0.54 (Renzetti et al., 1966). Semmens (1971) found right ventricular hypertrophy in every patient with COPD whose hematocrit was greater than 0.51. Hyperviscosity due to a raised hematocrit may cause symptoms such as lethargy, somnolence, and headache (York et al., 1980). In COPD, secondary polycythemia has been attributed both to chronic hypoxemia (Hurtado, 1945; Weil et al., 1968) and to elevated levels of carboxyhemoglobin in smokers (Smith and Landaw, 1978; Sagone and Balcerzak, 1975).

What can be done to treat secondary polycythemia? First, symptoms improve and the hematocrit falls with cessation of smoking (Sagone and Balcerzak, 1975; Smith and Landaw, 1978). Second, long-term oxygen therapy has been reported to lower the hematocrit in hypoxemic patients (Foster et al., 1978; Calverly et al., 1982b). However, incomplete response (Foster et al., 1978) or no response at all (Calverley, 1982b) occurs in patients on long-term oxygen therapy who continue to smoke. Furthermore, the MRC and NOTT studies reported no change in hemoglobin concentration and only small changes in the hematocrit during long-term home oxygen therapy.

Phlebotomy improves symptoms in patients whose hematocrit is higher than 0.55 (Dayton et al., 1975). However, there is no improvement in pulmonary function or gas exchange. Conflicting reports on the effect on exercise tolerance have been published (Dayton et al., 1975; Chetty et al., 1983). Thus, phlebotomy may be beneficial for symptomatic patients but has not been proven to improve prognosis, quality of life, or exercise tolerance.

D. Respiratory Infection

In patients with COPD, an increased volume of purulent sputum associated with worsening dyspnea and wheeze is suggestive of bronchial infection. *Haemophilus influenzae* and *Streptococcus pneumoniae* are possible causative organisms, but they are frequently isolated from patients with chronic bronchitis, regardless of the presence of symptoms of infection (Schreiner et al., 1978; Gump et al., 1976). Viruses have also been implicated as causes of bronchial infection in patients with chronic bronchitis, paticularly influenza and parainfluenza viruses, respiratory syncytial virus, and adenovirus (McHardy et al., 1980; Tager and Speizer, 11975; Monto and

Cavallaro, 1971). Asthma with sputum eosinophilia may mimic bronchial infection. Thus, a change in symptom may suggest bronchial infection, but this may be difficult to confirm by bacteriological or virological methods.

Antibiotics

It has been difficult to establish that antibiotics are efficacious in the treatment of exacerbations of chronic bronchitis. However, two well-designed, controlled studies have recently provided valuable evidence on this topic. Anthonisen and associates (1987b) studied 173 patients during 382 exacerbations of chronic bronchitis over 3.5 years. One hundred and eighty exacerbations were treated with placebo and 182 with broad-spectrum antibiotics (trimethoprim–sulfamethoxazole, amoxicillin, or doxycycline). There was a higher success rate with antibiotic therapy (68%) than with placebo (55%). The condition of 19% of placebo-treated patients deteriorated during treatment compared with 10% of antibiotic-treated patients. Peak flow recovered more rapidly with antibiotic treatment than with placebo. In the subgroup with increased dyspnea, increased sputum volume, and sputum purulence, 31% of placebo-treated patients deteriorated compared with 14% of antibiotic-treated patients. Thus, this study demonstrated definite benefit from the use of broad-spectrum antibiotics to treat exacerbations of chronic bronchitis. Side effects were uncommon and did not differ between patients receiving antibiotics and placebo.

Nicotra and associates (1982) studied 40 patients in a double-blind, randomized comparison of tetracycline and placebo in the treatment of acute exacerbations of chronic bronchitis. They found that sputum volumes were reduced by 32% in the treated group compared to 21% in the placebo group. Bacteriological evaluation showed a greater reduction in bacterial pathogens in the treated group. The alveolar–arterial oxygen gradient improved in both groups, but this was statistically significant only in the treated groups. Although none of the differences between placebo- and tetracycline-treated groups achieved statistical significance, this may have been because of the small number of patients studied. Certainly there were trends in favor of the treatment.

Thus, antibiotics seem efficacious in treating exacerbations of chronic bronchitis, particularly in those patients who have increased sputum volume and purulence together with increased symptoms of airflow obstruction.

Pneumococcal Vaccination

Pneumococcal vaccine has the potential to reduce the morbidity and mortality associated with pneumococcal infections in patients with COPD, but the results of two recent trials are not encouraging. A 14-valent pneumococcal capsular vaccine was compared to placebo treatment in 2295 high-risk patients in a Veterans Administration cooperative study (Simberkoff et al., 1986). There were 267 patients with chronic pulmonary disease in the placebo group and 272 similar patients in the vaccine group. Pneumococcal infections occurred more frequently in the patients with chronic pulmonary disease than in the other high-risk patients. However, the vaccine was not efficacious in preventing pneumonia or bronchitis in the treated group. A recent study by Davis and colleagues (1987) examined 63 patients with COPD who were randomly assigned to vaccination with 14-valent pneumococcal vaccine or placebo and then evaluated for 2 years. There was no reduction in the rate of pneumonia in the vaccinated group. Seventy-three percent of pneumonias were due to nonpneumococcal causes. Larger studies with longer follow-up are required before it can be concluded that pneumococcal vaccine is not efficacious in patients with COPD.

Influenza Vaccination

Allowing for the variations in the methods used in the large number of trials of influenza vaccination and for the problem of matching the vaccine strain with the wild one in the succeeding winter, it is estimated that influenza vaccine has an efficacy of 60–70% (Office of Technology Assessment, 1981). Although annual influenza vaccination is recommended for patients with COPD (National Health and Medical Research Council of Australia, 1986; Centers for Disease Control, 1987), the evidence for its efficacy in patients with COPD has not been studied as extensively as the major high-risk group—the elderly, especially those in nursing homes. Studies of efficacy in patients with chronic bronchitis have given variable results due, at times, to obvious reasons such as vaccination during or after the influenza outbreak (Medical Research Council, 1959). Overall, the methods used in these studies were poor, especially the failure to validate whether exacerbations of COPD were due to influenza infection (Medical Research Council, 1964).

Allowing for an efficacy of 60–70%, a cost–effectiveness analysis of influenza vaccination has been carried out by the Office of Technology Assessment (OTA). It was found that the cost per quality adjusted life year saved (QALYS) by influenza vaccination was lower the older the patient and the higher the risk group, to the extent that money was saved by vaccination in the age group older than 65. The economic analysis is much less impressive if the cost of subsequent medical and hospital care is added to the overall cost of the vaccine program. Whether these costs are added reflects to some extent the difference in perspective about funding of health care between clinicians who are satisfied to prevent death from an acute exacerbation of COPD and health economists who, while pleased that one episode of health care cost has been avoided, realize that the person saved, if elderly and sick, will generate many more costs.

In summary, while the evidence for the efficacy and effectiveness of influenza vaccination for the prevention of morbidity and mortality in patients with COPD is not as good as would be preferred, the vaccine appears to be worth using on an annual basis for patients with COPD.

VI. Ventilatory Stimulants

Respiratory stimulants have been used in patients with ventilatory failure due to COPD to reduce hypercapnia and improve hypoxemia. In 1970, Woolf advocated the use of central nervous system stimulants such as nikethamide and ethamivan for this purpose. However, these drugs may cause tremor, sweating, itching, nausea, and vomiting. In some cases, hypercapnia actually worsens with treatment. These drugs are contraindicated in patients with asthma and ventilatory failure due to respiratory muscle weakness. Furthermore, in a review of the efficacy of respiratory stimulants, Bickerman and Chusid (1970) pointed out the absence of suitably controlled clinical trials.

Doxapram is a respiratory stimulant that blunts the rise in $PaCO_2$ that occurs in patients with COPD upon commencement of supplemental oxygen (Riordan et al., 1975). However, there is no evidence that doxapram reduces hospital stay, improves mortality, relieves dyspnea, or improves exercise tolerance.

Medroxyprogesterone acetate improves chronic hypercapnia and hypoxemia in patients with COPD (Skatrud et al., 1980). When used during sleep in these patients, it improves arterial oxygen saturation and reduces $PaCO_2$ in non-REM sleep (Skatrud et al., 1981). However, the effects on quality of sleep, quality of life, and mortality have not been studied. In awake ambulatory patients with COPD, medroxyprogesterone does not improve dyspnea or exercise tolerance (Al-Damluji, 1986).

Almitrine is a recently developed agent that increases PaO_2 by improving $\dot{V}/\dot{Q}$ matching, probably by increasing hypoxic pulmonary vasoconstriction in lung regions with low V/Q ratios. When used in high doses it also increases the sensitivity of the carotid body to hypoxemia (Marmo, 1986). In patients with COPD, almitrine in a dosage of 100 mg/day increased PaO_2 by an average of 12 mmHg (Johanson et al., 1986), with no change in $PaCO_2$ or FEV_1. There was also improvement in breathlessness during treatment (Bourgouin-Karaouni et al., 1986). Both dyspnea and exercise tolerance were improved in 415 patients in an uncontrolled study reported by Marsac (1986). No studies have reported on quality of life.

The Vectarion International Multicentre Study Group (VIMS) recently presented evidence of the beneficial effects of almitrine in patients with COPD (Howard et al., 1987). This group studied 701 patients in a double-blind trial in which patients were randomly assigned to receive placebo or almitrine in a dosage of 100 mg/per day. Treatment was continued for 1 year. PaO_2 was improved only in patients taking the active compound; $PaCO_2$ was unchanged. Patients in the group receiving treatment were hospitalized less, and had less edema during the study period. Improvement in polycythemia was also noted. Effects on breathlessness, exercise tolerance, and quality of life were not reported. In an earlier report from the same group, there was no significant improvement in mortality in the treated group (Ansquer, 1986).

Not all patients respond to treatment with almitrine. The VIMS group (Howard et al., 1987) noted that PaO_2 did not increase with therapy in 23% of patients receiving almitrine. Fifteen percent of the group receiving almitrine in Ansquer's report (1986) were noncompliant with treatment, compared with 7% of the placebo group. Fourteen percent of the group receiving treatment had to discontinue it because of side effects, compared with only 4% of the placebo group. Reasons for stopping treatment included gastrointestinal intolerance, dyspnea, rash, and peripheral neuropathy (Marsac, 1986). Several cases of hyperesthetic polyneuropathy beginning 2–10 months after commencement of therapy have been reported (Gerard et al., 1986). However, subclinical peripheral neuropathy is common in patients with COPD (Lerebours et al., 1986) and did not worsen during treatment with almitrine in the study by Paramelle and associates (1986). Almitrine produces a small, significant increase in mean pulmonary artery pressure, both at rest and during exercise (Simonneau et al., 1986; MacNee et al., 1986). Whether this has any adverse effect on exercise tolerance or prognosis has not yet been determined.

Almitrine may be efficacious in patients with COPD who have chronic respiratory failure. However, not all patients respond to treatment, we cannot predict which patients will respond, and side effects may be significant.

VII. Conclusion

All forms of therapy for COPD may cause significant side effects and thus the potential for gain must be balanced against the potential for harm. It is important that therapy be individualized to provide maximum benefit for minimum harm. One potentially useful method of individualizing therapy is to perform a randomized trial with individual patients (Guyatt et al., 1986). In this method a patient is prescribed active therapy or an identical placebo for alternating periods of 1–2 weeks, and symptoms are recorded in a diary. Objective measurements of pulmonary function and exercise tolerance are also carried out. Thus, the efficacy of any single therapy can be assessed in any individual. Other treatments can then be added, one at a time, with appropriate placebo controls. No treatment needs to be continued unless it can be shown to provide clinically important benefit for the individual patient. This system requires the active participation of the pharmacy service in the preparation and dispensing of active and placebo treatments.

Quality of life is an important patient outcome that has been difficult to quantitate in clinical trials. Recently Guyatt and associates (1987b) developed a questionnaire for measuring quality of life in patients with COPD. They showed it to be precise and valid. It seems an ideal method of measuring symptomatic response to therapy in randomized trials in patients with COPD.

Another problem in assessing efficacy is deciding whether a finding of "no difference" is conclusive. The small sample size of many studies may explain why some authors failed to demonstrate the efficacy of therapy under evaluation. This problem may be overcome by performing meta-analysis of combined studies (Yusuf et al., 1985). We have not performed such an analysis because the patient outcomes chosen to demonstrate efficacy have varied greatly from study to study. In the future, uniform, meaningful patient outcomes would permit meta-analysis to be carried out.

In our examination of the efficacy of treatment for COPD, we used criteria developed by Sackett and associates (1981). This enabled us to assign a "trial design score" to each study. Some excellent studies demonstrated the efficacy of beta-adrenergic agents, theophylline, and antibiotics. Of the anticholinergic agents, there is little evidence that ipratropium bromide is useful addition for patients already using beta-adrenergic agents, and use of the more powerful atropine derivatives is limited by side effects. The benefits of corticosteroids appear to have been overestimated because response has been improperly defined as 15% improvement in FEV_1 over baseline. No properly conducted, prospective study of the long-term side effects of corticosteroids in COPD has been reported. Vasodilator therapy for patients with cor pulmonale is not efficacious and may be dangerous. Home oxygen therapy improves prognosis and stabilizes pulmonary hypertension and secondary polycythemia, but it is expensive and entails considerable restrictions in patients' lifestyles. Almitrine improves oxygenation, symptoms, exercise tolerance, and edema, reduces hospitalization and secondary polycythemia, but does not improve prognosis.

Our review of the literature suggests that quality of life in patients with COPD should be improved by thoughtful, critical, individualized treatment.

Acknowledgment

We thank Dr. R. J. Pierce for his helpful review of the manuscript and Mrs. J. Peate for preparation of the manuscript.

References

Albert, R. K., Martin, T. R., and Lewis, S. W. (1980). Controlled clinical trial of methylprednisolone in patients with chronic bronchitis and acute respiratory insufficiency. *Ann. Intern. Med.* **92**:753–758.

Al-Damluji, S. (1986). The effect of ventilatory stimulation with medroxy-progesterone on exercise performance and the sensation of dyspnoea in hypercapnic chronic bronchitis. *Br. J. Dis. Chest.* **80**:273–279.

Alexander, M. R., Dull, W. L., and Kasik, J. E. (1980). Treatment of chronic obstructive pulmonary disease with orally administered theophylline. A double-blind, controlled study. *J.A.M.A.* **244**:2286–2290.

Altose, M. D., Kendis, C., Connors, A. F., and DiMarco, A. F. (1986). Comparison of the effects of inspiratory muscle training and physical reconditioning on exercise capacity and dyspnoea in chronic obstructive lung disease (COLD). *Am. Rev. Respir. Dis.* **133**:A102.

Anderson, J. B., Dragsted, L., Kann, T., Johansen, S. H., Nielsen, K. B., Karbo, E., and Bentzen, L. (1979). Resistive breathing training in severe chronic obstructive pulmonary disease. A pilot study. *Scand. J. Respir. Dis.* **60**:151–156.

Ansquer, J. C. (1986). A one year double-blind, placebo-controlled study of the efficacy and safety of almitrine bismesylate in hypoxic COLD patients. *Eur. J. Respir. Dis.* **69**(Suppl.146):703–712.

Anthonisen, N. R. (1985). Home oxygen therapy. In *Harrison's Principles of Internal Medicine, Update VI*. Edited by K. J. Isselbacher, R. D. Adams, E. Braunwald, J. B. Martin, R. G. Petersdorf, and J. Wilson. New York, McGraw Hill, pp. 203–213.

Anthonisen, N. R., Wright, E. C., Hodgkin, J. E., and the IPPB Trial Group. (1986a). Prognosis in chronic obstructive pulmonary disease. *Am. Rev. Respir. Dis.* **133**:14–20.

Anthonisen, N. R., Wright, E. C., and the IPPD Trial Group (1986b). Bronchodilator response in chronic obstructive pulmonary disease. *Am. Rev. Respir. Dis.* **133**:814–819.

Anthonisen, N. R., Block, A. J., Kvale, P., and Petty, T. L. (1987a). Standards for the diagnosis and care of patients with chronic obstructive pulmonary disease (COPD) and asthma. Oxygen therapy. *Am. Rev. Respir. Dis.* **136**:235–236.

Anthonisen, N. R., Manfreda, J., Warren, C. P. W., Hershfield, E. S., Harding, G. K. M., and Nelson, N. A. (1987b). Antibiotic therapy in exacerbations of chronic obstructive pulmonary disease. *Ann. Intern. Med.* **106**:196–204.

Ashutosh, K., and Dunsky, M. (1987). Non-invasive tests of responsiveness of pulmonary hypertension to oxygen: prediction of survival in patients with chronic obstructive lung disease and cor pulmonale. *Chest* **92**:393–399.

Astin, T. W. (1972). Reversibility of airways obstruction in chronic bronchitis. *Clin. Sci.* **42**:725–733.

Barber, P. V., Chatterjee, S. S., and Scott, R. (1977). A comparison of ipratropium bromide, deptropine citrate and placebo in asthma and chronic bronchitis. *Br. J. Dis. Chest* **71**:101–104.

Barter, C. E., and Campbell, A. H. (1976). Relationship of constitutional factors and cigarette smoking to decrease in 1-second forced expiratory volume. *Am. Rev. Respir. Dis.* **113**:305–314.

Barter, C. E., Campbell, A. H., and Tandon, M. K. (1974). Factors affecting the decline of FEV_1 in chronic bronchitis. *Aust. N.Z. J. Med.* **4**:339–345.

Bellamy, D., and Hutchinson, D. C. S. (1981). The effects of salbutamol aerosol on lung function in patients with pulmonary emphysema. *Br. J. Dis. Chest* **75**:190–196.

Belman, M. J., and Mittman, C. (1980). Ventilatory muscle training improves exercise capacity in chronic obstructive pulmonary disease patients. *Am. Rev. Respir. Dis.* **121**:273–280.

Belman, M. J., and Kendregan, B. A. (1982). Physical training fails to improve ventilatory muscle endurance in patients with chronic obstructive pulmonary disease. *Chest* **81**:440–443.

Belman, M. J., Sieck, G. C., and Mazare, A. (1985). Aminophylline and its influence on ventilatory endurance in humans. *Am. Rev. Respir. Dis.* **131**:226–229.

Bickerman, H. A., and Chusid, E. L. (1970). The case against the use of respiratory stimulants. *Chest* **58**:53–56.

Bjerre-Jepson, K., Secher, N. H., and Kok-Jenson, A. (1981). Inspiratory resistance training in severe chronic obstructive pulmonary disease. *Eur. J. Respir. Dis.* **62**:405–411.

Blair, G. P., and Light, R. W. (1984). Treatment of chronic obstructive pulmonary disease with corticosteroids. Comparison of daily vs alternate-day therapy. *Chest* **86**:524–528.

Bourgouin-Karaouni, D., Mercier, J., and Prefaut, C. H. (1986). Long term studies on almitrine bismesylate in COPD patients. *Eur. J. Respir. Dis.* **69**(Suppl. 146):695–701.

Brown, I. G., Chan, C. S., Kelly, C. A., Dent, A. G., and Zimmerman, P. V. (1984a). Assessment of the clinical usefulness of nebulised ipratropium bromide in patients with chronic airflow limitation. *Thorax* **39**:272–276.

Brown, S. E., Pakron, F. J., Milne, N., Linden, G. S., Stansbury, D. W., Fischer, C. E., and Light, R. W. (1984b). Effects of digoxin on exercise capacity and right ventricular function during exercise in chronic airflow obstruction. *Chest* **85**:187–191.

Brown, S. E., Prager, R. S., Shinto, R. A., Fischer, C. E., Stansbury, D. W., and Light, R. W. (1986). Cardiopulmonary responses to exercise in chronic airflow obstruction. Effects of inhaled atropine sulphate. *Chest* **89**:7–11.

Buist, A. S., Sexton, G. J., Nagy, J. M., and Ross, B. B. (1976). The effect of smoking cessation and modification on lung function. *Am. Rev. Respir. Dis.* **114**:115–122.

Burrows, B. (1974). Arterial oxygenation and pulmonary hemodynamics in patients with chronic airways obstruction. *Am. Rev. Respir. Dis.* **110**:64–70.

Burrows, B., Kettel, L. S., Niden, A. H., Rabinowitz, M., and Diener, C. F. (1972). Patterns of cardiovascular dysfunction in chronic obstructive lung disease. *N. Engl. J. Med.* **286**:912–918.

Burrows, B., Bloom, J. W., Traver, G. A., and Cline, M. G. (1987). The course and prognosis of different forms of chronic airways obstruction in a sample from the general population. *N. Engl. J. Med.* **317**:1309–1314.

Bye, P. T., Esau, S. A., Walley, K. R., Macklem, P. T., and Pardy, R. L. (1984). Ventilatory muscles during exercise in air and oxygen in normal men. *J. Appl. Physiol.* **56**:464–471.

Bye, P. T., Esau, S. A., Levy, R. D., Shiner, R. J., Macklem, P. T., Martin, J. G., and Pardy, R. L. (1985). Ventilatory muscle function during exercise in air and oxygen in patients with chronic air-flow limitation. *Am. Rev. Respir. Dis.* **132**:236–240.

Calverley, P. M. A., Brezinova, V., Douglas, N. J., Catterall, J. R., and Flenley, D. C. (1982a). The effect of oxygenation on sleep quality in chronic bronchitis and emphysema. *Am. Rev. Respir. Dis.* **126**:206–210.

Calverley, P. M. A., Leggett, R. J., McElderry, L., and Flenley, D. C.

(1982b). Cigarette smoking and secondary polycythemia in hypoxic cor pulmonale. *Am. Rev. Respir. Dis.* **125**:507–510.

Campbell, E. J. M. (1960). A method of controlled oxygen administration which reduces the risk of carbon dioxide retention. *Lancet* **2**:12–14.

Campbell, A. H., Barter, C. E., O'Connell, J. M., and Huggins, R. (1985). Factors affecting the decline of ventilatory function in chronic bronchitis. *Thorax* **40**:741–748.

Centers for Disease Control. (1987). Prevention and control of influenza. *Morbid. Mortal. Weekly Rep.* **36**:373–380, 385–387.

Chan, C. S., Brown, I. G., Kelly, C. A., Dent, A. G., and Zimmerman, P. V. (1984). Bronchodilator responses to nebulised ipratropium and salbutamol singly and in combination in chronic bronchitis. *Br. J. Clin. Pharmacol.* **17**:103–105.

Chen, H., Dukes, R., and Martin, B. J. (1985). Inspiratory muscle training in patients with chronic obstructive pulmonary disease. *Am. Rev. Respir. Dis.* **131**:251–255.

Chester, E. H., Belman, M. J., Bahler, R. C., Baum, G. L., Schey, G., and Buch, P. (1977). Multidisciplinary treatment of chronic pulmonary insufficiency. 3. The effect of physical training on cardiopulmonary performance in patients with chronic obstructive pulmonary disease. *Chest* **72**:695–702.

Chervinsky, P. (1977). Double-blind study of ipratropium bromide, a new anticholinergic bronchodilator. *J. Allergy Clin. Immunol.* **59**:22–30.

Chetty, K. G., Brown, S. E., and Light, R. W. (1983). Improved exercise tolerance of the polycythemic lung patient following phlebotomy. *Am. J. Med.* **74**:415–420.

Chick, T. W., and Jenne, J. W. (1977). Comparative bronchodilator responses to atropine and terbutaline in asthma and chronic bronchitis. *Chest* **72**:719–725.

Cockcroft, A. E., Saunders, M. J., and Berry, G. (1981). Randomised controlled trial of rehabilitation in chronic respiratory disability. *Thorax* **36**:200–203.

Connaughton, J. J., Catterall, J. R., Wraith, P. K., Flenley, D. C., and Douglas, N. J. (1986). The clinical value of studies of breathing and oxygenation during sleep in patients with chronic bronchitis and emphysema. *Am. Rev. Respir. Dis.* **133**:A149.

Connaughton, J. J., Catterall, J. R., and Douglas, N. J. (1987). Do sleep studies contribute to the clinical management of chronic bronchitis? *Thorax* **42**:217 (abstract).

Connellan, S. J., and Gough, S. E. (1982). The effects of nebulized salbutamol on lung function and exercise tolerance in patients with severe airflow obstruction. *Br. J. Dis. Chest* **76**:135–142.

Corris, P. A., Neville, E., Nariman, S., and Gibson, G. J. (1983). Dose-response study of inhaled salbutamol powder in chronic airflow obstruction. *Thorax* **38**:292–296.

Cooper, C. B., Smith, C. M., and Cameron, I. R. (1985a). Respiratory muscle training compared with physiotherapy in chronic obstructive airways disease. *Thorax* **40**:717 (abstract).

Cooper, C. B., Waterhouse, J., Nicholl, J. P., Suggett, A. J., and Howard, P. (1985b). Survival of patients with hypoxic cor pulmonale given domiciliary oxygen therapy. *Thorax* **41**:235 (abstract).

Crockett, A. J., Alpers, J. H., and Chalmers, J. P. (1986). Cost centre management: how it helped reduce home oxygen costs. *Aust. Health Rev.* **9**:38–42.

Crompton, G. K. (1968). A comparison of responses to bronchodilator drugs in chronic bronchitis and chronic asthma. *Thorax* **23**:46–55.

Curzon, P. G. D., Martin, M. A., Cooke, N. J., and Muers, M. F. (1983). Effect of oral prednisolone on response to salbutamol and ipratropium bromide aerosols in patients with chronic airflow obstruction. *Thorax* **38**:601–604.

Davidson, A. C., Cooper, C. B., and Cameron, I. R. (1984). Does aminophylline improve exercise tolerance in chronic obstructive pulmonary disease? *Thorax* **39**:226–227 (abstract).

Davis, A. L., Aranda, C. P., Schiffman, G., and Christianson, L. C. (1987). Pneumococcal infection and immunologic response to pneumococcal vaccine in chronic obstructive pulmonary disease. A pilot study. *Chest* **92**:204–212.

Dayton, L. M., McCullough, R. E., Scheinhorn, D. J., and Weil, J. V. (1975). Symptomatic and pulmonary response to acute phlebotomy in secondary polycythaemia. *Chest* **68**:785–790.

Department of Clinical Epidemiology and Biostatistics, McMaster University (1981). How to read clinical journals: V: To distinguish useful from useless or even harmful therapy. *Can. Med. Assoc. J.* **124**:1156–1162.

Douglas, N. J., Davidson, I., Sudlow, M. F., and Flenley, D. C. (1979). Bronchodilatation and the site of airway resistance in severe chronic bronchitis. *Thorax* **34**:51–56.

Dull, W. L., Alexander, M. R., and Kasik, J. E. (1981). Isoproterenol challenge during placebo and oral theophylline therapy in chronic obstructive pulmonary disease. *Am. Rev. Respir. Dis.* **123**:340–342.

Dull, W. L., Alexander, M. R., Sadoul, P., and Woolson, R. F. (1982). The efficacy of isoproterenol inhalation for predicting the response to orally administered theophylline in chronic obstructive pulmonary disease. *Am. Rev. Respir. Dis.* **126**:656–659.

Dullinger, D., Kronenberg, R., and Niewoehner, D. E. (1986). Efficacy of inhaled metaproterenol and orally-administered theophylline in patients with chronic airflow obstruction. *Chest* **89**:171-173.

Easton, P. A., Jadue, C., Dhingra, S., and Anthonisen, N. R. (1986). A comparison of the bronchodilating effects of a beta-2 adrenergic agent (albuterol) and an anticholinergic agent (ipratropium bromide), given by aerosol alone or in sequence. *N. Engl. J. Med.* **315**:735-739.

Eaton, M. L., Green, B. A., Church, T. R., McGowan, T., and Niewochner, D. E. (1980). Efficacy of theophylline in "irreversible" airflow obstruction. *Ann. Intern. Med.* **92**:758-761.

Eaton, M. L., MacDonald, F. M., Church, T. R., and Niewoehner, D. E. (1982). Effects of theophylline on breathlessness and exercise tolerance in patients with chronic airflow obstruction. *Chest* **82**:538-542.

Eliasson, O., and Degraff, A. C. (1985). The use of criteria for reversibility and obstruction to define patient groups for bronchodilator trials. Influence of clinical diagnosis, spirometric and anthropometric variables. *Am. Rev. Respir. Dis.* **132**:858-864.

Eliasson, O., Hoffman, J., Trueb, D., Frederick, D., and McCormick, J. R. (1986). Corticosteroids in COPD. A clinical trial and reassessment of the literature. *Chest* **89**:484-490.

Emirgil, C., Sobol, B. J., Norman, J., Moskowitz, E., Goyal, P., Wadhwani, B., with the assistance of Varble, A., Waldie, J., and Weinheimer, R. (1969). A study of the long-term effect of therapy in chronic obstructive pulmonary disease. *Am. J. Med.* **47**:367-377.

Evans, J. A., Morrison, I. M., and Saunders, K. B. (1974). A controlled trial of prednisone, in low dosage, in patients with chronic airways obstruction. *Thorax* **29**:401-406.

Evans, T. W., Waterhouse, J. C., Carter, A., Nicholl, J. F., and Howard, P. (1986). Short burst oxygen treatment for breathlessness in chronic obstructive airways disease. *Thorax* **41**:611-615.

Evans, W. V. (1984). Plasma theophylline concentrations, six minute walking distances, and breathlessness in patients with chronic airflow obstruction. *Br. Med. J.* **289**:1649-1651.

Filuk, R. B., Easton, P. A., and Anthonisen, N. R. (1985). Responses to large doses of salbutamol and theophylline in patients with chronic obstructive pulmonary disease. *Am. Rev. Respir. Dis.* **132**:871-874.

Fishman, A. P. (1980). *Pulmonary Diseases and Disorders*, 1st. ed. New York, McGraw-Hill, p. 853.

Fleetham, J., West, P., Mezon, B., Conway, W., Roth, T., and Kryger, M. (1982). Sleep, arousals, and oxygen desaturation in chronic obstructive pulmonary disease. The effect of oxygen therapy. *Am. Rev. Respir. Dis.* **126**:429-433.

Flenley, D. C. (1985). Sleep in chronic obstructive lung disease. In *Clinics in Chest Medicine.* Symposium on Sleep Disorders, volume 6. Edited by M. H. Kryger. Philadelphia, W. B. Saunders, pp. 651–661.

Flynn, M. G., Barter, C. E., Nosworthy, J. C., Pretto, J. S., Rochford, P. O., and Pierce, R. J. (1988). Threshold pressure training, breathing pattern and exercise performance in chronic airflow obstruction. *Chest* (in press).

Foster, L. J., Corrigan, K., and Goldman, A. L. (1978). Effectiveness of oxygen therapy in hypoxic polycytaemic smokers. *Chest* **73**:572–576.

Fourrier, F., Chopin, C., Durocher, A., Dubois, D., and Wattel, F. (1982). Intravenous nitroglycerin in acute respiratory failure of patients with chronic obstructive lung disease, secondary pulmonary hypertension and cor pulmonale. *Intensive Care Med.* **8**:85–88.

Frith, P. A., Jenner, B., Dangerfield, R., Atkinson, J., and Drennan, C. (1986). Oxitropium bromide: dose–response and time–response study of a new anticholinergic bronchodilator drug. *Chest* **89**:249–253.

Gerard, M., Leger, P., Couturier, J. C., and Robert, D. (1986). Ten cases of peripheral neuropathy during treatment with almitrine in COPD patients. *Eur. J. Respir. Dis.* **69**(Suppl.146):591–596.

Gertz, I., Hedenstierna, G., and Wester, P. O. (1979). Improvement in pulmonary function with diuretic therapy in the hypervolemic and polycythemic patient with chronic obstructive pulmonary disease. *Chest* **75**:146–151.

Gilman, A. G., Goodman, L. S., and Gilman, A. (1980). *The Pharmacological Basis of Therapeutics*, 6th ed. New York, Macmillan, pp. 592–607.

Goldstein, R. S., Allen, L. C., Thiessen, J. J., Michalko, K., Dayneka, N., and Woolf, C. R. (1986). Daily maintenance dose of a long-acting theophylline from a single theophylline serum level. *Chest* **89**:103–108.

Goldstein, R. S., Ramcharan, V., Bowes, G., McNicholas, W. T., Bradley, D., and Phillipson, E. A. (1984). Effect of supplemental nocturnal oxygen on gas exchange in patients with severe obstructive lung disease. *N. Engl. J. Med.* **310**:425–429.

Gross, J. N., and Skorodin, M. S. (1984). Role of the parasympathetic nervous system in airway obstruction due to emphysema. *N. Engl. J. Med.* **311**:421–425.

Gump, D. W., Phillips, C. A., Forsyth, B. R., McIntosh, K., Lamborn, K. R., and Stouch, W. H. (1976). Role of infection in chronic bronchitis. *Am. Rev. Respir. Dis.* **113**:465–474.

Guyatt, G., Sackett, D., Taylor, D. W., Chong, J., Roberts, R., and Pugsley, S. (1986). Determining optimal therapy—randomized trials in individual patients. *N. Engl. J. Med.* **314**:889–892.

Guyatt, G. H., Townsend, M., Pugsley, S. O., Keller, J. L., Short, H. D.,

Taylor, D. W., and Newhouse, M. T. (1987a). Bronchodilators in chronic airflow limitation. Effects on airway function, exercise capacity and quality of life. *Am. Rev. Respir. Dis.* **135**:1069-1074.

Guyatt, G. H., Berman, L. B., Townsend, M., Pugsley, S. O., and Chambers, L. W. (1987b). A measure of quality of life for clinical trials in chronic lung disease. *Thorax* **42**:773-778.

Harding, S. M., and Freedman, S. (1978). A comparison of oral and inhaled steroids in patients with chronic airflow obstruction: features determining response. *Thorax* **33**:214-218.

Hogg, J. C., Macklem, P. T., and Thurlbeck, W. M. (1968). Site and nature of airway obstruction in chronic obstructive lung disease. *N. Engl. J. Med.* **278**:1355-1360.

Howard, P., Voisin, C., and Ansquer, J. C. (1987). Long term trial of almitrine bismesylate in chronic obstructive airways disease. Vectarion International Multicentre Study Group (VMS). *Am. Rev. Respir. Dis.* **135**:A277.

Hruby, J., and Butler, J. (1975). Variability of routine pulmonary function tests. *Thorax* **30**:548-553.

Hughes, J. A., Hutchison, D. C. S., Bellamy, D., Dowd, D. E., Ryan, K. C., and Hugh-Jones, P. (1981). The influence of cigarette smoking and its withdrawal on the annual change of lung function in pulmonary emphysema. *Q. J. Med.* **51**:115-124.

Hughes, J. A., Tobin, M. J., Bellamy, D., and Hutchinson, D. C. S. (1982). Effects of ipratropium bromide and fenoterol aerosols in pulmonary emphysema. *Thorax* **37**:667-670.

Hunt, J. M., Pierce, R. J., Barter, C. E., and Rochord, P. O. (1988). The non-invasive assessment of the acute effects of oxygen breathing in patients with hypoxaemic chronic obstructive pulmonary disease. *Thorax* **42**(9):742.

Hunter, C. C. (1967). Errors in management of patients dying of chronic obstructive lung disease. *J.A.M.A.* **199**:488-491.

Hurtado, A., Merino, C., and Delgado, E. (1945). Influence of anoxemia on the hemopoietic activity. *Arch. Intern. Med.* **75**:284-323.

Jenkins, C. R., Chow, C. M., Fisher, B. L., and Marlin, G. E. (1981). Comparison of ipratropium bromide and salbutamol by aerosolized solution. *Aust. N. Z. J. Med.* **11**:513-516.

Jenne, J. W., Siever, J. R., Druz, W. S., Solano, J. V., Cohen, S. M., and Sharp, J. T. (1984). The effect on maintenance theophylline therapy on lung work in severe chronic obstructive pulmonary disease while standing and walking. *Am. Rev. Respir. Dis.* **130**:600-605.

Johanson, W. G., Mullins, R. C., Bell, R. C., West, L. G., and Bachand, R. T. (1986). The efficacy of almitrine in improvement of hypoxaemia in patients with COPD. *Eur. J. Respir. Dis.* **69**(Suppl.146):663 (abstract).

Kearley, R., Wynne, J. W., Block, A. J., Boysen, P. G., Lindsey, S., and Martin, C. (1980). The effect of low flow oxygen on sleep-disordered breathing and oxygen desaturation. A study of patients with chronic obstructive lung disease. *Chest* **78**:682–685.

Keens, T. G., Krastins, I. R. B., Wannamaker, E. M., Levison, H., Crozier, D. N., and Bryan, A. C. (1977). Ventilatory muscle endurance training in normal subjects and patients with cystic fibrosis. *Am. Rev. Respir. Dis.* **116**:853–860.

Kirby, J., McNicol, M. W., and Tattersfield, A. E. (1970). Arrhythmias, digitalis, and respiratory failure. *Br. J. Dis. Chest* **64**:212–219.

Klein, R. C., Salvaggio, J. E., and Kundur, V. G. (1969). The response of patients with "idiopathic" obstructive pulmonary disease and "allergic" obstructive bronchitis to prednisone. *Ann. Intern. Med.* **71**:711–718.

Klock, L. E., Miller, T. D., Morris, A. H., Watanabe, S., and Dickman, M. (1975). A comparative study of atropine sulfate and isoproterenol hydrochloride in chronic bronchitis. *Am. Rev. Respir. Dis.* **112**:371–376.

Lam, W. K., So, S. Y., and Yu, D. Y. C. (1983). Response to oral corticosteroids in chronic airflow obstruction. *Br. J. Dis. Chest* **77**:189–198.

Larson, J. L., Kim, M. J., and Sharp, J. T. (1986). Inspiratory muscle training with a threshold resistive breathing device in patients with chronic obstructive pulmonary disease. *Am. Rev. Respir. Dis.* **133**:A100.

Lefcoe, N. M., Toogood, J. H., Blenner-Lassett, G., Baskerville, J., and Paterson, N. A. M. (1982). The addition of an aerosol anticholinergic to an oral beta-agonist plus theophylline in asthma and bronchitis. A double-blind single dose study. *Chest* **82**:300–305.

Lerebours, C., Ozenne, G., Senant, J., Moore, N., David, P. H., and Nouvet, G. (1986). Abnormalities in the electrophysiological examination of patients with chronic obstructive lung disease: a preliminary study of the effects of almitrine. *Eur. J. Respir. Dis.* **69**:713–714.

Leitch, A. G., Hopkin, J. M., Ellis, D. A., Merchant, S., and McHardy, G. J. R. (1978). The effect of aerosol ipratropium bromide and salbutamol on exercise tolerance in chronic bronchitis. *Thorax* **33**:711–713.

Leitch, A. G., Morgan, A., Ellis, D. A., Bell, G., Haslett, C., and McHardy, G. J. R. (1981). Effect of oral salbutamol and slow-release aminophylline on exercise tolerance in chronic bronchitis. *Thorax* **36**:787–789.

Lightbody, I. M., Ingram, C. G., Legge, J. S., and Johnston, R. N. (1978). Ipratropium bromide, salbutamol and prednisolone in bronchial asthma and chronic bronchitis. *Br. J. Dis. Chest* **72**:181–186.

Lulling, J., Delwiche, J. P., Ledent, C., and Prignot, J. (1980). Controlled trial of the effect of repeated administration of ipratropium bromide on ventilatory function of patients with severe chronic airways obstruction. *Br. J. Dis. Chest* **74**:135–141.

Lupi-Herrera, Seoane, M., and Verdejo, J. (1984). Hemodynamic effect of hydrallazine in advanced, stable chronic obstructive pulmonary disease with cor pulmonale. Immediate and short-term evaluation at rest and during exercise. *Chest* **85**:156–163.

McGavin, C. R., Gupta, S. P., Lloyd, E. L., and McHardy, G. J. R. (1977). Physical rehabilitation for the chronic bronchitic: results of a controlled trial of exercises in the home. *Thorax* **32**:307–311.

McGavin, C. R., Artvinli, M., Naoe, H., and McHardy, G. J. R. (1978). Dyspnoea, disability and distance walked: comparison of estimates of exercise performance in respiratory disease. *Br. Med. J.* **2**:241–243.

McHardy, V. U., Inglis, J. M., Calder, M. A., Crofton, J. W., Gregg, I., Ryland, D. A., Taylor, P., Chadwick, M., Coombs, D., and Riddell, R. W. (1980). A study of infective and other factors in exacerbations of chronic bronchitis. *Br. J. Dis. Chest* **74**:228–238.

McKeon, J. L., Turner, J., Kelly, C., Dent, A., and Zimmerman, P. V. (1986a). The effect of inspiratory resistive training on exercise capacity in optimally treated patients with severe COPD. *Aust. N. Z. J. Med.* **16**:648–652.

McKeon, J. L., Tomlinson, J. C., Tarrant, P. E., and Mitchell, C. (1986b). The assessment of portable oxygen in patients with chronic obstructive lung disease. *Aust. N. Z. J. Med.* **16**:621 (abstract).

McKeon, J. L., Saunders, N. A., and Murree-Allen, K. (1987). Domiciliary oxygen: rationalization of supply in the Hunter Region from 1982–1986. *Med. J. Aust.* **146**:73–78.

McKeon, J. L., Murree-Allen, K., and Saunders, N. A. (1988a). The effects of breathing supplemental oxygen before progressive, maximal exercise in patients with chronic obstructive pulmonary disease. *Thorax* **43**:53–60.

McKeon, J. L., Murree-Allen, K., and Saunders, N. A. (1988b). Prediction of oxygenation during sleep in patients with chronic obstructive pulmonary disease. *Thorax* **43**:312–317.

MacNee, W., Connaughton, J. J., Rhind, G. B., Hayhurst, M. D., Douglas, N. J., Muir, A. L., and Flenley, D. C. (1986). A comparison of the effects of almitrine or oxygen breathing on pulmonary arterial pressure and right ventricular ejection fraction in hypoxic chronic bronchitis and emphysema. *Am. Rev. Respir. Dis.* **134**:559–565.

MacNee, W., Wathen, C. G., Hannan, W. J., Flenley, D. C., and Muir, A. L. (1983). Effects of pirbuterol and sodium nitroprusside on pulmonary hemodynamics in hypoxic cor pulmonale. *Br. Med. J.* **287**:1169–1172.

Madsen, F., Secher, N. G., Kay, L., Kok-Jensen, A., and Rube, N. (1985). Inspiratory resistance versus general physical training in patients with chronic obstructive pulmonary disease. *Eur. J. Respir. Dis.* **67**:167–176.

Mahler, D. A., Matthay, R. A., Snyder, P. E., Wells, C. K., and Loke, J.

(1985). Sustained-release theophylline reduces dyspnoea in nonreversible obstructive airway disease. *Am. Rev. Respir. Dis.* **131**:22–25.

Marsac, J. (1986). The assessment of almitrine bismiselate in the long-term treatment of chronic obstructive bronchitis. *Eur. J. Respir. Dis.* **69**(Supple.146):685–693.

Marvin, P. M., Baker, B. J., Dutt, A. K., Murphy, M. L., and Bone, R. C. (1983). Physiological effects of oral bronchodilators during rest and exercise in chronic obstructive pulmonary disease. *Chest* **84**:684–689.

Mann, J. S., Howarth, P. H., and Holgate, S. T. (1984). Bronchoconstriction induced by ipratropium bromide in asthma: relation to hypotonicity. *Br. Med. J.* **289**:469.

Marmo, E. (1986). The pharmacological properties of almitrine bismesylate. *Eur. J. Respir. Dis.* **69**(Suppl.146):619–632.

Mathur, P. N., Powles, P., Pugsby, S. O., McEwan, M. P., and Campbell, E. J. M. (1981). Effect of digoxin on right ventricular function in severe chronic airflow obstruction. A controlled clinical trial. *Ann. Intern. Med.* **95**:283–288.

Mathur, P. N., Powles, A. C. P., Pugsley, S. O., McEwan, M. P., and Campbell, E. J. M. (1985). Effects of long-term administration of digoxin on exercise performance in chronic airflow obstruction. *Eur. J. Respir. Dis.* **66**:273–283.

Medical Research Council Committee on Influenza and Other Respiratory Virus Vaccines (1959). Field trial of influenza virus vaccine in patients with chronic bronchitis during the winter 1957-8. *Br. Med. J.* **2**:905–908.

Medical Research Council Committee on Influenza and Other Respiratory Virus Vaccines (1964). Clinical trials of oil-adjuvant influenza vaccines, 1960-5. *Br. Med. J.* **2**:267–271.

Medical Research Council Working Party (1981). Long term domiciliary oxygen therapy in chronic hypoxic cor pulmonale complicating chronic bronchitis and emphysema. *Lancet* **1**:681–686.

Melot, C., Hallemans, R., Naeije, R., Molls, P., and Lejeune, P. (1984). Deleterious effect of nifedipine on pulmonary gas exchange in chronic obstructive pulmonary disease. *Am. Rev. Respir. Dis.* **130**:612–616.

Mendella, L. A., Manfreda, J., Warren, C. P. W., and Anthonisen, N. R. (1982). Steroid response in stable chronic obstructive pulmonary disease. *Ann. Intern. Med.* **96**:17–21.

Mitchell, R. S., Stanford, R. E., Johnson, J. M., Silvers, G. W., Dart, G., and George, M. S. (1976). The morphologic features of the bronchi, bronchioles, and alveoli in chronic airway obstruction: a clinicopathological study. *Am. Rev. Respir. Dis.* **114**:137–145.

Mitchell, R. S., Webb, N. C., and Filley, G. F. (1964). Chronic obstructive bronchopulmonary disease: III. Factors influencing prognosis. *Am. Rev. Respir. Dis.* **89**:878–896.

Mitchell, D. M., Rehahn, M., Gildeh, P., Dimond, A. H., and Collins, J. V. (1984a). Effects of prednisolone in chronic airflow limitation. *Lancet* 2:193–196.

Mitchell, D. M., Gildeh, P., Rehahn, M., Dimond, A. H., and Collins, J. V. (1984b). Psychological changes and improvement in chronic airflow limitation after corticosteroid treatment. *Thorax* 39:924–927.

Monto, A. S., and Cavallaro, J. J. (1971). The Tecumseh study of respiratory illness: II. Patterns of occurrence of infection with respiratory pathogens. *Am. J. Epidemiol.* 94:280–289.

Moore-Gillon, J. C., Treacher, D. F., Gaminara, E. J., Pearson, T. C., and Cameron, I. R. (1986). Intermittent hypoxia in patients with unexplained polycythaemia. *Br. Med. J.* 293:588–590.

Morley, T. F., Zappasodi, S. J., Belli, A., and Giudice, J. C. (1987). Pulmonary vasodilator therapy for chronic obstructive pulmonary disease and cor pulmonale. Treatment with nifedipine, nitroglycerin and oxygen. *Chest* 92:71–76.

Mungall, I. P. F., and Hainsworth, R. (1979). Assessment of respiratory function in patients with chronic obstructive airways disease. *Thorax* 34:254–258.

Murciano, D., Aubier, M., Lecocguic, Y., and Pariente, R. (1984). Effects of theophylline on diaphragmatic strength and fatigue in patients with chronic obstructive pulmonary disease. *N. Engl. J. Med.* 311:349–353.

Nicholas, J. J., Gilbert, R., Gabe, R., and Auchincloss, J. H. (1970). Evaluation of an exercise therapy programme for patients with chronic obstructive pulmonary disease. *Am. Rev. Respir. Dis.* 102:1–9.

Nicotra, M. B., Rivera, M., and Awe, R. J. (1982). Antibiotic therapy of acute exacerbations of chronic bronchitis. *Ann. Intern. Med.* 97:18–21.

Nocturnal Oxygen Therapy Trial Group. (1980). Continuous or nocturnal oxygen therapy in hypoxaemic chronic obstructive lung disease. A clinical trial. *Ann. Intern. Med.* 93:391–398.

Office of Technology Assessment (1981). Cost effectiveness of influenza vaccination. Washington, D.C., Congress of the United States.

O'Reilly, J. F., Shaylor, J. M., Fromings, K. M., and Harrison, B. D. W. (1982). The use of the 12 minute walking test in assessing the effect of oral steroid therapy in patients with chronic airways obstruction. *Br. J. Dis. chest* 76:374–382.

Oppenheimer, E. A., Rigatto, M., and Fletcher, C. M. (1968). Airways obstruction before and after isoprenaline, histamine, and prednisolone in patients with chronic obstructive bronchitis. *Lancet* 1:552–557.

Packer, M., Greenberg, B., Massie, B., and Dash, H. (1982). Deleterious effects of hydralazine in patients with pulmonary hypertension. *N. Engl. J. Med.* 306:1326–1331.

Paez, P. N., Phillipson, E. A., Masangkay, P. M., and Sproule, B. J. (1967). The physiological basis of training patients with emphysema. *Am. Rev. Respir. Dis.* **95**:944–953.

Papiris, S., Galavotti, V., and Sturani, C. (1986). Effects of beta-agonists on breathlessness and exercise tolerance in patients with chronic obstructive pulmonary disease. *Respiration* **49**:101–108.

Paramelle, B., Vila, A., Stoebner, P., Muller, P., Gavelle, D., Lesbros, J., and Brambilla, C. (1986). Peripheral neuropathics and chronic hypoxemia in chronic obstructive lung disease. *Eur. J. Respir. Dis.* **69**:715 (abstract).

Pardy, R. L., Rivington, R. N., Despas, P. J., and Macklem, P. T. (1981). Inspiratory muscle training compared with physiotherapy in patients with chronic air-flow limitation. *Am. Rev. Respir. Dis.* **123**:421–425.

Peacock, A., Busst, C., Dawkins, K., and Denison, D. M. (1983). Response of pulmonary circulation to oral pirbuterol in chronic airflow obstruction. *Br. Med. J.* **287**:1178–1180.

Pennock, B. E., and Rogers, R. M. (1978). An evaluation of tests used to measure bronchodilator drug response. *Chest* **73**(suppl):988–989.

Peterson, D. I., Lonergan, L. H., and Hardinge, M. G. (1968). Smoking and pulmonary function. *Arch. Environ. Health* **16**:215–218.

Petrie, G. R., and Palmer, K. N. V. (1975). Comparison of aerosol ipratropium bromide and salbutamol in chronic bronchitis and asthma. *Br. Med. J.* **1**:430–432.

Petty, T. L., Brink, G. A., Miller, M. W., and Corsello, P. R. (1970). Objective functional improvement in chronic airway obstruction. *Chest* **57**:216–223.

Pierce, R. J., Holmes, P. W., and Campbell, A. H. (1982). Use of ipratropium bromide in patients with severe airways obstruction. *Aust. N.Z. J. Med.* **12**:38–43.

Pineda, H., Haas, F., Axen, K., and Haas, A. (1984). Accuracy of pulmonary function tests in predicting exercise tolerance in chronic obstructive pulmonary disease. *Chest* **86**:564–567.

Poppius, H., and Salorinne, Y. (1973). Comparative trial of a new anticholinergic bronchodilator Sch1000, and salbutamol in chronic bronchitis. *Br. Med. J.* **4**:134–136.

Postma, D. S., Steenhuis, E. J., van der Weele, L. Th., and Sluiter, H. J. (1985). Severe chronic airflow obstruction: can corticosteroids slow down progression? *Eur. J. Respir. Dis.* **67**:56–64.

Postma, D. S., De Vries, K., Koeter, G. H., and Sluiter, H. J. (1986). Independent influences of reversibility of airflow obstruction and non-specific hyperreactivity in the long term course of lung function in chronic airflow obstruction. *Am. Rev. Respir. Dis.* **134**:276–280.

Renzetti, A. D., McClement, J. H., and Litt, B. D. (1966). The Veterans Administration co-operative study of pulmonary function. III. Mortality in relation to respiratory function in chronic obstructive pulmonary disease. *Am. J. Med.* **41**:115–129.

Report to the Medical Research Council by the Subcommittee on Clinical Trials in Asthma. (1956). Controlled trial of effects of cortisone acetate in chronic asthma. *Lancet* **2**:798–803.

Rhind, C. B., Prince, K. L., Scott, W., and Flenley, D. C. (1986). Symptomatic oxygen therapy in hypoxic chronic bronchitis. *Thorax* **41**:245 (abstract).

Riordan, J. F., Sillett, R. W., and McNicol, M. W. (1975). A controlled trial of doxapram in acute respiratory failure. *Br. J. Dis. Chest* **69**:57–62.

Sagone, A. L., and Balcerzak, S. P. (1975). Smoking as a cause of erythrocytosis. *Ann. Intern. Med.* **82**:512–515.

Schreiner, A., Bjerkestrand, G., Digranes, A., Halvorsen, F. J., and Kommedal, T. M. (1978). Bacteriological findings in the transtracheal aspirate from patients with acute exacerbation of chronic bronchitis. *Infection* **6**:54–56.

Semmens, J. M. (1971). The pulmonary artery in the aged and diseased lung; its muscularity and its relation to hypertrophy of the right ventricle. London, M. D. thesis.

Shim, C., Stover, D. E., and Williams, M. H. (1978). Response to corticosteroids in chronic bronchitis. *J. Allergy Clin. Immunol.* **62**:363–367.

Shim, C. S., and Williams, M. H. (1983). Bronchodilator response to oral aminophylline and terbutaline versus aerosol albuterol in patients with chronic obstructive pulmonary disease. *Am. J. Med.* **75**:697–701.

Shim, C. S., and Williams, M. H. (1985). Aerosol beclomethasone in patients with steroid-responsive chronic obstructive pulmonary disease. *Am. J. Med.* **78**:655–658.

Simberkoff, M. S., Cross, A. P., Al-Ibrahim, M., Baltch, A. L., Geisler, P. J., Nadler, J., Richmond, A. S., Smith, R. P., Schiffman, G., Shepard, D. S., and Nan Eckhout, J. P. (1986). Efficacy of pneumococcal vaccine in high-risk patients. Results of a Veterans Administration Co-operative Study. *N. Engl. J. Med.* **315**:1318–1327.

Simonneau, G., Meignan, M., Denjean, A., Raffestin, B., Harf, A., and Prost, J. F. (1986). Cardiopulmonary effects of a single oral dose of almitrine at rest and on exercise in patients with hypoxic chronic airflow obstruction. *Chest* **89**:174–179.

Sinclair, D. J. M., and Ingram, C. C. (1980). Controlled trial of supervised exercise training in chronic bronchitis. *Br. Med. J.* **280**:519–521.

Skatrud, J. B., Dempsey, J. A., Bhansali, P., and Irwin, C. (1980). Determinants of chronic carbon dioxide retention and its correction in humans. *J. Clin. Invest.* **65**:813–821.

Skatrud, J. B., Dempsey, J. A., Iber, C., and Berssenbrugge, A. (1981). Correction of CO_2 retention during sleep in patients with chronic obstructive pulmonary diseases. *Am. Rev. Respir. Dis.* **124**:260–268.

Smith, J. R., and Landaw, S. A. (1978). Smokers' polycythaemia. *N. Engl. J. Med.* **298**:6–10.

Sonne, L. J., and Davis, J. A. (1982). Increased exercise performance in patients with severe COPD following inspiratory resistive training. *Chest* **81**:436–439.

Starke, I. D., Parker, R. A., and Turner-Warwick, M. (1982). Atropine methonitrate and salbutamol in chronic airways obstruction: peak effect and duration of action. *Respiration* **43**:51–56.

Stein, D. A., Bradley, B. L., and Miller, W. C. (1982). Mechanisms of oxygen effects on exercise in patients with chronic obstructive pulmonary disease. *Chest* **81**:6–10.

Stokes, T. C., Shaylor, J. M., O'Reilly, J. F., and Harrison, B. D. W. (1982). Assessment of steroid responsiveness in patients with chronic airflow obstruction. *Lancet* **2**:345–348.

Stradling, J. R. (1986). Hypercapnia during oxygen therapy in airways obstruction: a reappraisal. *Thorax* **41**:897–902.

Stradling, J. R., Cookson, W. D. C. M., Warby, A. R. H., and Lane, D. J. (1987). The effect of nocturnal hypoxaemia on survival of patients with chronic obstructive airways obstruction. *Thorax* **42**:216 (abstract).

Strain, D. S., Kinasewitz, G. T., Franco, D. P., and George, R. B. (1985). Effect of steroid therapy on exercise performance in patients with irreversible chronic obstructive pulmonary disease. *Chest* **88**:718–721.

Stretton, T. B. (1985). Provision of long term oxygen therapy. *Thorax* **40**: 801–805.

Sturani, C., Bassein, L., Schiavina, M., and Gunella, G. (1983). Oral nifedipine in chronic cor pulmonale secondary to severe chronic obstructive pulmonary disease (COPD). Short and long-term hemodynamic effects. *Chest* **84**:135–142.

Swinburn, C. R., Wakefield, J. M., and Jones, P. W. (1984). Relationship between ventilation and breathlessness during exercise in chronic obstructive airways disease is not altered by prevention of hypoxaemia. *Clin. Sci.* **67**:515–519.

Tager, I., and Speizer, F. E. (1975). Role of infection in chronic bronchitis. *N. Engl. J. Med.* **292**:563–571.

Taylor, D. R., Buick, B., Kinney, C., Lowry, R. C., and McDevitt, D. G. (1985). The efficacy of orally administered theophylline, inhaled salbutamol, and a combination of the two as chronic therapy in the management of chronic bronchitis with reversible air-flow obstruction. *Am. Rev. Respir. Dis.* **131**:747–751.

Teule, G. J. J., and Majid, P. A. (1980). Haemodynamic effects of terbutaline in chronic obstructive airways disease. *Thorax* **35**:536–542.

Tobin, M. J., Hughes, J. A., and Hutchinson, D. C. S. (1984). Effects of ipratropium bromide and fenoterol aerosols on exercise tolerance. *Eur. J. Respir. Dis.* **65**:441–446.

Trinquet, G., Duchier, J., and Jacquet, C. (1975). The bronchodilating effect of Sch 1000 MDI and inhalations of atropine methsulphate in patients suffering from bronchial asthma or from chronic bronchitis and emphysema. *Postgrad. Med. J.* Suppl. 7:119–120.

Tweeddale, P. M., Alexander, F., and McHardy, G. J. R. (1987). Short term variability in FEV_1 and bronchodilator responsiveness in patients with obstructive ventilatory defects. *Thorax* **42**:487–490.

Tydeman, D., Chandler, A., Culot, A., Graveling, B., and Harrison, B. (1984). How long is exercise training required to produce and maintain improvement in patients with chronic airways obstruction? *Thorax* **39**:226 (abstract).

Vyas, M. N., Banister, E. W., Morton, J. W., and Grzybowski, S. (1971a). Response to exercise in patients with chronic airway obstruction. 1. Effects of exercise training. *Am. Rev. Respir. Dis.* **103**:390–399.

Vyas, M. N., Banister, E. W., and Morton, J. W. (1971b). Response to exercise in patients with chronic airway obstruction. II. Effects of breathing 40% oxygen. *Am. Rev. Respir. Dis.* **103**:401–412.

Waterhouse, J. C., and Howard, P. (1983). Breathlessness and portable oxygen in chronic obstructive airways disease. *Thorax* **38**:302–306.

Weil, J. V., Jamieson, G., Brown, D. W., Grover, R. F., Balchum, O. J., and Murray, J. F. (1968). The red cell mass-arterial oxygen relationship in normal man. Application to patients with chronic obstructive airways disease. *J. Clin. Invest.* **47**:1627.

Weitzenblum, E., Hirth, C., Ducolone, A., Mirhom, R., Rasaholinjanahary, J., and Ehrhart, M. (1981). Prognostic value of pulmonary artery pressure in chronic obstructive pulmonary disease. *Thorax* **36**:752–758.

Weitzenblum, E., Sautegeau, A., Ehrhart, M., Mammosser, M., and Pelletier, A. (1985). Long-term oxygen therapy can reverse the progression of pulmonary hypertension in patients with chronic obstructive pulmonary disease. *Am. Rev. Respir. Dis.* **131**:493–498.

Whitaker, W. (1954). Pulmonary hypertension in congestive heart failure complicating chronic lung disease. *Q. J. Med.* **23**:57–72.

Williams, I. P., and McGavin, C. R. (1980). Corticosteroids in chronic airways obstruction: can the patient's assessment be ignored? *Br. J. Dis. Chest* **74**:142–148.

Wilhelmsen, L. (1967). Effects on broncho-pulmonary symptoms, ventilation, and lung mechanics of abstinence from tobacco smoking. *Scand. J. Respir. Dis.* **48**:407–414.

Winter, J. H., Carter, R., and Moran, F. (1985). Bronchial reactivity following prednisolone in chronic obstructive pulmonary disease. *Thorax* **41**:240 (abstract).

Woodcock, A. A., Gross, E. R., and Geddes, D. M. (1981). Oxygen relieves breathlessness in "pink puffers." *Lancet* **1**:907–909.

Woolf, C. R. (1970). The use of "respiratory stimulant" drugs. *Chest* **58**: 49–53.

York, E. L., Jones, R. L., Menon, D., and Sproule, B. J. (1980). Effects of secondary polycythaemia on cerebral blood flow in chronic obstructive pulmonary disease. *Am. Rev. Respir. Dis.* **121**:813.

Yusuf, S., Peto, R., Lewis, J. A., Collins, R., and Sleight, P. (1985). Beta-blockade during and after myocardial infarction. *Prog. Cardiovasc. Dis.* **27**:335–371.

Zielinski, J., Hawrylkiewicz, I., Gorecka, D., Gluskowski, J., and Koscinska, M. (1986). Captopril effects on pulmonary and systemic hemodynamics in chronic cor pulmonale. *Chest* **90**:562–565.

AUTHOR INDEX

Italic numbers give the page on which the complete reference is listed.

SUBJECT INDEX

A

Acetylcholine, 188
Acid aerosol chemistry, 202–205
Acid air pollution, 201–221 (*see also* Air pollution)
  controlled exposure studies of, 214–219
  COPD and 201–221
  population-based studies of, 205–214
    Donora, Pennsylvania, 208
    London, England, 208–210
    Meuse Valley, Belgium, 206
    Ontario, Canada, 210–212
    Yokkaichi, Japan, 212–214
Adenosine deaminase, 151
Air pollution (*see also* Acid air pollution)
  asthma admissions and, 211–212
  asthma mortality and, 212–213
  chronic bronchitis mortality and, 212–213
  episodes and respiratory symptoms, 206–210
  hospital admissions and, 210–212
  mortality rates and, 208–210
  respiratory admissions and, 211–212

Airflow obstruction, 67 (*see also* Small airways disease)
  K in smokers, 70
  role of small airways in, 61–63
Airway hyperreactivity, 169–172 (*see also* Airway responsiveness)
  asthma and, 172
  atopy and, 184
  eosinophilia and, 187
  IgE and, 187
  mucus hypersecretion and, 189
  in the newborn, 151–152
  ozone and, 172
  prevalence of asthma and, 186
  smoking and, 186–190
  viral infections and, 172
Airway responsiveness
  allergy and, 150, 151
  alpha-adrenergic hyperresponsiveness, 171
  atopy and, 184
  autonomic nervous system in, 152
  baseline lung function and, 187–188
  beta-adrenergic hyporesponsiveness, 171
  breast feeding and, 156
  bronchial irritability, 174